Applied Methods of Cost-effectiveness Analysis in Health Care

T0202216

Handbooks in Health Economic Evaluation Series

Series editors: Alastair M. Gray and Andrew Briggs

Existing volumes in the series:

Decision Modelling for Health Economic Evaluation
Andrew Briggs, Mark Sculpher, and Karl Claxton

Economic Evaluation in Clinical Trials
Henry A. Glick, Jalpa A. Doshi, Seema S. Sonnad, and Daniel Polsky

Applied Methods of Cost–Benefit Analysis in Health Care
Emma McIntosh, Philip M. Clarke, Emma Frew, and Jordan Louviere

Applied Methods of Cost-effectiveness Analysis in Health Care

Alastair M. Gray

Philip M. Clarke

Jane L. Wolstenholme

Sarah Wordsworth

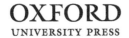

OXFORD
UNIVERSITY PRESS

OXFORD
UNIVERSITY PRESS

Great Clarendon Street, Oxford OX2 6DP

Oxford University Press is a department of the University of Oxford.
It furthers the University's objective of excellence in research, scholarship,
and education by publishing worldwide in

Oxford New York

Auckland Cape Town Dar es Salaam Hong Kong Karachi
Kuala Lumpur Madrid Melbourne Mexico City Nairobi
New Delhi Shanghai Taipei Toronto

With offices in

Argentina Austria Brazil Chile Czech Republic France Greece
Guatemala Hungary Italy Japan Poland Portugal Singapore
South Korea Switzerland Thailand Turkey Ukraine Vietnam

Oxford is a registered trade mark of Oxford University Press
in the UK and in certain other countries

Published in the United States
by Oxford University Press Inc., New York

© Oxford University Press 2011

British Library Cataloguing in Publication Data
Data available

Library of Congress Cataloging in Publication Data
Data available

Typeset in Minion by Glyph International, Bangalore, India

ISBN 978-0-19-922728-0

Series preface

Economic evaluation in health care is a thriving international activity that is increasingly used to allocate scarce health resources, and within which applied and methodological research, teaching, and publication are flourishing. Several widely respected texts are already well established in the market, so what is the rationale for not just one more book, but for a series? We believe that the books in the series *Handbooks in Health Economic Evaluation* share a strong distinguishing feature, which is to cover as much as possible of this broad field with a much stronger practical flavour than existing texts, using plenty of illustrative material and worked examples. We hope that readers will use this series not only for authoritative views on the current practice of economic evaluation and likely future developments, but for practical and detailed guidance on how to undertake an analysis. The books in the series are textbooks, but first and foremost they are handbooks.

Our conviction that there is a place for the series has been nurtured by the continuing success of two short courses we helped develop—Advanced Methods of Cost-Effectiveness Analysis, and Advanced Modelling Methods for Economic Evaluation. Advanced Methods was developed in Oxford in 1999 and has run several times a year ever since, in Oxford, Canberra, and Hong Kong. Advanced Modelling was developed in York and Oxford in 2002 and has also run several times a year ever since, in Oxford, York, Glasgow, and Toronto. Both courses were explicitly designed to provide computer-based teaching that would take participants not only through the theory but also through the methods and practical steps required to undertake a robust economic evaluation or construct a decision analytic model to current standards. The proof of concept was the strong international demand for the courses—from academic researchers, government agencies, and the pharmaceutical industry—and the very positive feedback on their practical orientation.

Therefore the original concept of the Handbook series, as well as many of the specific ideas and illustrative material, can be traced to these courses. The Advanced Modelling course is in the phenotype of the first book in the series, *Decision Modelling for Health Economic Evaluation*, which focuses on the role and methods of decision analysis in economic evaluation. The Advanced Methods course has been an equally important influence on *Applied Methods of Cost-effectiveness Analysis in Health Care*, the third book in the series which sets out the key elements of analysing costs and outcomes, calculating cost-effectiveness, and reporting results. The concept was then extended to cover several other important topic areas. Firstly, the design, conduct, and analysis of economic evaluations alongside clinical trials have become a specialized area of activity with distinctive methodological and practical issues, and their own debates and controversies. It seemed worthy of a dedicated volume—hence the second book in the series, *Economic Evaluation in Clinical Trials*. Next, while the use of cost–benefit analysis in health care has spawned a substantial literature, this is mostly theoretical, polemical, or focused on specific issues such as willingness to pay. We believe that the fourth book in the series, *Applied Methods of Cost–Benefit Analysis in Health Care*, fills an important gap in the literature by providing a comprehensive guide not only to the theory but also to the practical conduct of cost–benefit analysis, again with copious illustrative material and worked out examples.

Each book in the series is an integrated text prepared by several contributing authors, widely drawn from academic centres in the UK, the USA, Australia, and elsewhere. Part of our role as editors has been to foster a consistent style, but not to try to impose any particular line. That would have been unwelcome and also unwise amidst the diversity of an evolving field. News and information about the series, as well as supplementary material for each book, can be found at the series website (http://www.herc.ox.ac.uk/books).

Oxford   Alastair Gray
Glasgow   Andrew Briggs
                                                                          July 2006

Acknowledgements

Many people have been involved directly and indirectly in this book, reflecting the fact that the Advanced Methods of Cost-Effectiveness short course from which it has grown has always been a team effort. The course was originally conceived and developed by Andy Briggs, Philip Clarke, Alastair Gray, Kathy Johnston, and Jane Wolstenholme. Almost every member of the Health Economics Research Centre has subsequently been involved in teaching or tutoring, and many incremental changes to material have resulted. We are grateful to all of these present and past colleagues, and to the many hundreds of students who have so far attended the course, providing valuable feedback and insight, and challenging us to express ideas as clearly as possible.

During the preparation of this book a number of individuals contributed significantly, providing detailed comments on the text of the book or the exercises. We would like to thank in particular Maria Alva, James Buchanan, Helen Campbell, Helen Dakin, Boby Mihaylova, Judit Simon, and Elizabeth Stokes. We would also like to thank Alison Hayes and Tom Lung from the University of Sydney for their comments on Chapters 3 and 4. In addition, Jose Leal, Ramon Luengo-Fernandez, and Oliver Rivero-Arias made valuable contributions to the chapters on modelling, costing, and presenting results, and to the development and testing of the exercises. For many years Alison Gater has played an invaluable role in both sustaining and organising the course, and has dealt with permissions and many other administrative matters related to the manuscript. In addition to his key role in getting the course off the ground, we are grateful to Andy Briggs for his comments and support in his role as series co-editor. Finally, we would like to thank Charlotte, Andy, and Dave for repairing the many domestic disruptions involved in producing a book.

Contents

Abbreviations and acronyms

ACER	average cost-effectiveness ratio	MAUS	multi-attribute utility systems
AIC	Akaike information criterion	OLS	ordinary least-squares
CBA	cost-benefit analysis	PCI	pay cost index
CCA	cost-consequence analysis	PPP	purchasing power parity
CEA	cost-effectiveness analysis	PSA	probabilistic sensitivity analysis
CI	confidence interval	QALE	quality-adjusted life-expectancy
CM	choice modelling	QALY	quality-adjusted life-year
CMA	cost-minimization analysis	QAS	quality-adjusted survival time
CPI	consumer price index	RCI	Reference Cost Index
CUA	cost-utility analysis	RCT	randomized controlled trial
CV	contingent valuation	RR	relative risk
DALY	disability-adjusted life-year	RS	rating scale
DRG	diagnosis-related group	SD	standard deviation
FCA	friction cost approach	SE	standard error
GDP	gross domestic product	SG	standard gamble
GLM	generalized linear model	SMAC	Standing Medical Advisory Committee
HCA	human capital approach		
HSCI	health service cost index	SP	stated preference
HUI	Health Utility Index	STPR	social time preference rate
ICER	incremental cost-effectiveness ratio	TTO	time trade-off
		WHO	World Health Organization
IPW	inverse probability weighting	YLD	years of life with a disability
KM	Kaplan–Meier	YLL	years of life lost
KMSA	Kaplan–Meier sample average		

Other abbreviations are defined where they occur in the text.

Chapter 1

Introduction

The British economist Lionel Robbins famously defined economics as '...a science which studies human behaviour as a relationship between ends and scarce means which have alternative uses' (Robbins 1932). The concepts of scarcity and choice will have resonance for anyone involved in the planning and provision of health care: the available resources are never sufficient to allow all available health interventions to be provided, and so choices have to be made, which sometimes involve very difficult decisions. How scarce resources can best be allocated in order to best satisfy human wants is in fact the basic economic problem, and it is encountered whether the context is sub-Saharan Africa or North America, even though the absolute level of resources available may differ enormously.

In health care, this problem can be restated as 'How can the scarce health resources allocated to health care best be used in order to maximise the health gain obtained from them?' This is not to assert that maximizing health gain is the only objective of a health care system—it may also have interests in the fairness with which resources are used, or in other objectives such as education, training, and research. But maximizing health gain—the efficiency objective—is clearly important, and since the 1970s a set of analytical methods of economic evaluation has been developed to help decision-makers address this problem.

1.1 Origins of the book

The origins of this book can be traced to the course 'Advanced Methods of Cost-Effectiveness Analysis', which was developed by a team at the Health Economics Research Centre, University of Oxford, and first presented in 1999. Since then it has been run at least twice annually, including in Hong Kong and Australia. The idea behind the course was to provide a somewhat more advanced study of the methods of cost-effectiveness analysis for health-care interventions than was then routinely available elsewhere, to give participants 'hands on' experience of methods by extensive use of computer-based exercises and data handling, and to broaden the knowledge base of researchers and users through the use of practical examples and problems.

This book is built directly on the teaching material developed for that course and on the accumulated experience of teaching it. The intention is not that it will replace or supplant the several excellent general textbooks already available, which give a comprehensive treatment of the methodological principles of economic evaluation in health care (e.g. Drummond *et al.* 2005; Gold *et al.* 1996), but rather that it will provide the reader with a more detailed description and set of instructions on how to perform a cost-effectiveness analysis of a health intervention. Therefore it can be seen as a more practical handbook, in line with other volumes in the series *Handbooks in Health Economic Evaluation*, of which it is a part (Briggs *et al.* 2006; Glick *et al.* 2007; McIntosh *et al.* 2010).

1.2 **Rationale**

An important reason for devising the course, and now for translating it into a book, is that standards of best practice in economic evaluation have become more explicit and more demanding over time. From the early 1990s health technology assessment and reimbursement agencies began to produce and refine guides to the way they wished economic data to be analysed and presented, for example for Australia (Commonwealth of Australia 1995; Pharmaceutical Benefits Advisory Committee 2008), for Ontario (Ontario Ministry of Health 1994), for Canada as a whole (Canadian Coordinating Office for Health Technology Assessment 1997; Canadian Agency for Drugs and Technologies in Health 2006), and for England and Wales (NICE 2004, 2008).

Even without the spur of having to make formal reimbursement decisions, in 1993 the US Public Health Service became so frustrated by the lack of consensus in the techniques used to conduct cost-effectiveness analysis that it convened an expert group to make recommendations that would improve quality and enhance comparability. The result was an influential textbook, which included a strong plea for the use of a **reference case** or standard set of methodological practices which, if included by analysts when reporting their results (along with other scenarios if desired), would significantly increase comparability between studies (Gold *et al.* 1996).

This trend was followed by journals such as the *British Medical Journal* and the *New England Journal of Medicine*, which began to specify how they wanted economic evaluations to be presented, and how they expected referees to assess them (Kassirer and Angell 1994; Drummond and Jefferson 1996, on behalf of the *BMJ* Economic Evaluation Working Party). More specialized guidelines have also been produced, for example to improve standards in decision analytic modelling (Philips *et al.* 2006).

Another rationale for the course and this book is that health economists are becoming involved in more complex studies. For example, they may be conducting economic evaluations alongside large pragmatic trials running over a long period of time with multiple comparisons, multiple endpoints, and incomplete patient-specific data on resource use and quality of life. There has also been a dawning recognition that even the largest and longest clinical trials do not remove the need for modelling, which may be required before, during, after, and instead of trials (Buxton *et al.* 1997).

Finally, the title—when the course was conceived it seemed reasonable to call it 'Advanced Methods of Cost-Effectiveness Analysis', as the prevailing standards in the published literature often fell well short of best practice. When Briggs and Gray (1999) surveyed 492 studies published up to 1996 that reported results in terms of cost per life-year or cost per quality-adjusted life-year, they found that barely 10% had used patient-level data, that fewer than 1% reported a confidence interval for estimates of average cost, and that 20% did not report any measure of variance at all. However, in the time that has elapsed since then, and partly as a result of the various textbooks, guidelines, and courses mentioned above, methods have improved and the contents of this book are, or at least should be, considered standard practice. Therefore we have called this text 'Applied Methods of Cost-effectiveness Analysis in Health Care'.

1.3 Structure and content

Chapter 2 sets the scene by describing the different types of economic evaluation, introducing the cost-effectiveness plane, differentiating between incremental and average cost-effectiveness ratios, and exploring different ways of trying to identify the maximum willingness to pay for a quality-adjusted life-year. Chapter 3 then begins our treatment of health outcomes by focusing on estimating changes in life expectancy, including life-table methods, dealing with competing risks, and discounting methods for outcomes. Chapter 4 extends this to consider survival analysis, extrapolation, and quality-adjusted life expectancy when patient-level data are available. Chapter 5 rounds off the consideration of health outcomes by considering how quality adjustment can be done: it reviews the different types of outcome measures likely to be used in cost-effectiveness and cost-utility analyses, and how to use, interpret, and present them.

In Chapter 6 we turn to the cost side of the cost-effectiveness equation, setting out methods of defining, measuring, and valuing costs. Chapter 7 continues the treatment of costs by considering issues in the analysis of cost data, including handling missing and censored data and dealing with skewness.

Chapter 8 is the first of three chapters dealing with modelling. It introduces the rationale for modelling, and then deals with the construction and analysis of decision-tree models. Chapter 9 extends this to Markov models, explaining what they are, what they do, and the key steps involved in constructing and analysing a Markov model. Other modelling techniques such as discrete event simulation are also mentioned. Chapter 10 completes the material on modelling by exploring the methods used to take account of uncertainty, focusing in particular on the use of probabilistic sensitivity analysis (PSA) in evaluating cost-effectiveness models.

Chapter 11 pulls together the cost, outcome, and modelling elements of the book to review and demonstrate appropriate ways of presenting cost-effectiveness results. It illustrates the use of the cost-effectiveness plane, ellipses, the construction and interpretation of cost-effectiveness acceptability curves, and the advantages of the net benefit approach. The final chapter (Chapter 12) concludes the book by briefly reviewing its main themes and contemplating some future directions in the development of methods of cost-effectiveness analysis.

1.4 Exercises

As with other handbooks in this series, an important feature of this book is an emphasis on practical examples and exercises. Some of the exercises are stand-alone activities designed to provide experience of dealing with particular types of analysis or data issues, but running through the outcome, cost, and presenting results chapters is an integrated exercise which uses the same underlying dataset consisting of a set of hypothetical patients, with their associated characteristics, complications, costs, and outcomes.

The data were generated using the UK Prospective Diabetes Study Outcome Model (Clarke *et al.* 2004), a simulation model developed using patient-level data from a large prospective trial of therapies for type 2 diabetes. This exercise gradually builds on the solutions derived in previous chapters. More details are provided in the relevant place in each chapter. As with previous handbooks (Briggs *et al.* 2006), we have chosen to base these exercises largely on Microsoft Excel® software, which is widely available, transparent, and avoids the 'black-box' aspects of some other dedicated software. Some degree of familiarity with Excel is assumed, but the step-by-step guides should permit all readers to complete the exercises. The exercises in Chapters 8, 9, and 10 can be done using either Excel or TreeAge™ software. Again, detailed notes are provided, but readers will have to obtain a licensed copy of TreeAge if they do not have it already. The step-by-step guides can be found at the end of each chapter, and supplementary material including workbooks and solution files can also be found on the website www.herc.ox.ac.uk/books/applied that has been set up to support this book.

References

Briggs, A.H., Claxton, K., and Sculpher, M.J. (2006). *Decision Modelling for Health Economic Evaluation*. Oxford University Press.

Briggs, A.H. and Gray, A.M. (1999). Handling uncertainty in economic evaluations of healthcare interventions. *British Medical Journal*, **319**, 635–8.

Buxton, M.J., Drummond, M.F., Van, H.B., *et al.* (1997). Modelling in economic evaluation: an unavoidable fact of life [editorial]. *Health Economics*, **6**, 217–27.

Canadian Agency for Drugs and Technologies in Health (2006). *Guidelines for Economic Evaluation of Pharmaceuticals: Canada*. Canadian Agency for Drugs and Technologies in Health (CADTH), Ottawa.

Canadian Coordinating Office for Health Technology Assessment (1997). *Guidelines for the Economic Evaluation of Pharmaceuticals: Canada* (2nd edn). Canadian Coordinating Office for Health Technology Assessment (CCOHTA), Ottawa.

Clarke, P., Gray, A., Briggs, A., *et al.* (2004). A model to estimate the lifetime health outcomes of patients with type 2 diabetes: the United Kingdom Prospective Diabetes Study (UKPDS) Outcomes Model (UKPDS 68). *Diabetologia*, **47**, 1747–59.

Commonwealth of Australia (1995). *Guidelines for the Pharmaceutical Industry on Preparation of Submissions to the Pharmaceutical Benefits Advisory Committee: Including Economic Analyses*. Department of Health and Community Services, Canberra.

Drummond, M.F. and Jefferson, T.O. (1996). Guidelines for authors and peer reviewers of economic submissions to the *BMJ*. *British Medical Journal*, **313**, 275–83.

Drummond, M.F., Sculpher, M.J., Torrance, G.W., O'Brien, B.J., and Stoddart, G.L. (2005). *Methods for the Economic Evaluation of Health Care Programmes* (3rd edn). Oxford University Press.

Glick, H., Doshi, J.A., Sonnad, S.S., and Polsky, D. (2007). *Economic Evaluation in Clinical Trials*. Oxford University Press.

Gold, M.R., Siegel, J.E., Russell, L.B., and Weinstein, M.C. (1996). *Cost-Effectiveness in Health and Medicine*. Oxford University Press, New York.

Kassirer, J.P. and Angell, M. (1994). The journal's policy on cost-effectiveness analyses [editorial]. *New Engand Journal of Medicine*, **331**, 669–70.

McIntosh, E., Louviere, J.J., Frew, E., and Clarke, P.M. (2010). *Applied Methods of Cost–Benefit Analysis in Health Care.* Oxford University Press.

NICE (2004). *Guide to the Methods of Technology Appraisal.* National Institute for Health and Clinical Excellence, London.

NICE (2008). *Guide to the Methods of Technology Appraisal.* National Institute for Health and Clinical Excellence, London.

Ontario Ministry of Health (1994). *Ontario Guidelines for Economic Analysis of Pharmaceutical Products.* Ontario Ministry of Health, Toronto.

Pharmaceutical Benefits Advisory Committee (2008). *Guidelines for Preparing Submissions to the Pharmaceutical Benefits Advisory Committee (Version 4.3).* Australian Government, Department of Health and Ageing, Canberra.

Philips, Z., Bojke, L., Sculpher, M., Claxton, K., and Golder, S. (2006). Good practice guidelines for decision-analytic modelling in health technology assessment: a review and consolidation of quality assessment. *PharmacoEconomics,* **24**, 355–71.

Robbins, L. (1932). *An Essay on the Nature and Significance of Economic Science.* Macmillan, London.

Chapter 2

Economic evaluation in health care

In this chapter, we describe the different types of economic evaluation: cost-consequence analysis (CCA), cost-minimization analysis (CMA), cost-effectiveness analysis (CEA), cost-utility analysis (CUA), and cost-benefit analysis (CBA).

We then introduce the cost-effectiveness plane as a graphic device to aid understanding, analysis and presentation of results. The chapter then sets out and illustrates the difference between incremental and average cost-effectiveness ratios, and explores the concepts of dominance and extended dominance. A worked example is then presented to show how cost-effectiveness information could in principle be used to maximize health gain from an existing budget.

The second half of the chapter explores different ways of identifying the maximum willingness to pay for a health gain such as a quality-adjusted life-year: rule of thumb, league tables, revealed preference, and stated preference.

2.1 Methods of economic evaluation

Economic evaluation is based on the recognition that information on the effectiveness of interventions is necessary but not sufficient for decision-making; it is also necessary to explicitly consider the costs, and in particular the opportunity costs or benefits foregone, of different courses of action. The extent to which different methods of economic evaluation relate to underlying economic theory have been extensively debated, but it is a reasonable proposition that the economic approach offers a coherent, explicit, and theoretically based approach to measuring and valuing costs and outcomes, dealing with individual and social choice, and handling uncertainty (Weinstein and Manning 1997).

Economic evaluation can be defined as a comparison of alternative options in terms of their costs and consequences (Drummond *et al.* 2005). As such, all methods of economic evaluation involve some kind of comparison between alternative interventions, treatments, or programmes. Therefore we have two (or more) options to compare, and two dimensions (costs and consequences) along which to compare them. Costs can be thought of as the value of the resources involved in providing a treatment or intervention; this would invariably include health care resources, and might be extended to include social care resources, those provided by other agencies, and possibly the time and other costs incurred by patients and their families or other informal carers. Consequences can be thought of as the health effects of the intervention.

2.1.1 Cost-consequence analysis

The simplest way of reporting the costs and consequences of two interventions would be to calculate and report all the various costs and consequences in a separate and disaggregated way, leaving the reader or decision-maker to interpret and synthesize them in some way. This is sometimes described as a cost-consequence analysis. An example is a study by Ellstrom *et al.* (1998), who reported an assessment of the economic consequences and health status of women in Sweden who had been randomized to receive either a total laparoscopic hysterectomy or a total abdominal hysterectomy. Considering the costs first, they found that the hospital costs were slightly higher for patients undergoing laparoscopic rather than abdominal surgery, but the costs of time off work were about 50% lower. The authors then reported several different measures of the health consequences, in particular noting that there was no statistically significant difference in the complication rate between the two groups, but that health status as measured by the SF-36 Health Survey improved significantly faster postoperatively in the laparascopic group than in the abdominal group.

Reporting results in a disaggregated way is a positive attribute of cost-consequence studies, but by stopping at that point cost-consequence analysis shifts the burden of interpretation and synthesis onto the decision-maker and assumes that users can reliably and consistently process such information. They also assume that the users of the economic evaluation are the right people to decide what weights to put on different outcomes: for example, lower costs but poorer health consequences, or better long-term quality of life but more short-term complications. As a result, such studies are relatively uncommon.

2.1.2 Cost-minimization analysis

A second form of economic evaluation is sometimes described as cost-minimization analysis (Drummond *et al.* 2005). Again, both costs and health outcomes or consequences are of interest, but in this case it is assumed that the health outcomes of two or more options are identical, and so the option that has the lowest costs will be preferred: the objective has become minimization of cost.

A cost-minimization format is sometimes adopted when a prospective economic evaluation being conducted alongside a clinical trial fails to find any significant difference in the primary clinical outcome. However, this will seldom be the appropriate way to proceed (Briggs and O'Brien 2001). Firstly, failure to find a difference in a study designed and powered to test the hypothesis that two treatments differ in efficacy cannot be interpreted as evidence that no difference exists. Demonstrating equivalence or non-inferiority of clinical outcome typically requires much larger sample sizes and hence is a less common trial design. Second, the interest of the health economist is not in clinical differences alone, but in the joint distribution of cost and effect differences, which may indicate a weight of evidence favouring one treatment over another even where clinical equivalence has formally been demonstrated (this point is explored in more detail in Chapter 11). As a result of these shortcomings, the circumstances in which cost-minimization analysis will be an appropriate method are highly constrained and infrequent.

2.1.3 Cost-effectiveness analysis

In cost-effectiveness analysis we first calculate the costs and effects of an intervention and one or more alternatives, then calculate the differences in cost and differences in effect, and finally present these differences in the form of a ratio, i.e. the cost per unit of health outcome or effect (Weinstein and Stason 1977). Because the focus is on differences between two (or more) options or treatments, analysts typically refer to incremental costs, incremental effects, and the incremental cost-effectiveness ratio (ICER). Thus, if we have two options *a* and *b*, we calculate their respective costs and effects, then calculate the difference in costs and difference in effects, and then calculate the ICER as the difference in costs divided by the difference in effects:

$$\text{ICER} = \frac{\text{Cost}_a - \text{Cost}_b}{\text{Effect}_a - \text{Effect}_b} = \frac{\Delta\text{Cost}}{\Delta\text{Effect}}$$

The effects of each intervention can be calculated using many different types of measurement unit. Two diagnostic tests could be compared in terms of the cost per case detected, two blood pressure interventions by the cost per 1 mmHg reduction in systolic blood pressure, and two vaccination options by the cost per case prevented. However, decision-makers will typically be interested in resource allocation decisions across different areas of health care: for example, whether to spend more on a new vaccination programme or on a new blood pressure treatment. Consequently a measure of outcome that can be used across different areas is particularly useful, and the measure that has so far gained widest use is the quality-adjusted life-year (QALY).

2.1.4 Cost-utility analysis

The QALY attempts to capture in one metric the two most important features of a health intervention: its effect on survival measured in terms of life-years, and its effect on quality of life. Because the weights or valuations placed on particular health states are related to utility theory and frequently referred to as utilities or utility values, cost-effectiveness analyses which measure outcomes in terms of QALYs are sometimes referred to as cost-utility studies, a term coined by Torrance (1976) in 1976, but are sometimes simply considered as a subset of cost-effectiveness analysis. The use of a specific term for this type of evaluation has the benefit of highlighting the fact that such studies use a generic measure of health outcome that potentially permits comparison across all such studies (Drummond *et al.* 2005).

2.1.5 Cost-benefit analysis

Cost-effectiveness analysis places no monetary value on the health outcomes it is comparing. It does not measure or attempt to measure the underlying worth or value to society of gaining additional QALYs, for example, but simply indicates which options will permit more QALYs to be gained than others with the same resources, assuming that gaining QALYs is agreed to be a reasonable objective for the health care system. Therefore the cost-effectiveness approach will never provide a way of determining how much in total it is worth spending on health care and the pursuit of QALYs rather than on other social objectives such as education, defence, or private consumption. It does not permit us to say whether health care spending is too high or too low, but rather confines itself to the question of how any given level of spending can be arranged to maximize the health outcomes yielded.

In contrast, cost-benefit analysis (CBA) does attempt to place some monetary valuation on health outcomes as well as on health care resources. If a new surgical procedure reduces operative mortality by 5%, a cost-benefit approach would try to estimate whether each death averted had a value of £5000 or £500,000 or £5 million, and then assess whether the monetary value of the benefits was greater or less than the costs of obtaining these benefits.

CBA also holds out the promise of permitting comparisons not just within the health care budget, but between different areas of expenditure such as education, transport, and environment. Other claimed advantages of CBA are that it is more firmly based in welfare theory than cost-effectiveness analysis, and that it aims to include all benefits, and not just the health outcomes that cost-effectiveness analysis focuses on. Thus a CBA of a health intervention might try to measure not only the monetary value of any health benefits gained by the patient, but also the value to society of other consequences, such as the ability to take paid employment.

CBA is sometimes traced back to the 1939 US Flood Control Act, which stated that flood control projects should be supported 'if the benefits to whomsoever they may accrue are in excess of the estimated costs' (Pearce and Nash 1981). It has become firmly established in environmental and transport economics, and examples of its application to health problems go back at least to Weisbrod's (1971) examination of the costs and benefits of research expenditure on poliomyelitis. However, in health, cost-effectiveness analysis rapidly attained ascendancy in the applied literature (Warner and Hutton 1980) and to date this has been maintained (Elixhauser 1993, 1998).

The reasons for the more widespread use of cost-effectiveness analysis compared with cost-benefit analysis in health care are discussed extensively elsewhere, including in a companion volume to this book (McIntosh et al. 2010), but two main issues can be identified. Firstly, significant conceptual or practical problems have been encountered with the two principal methods of obtaining monetary valuations of life or quality of life: the human capital approach, which uses the present value of an individual's future earnings as a way of valuing the gains or losses from mortality and morbidity (as in Weisbrod's (1971) study of poliomyelitis), and the willingness to pay approach, which attempts to obtain valuations of health benefits by means of either revealed preferences (for example, willingness to pay for safety features in cars, or to travel for a health check (Clarke 1998)) or a stated preference or contingent valuation exercise, where respondents say how much they would hypothetically be willing to pay for an intervention or some other attribute of an intervention, such as speedier or more proximate access. Second, within the health care sector there remains a widespread and intrinsic aversion to the concept of placing explicit monetary values on health or on life. This may be related to the fact that those affected by health care resource allocation decisions are sometimes clearly identifiable small groups or individuals, who tend to be viewed, rightly or wrongly (Cookson et al. 2008), differently from the statistical lives that are the norm in environmental and transport policy-making.

2.1.6 Economic evaluation, efficiency, and welfare theory

It should be evident from the discussion above that the differences between cost-effectiveness analysis and cost-benefit analysis are not simply technical issues, but raise some quite fundamental questions about the theoretical foundations of these approaches. Cost-benefit analysis can be more directly traced to standard welfare economic theory, in which social welfare is the sum total of individual welfare or utility, and resource allocation decisions can be assessed in terms of whether they result in a net improvement in social welfare (Pearce and Nash 1981). If the gainers from a policy could in principle compensate any losers and still be better off in welfare terms, then net social welfare has increased (the Kaldor–Hicks criterion of potential Pareto improvement). In the context of health care, this has typically meant expressing all costs, health benefits, and health disbenefits in monetary terms to assess whether or not net social welfare has potentially increased.

In principle this approach should simplify the decision rule: if benefits outweigh costs it will be worth proceeding as there will be a net social benefit, while if costs outweigh benefits it will not. However, in practice, when there is a budget constraint, it will be necessary to order or prioritize different policies in terms of their cost-benefit ratio to make sure that the available resource are directed towards the policies offering the largest welfare improvements, and this procedure would then have similarities to ordering using cost-effectiveness ratios.

The cost-benefit approach should also, in principle, permit broad questions of **allocative efficiency** to be addressed. As the method is not restricted to welfare gains from health improvement, cost-benefit appraisals could be conducted across different sectors of the economy and used to determine how much should be allocated to health care, transport, education, or defence. In contrast, cost-effectiveness analysis can address questions of **productive** or **production efficiency**, where a specified good or service is being produced at the lowest possible cost—in this context, health gain using the health care budget. However, it cannot address the question of whether the amount of health gain being produced truly matches the individual preferences of society, i.e. whether we are allocating too little, too much, or the right amount to health care.

The contrasts between these positions are not necessarily as stark as suggested above. Some analysts have attempted to relate cost-effectiveness analysis directly to welfare theory (Garber and Phelps 1997; Weinstein and Manning 1997). Others have proposed an extension to welfare theory, termed 'extra-welfarism', which argues that utility is not the only relevant argument in the social welfare function, that health is the most important and relevant outcome when conducting normative analysis in the health sector, and that the sources of valuation of relevant outcomes may differ in health (Culyer 1989; Brouwer *et al.* 2008). From this perspective, cost-effectiveness becomes appropriate and theoretically based. It is also worth noting that many of the practical and methodological issues confronting cost-effectiveness, such as obtaining precise estimates of cost and effect differences, and handling and adequately reporting different forms of uncertainty, would also be confronted by cost-benefit analyses in health care (McIntosh *et al.* 2010).

2.2 **The cost-effectiveness plane**

Cost-effectiveness analysis inhabits a two-dimensional word of costs and effects, and this can be represented graphically in the form of the cost-effectiveness plane, which we will use extensively throughout this book (Figure 2.1).

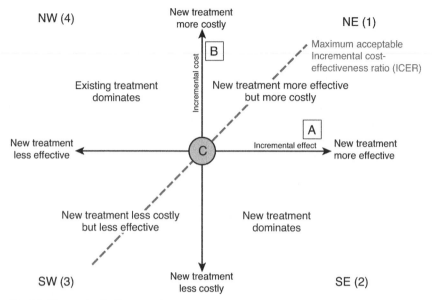

Fig. 2.1 The cost-effectiveness plane.

This graphic approach was first set out by Anderson *et al.* (1986), but rearranged and refined by Black (1990). The figure is used to plot the incremental cost and incremental benefit of the new intervention versus the comparator, which may be current treatment, no treatment, or some other specified alternative. Incremental effectiveness (relative to the comparator) is shown on the x-axis, while the y-axis shows the incremental cost and the origin of the graph (C) represents the point of comparison or control. Therefore, compared with this central point, the intervention of interest can be more effective or less effective, and can be more costly or less costly, and these combinations are represented by the four quadrants of the figure.

If the new intervention is found to be less costly and more effective, it will be in the south-east quadrant (quadrant 2 counting clockwise from the north-east), and decision-makers will have no difficulty in quickly opting to adopt this technology as they will be getting more health for less cost; the new treatment can be said to dominate the comparator. If it turns out to be less effective and more costly, it will be in the north-west quadrant (quadrant 4), and a decision to reject can equally readily be made; in this case the new treatment is dominated by the comparator. More interesting and typically more common situations arise in the north-east and south-west quadrants, where the new intervention is more effective but also more costly (the north-east quadrant, quadrant 1), or is less effective but also less costly (the south-west quadrant, or quadrant 3). In these areas of the figure, there is a trade-off between effect and cost: additional health benefit can be obtained but at higher cost (north-east), or savings can be made but only by surrendering some health benefit (south-west).

The question which then arises is whether or not the trade-off is acceptable, i.e. whether the health gain (or cost saving) is worth the additional cost (or health loss).

For example, within the north-east quadrant of the plane, it is possible to imagine a new therapy that is not very costly and is extremely effective in comparison with current treatment (region A). However, still in the same quadrant, a therapy could be marginally more effective than the existing treatment but cost a great deal more (region B). Note that the coordinates of each of these points are the difference in cost and difference in effect, or ΔCost/ΔEffect, and so the slope of the line running from the origin of the figure to these points is the incremental cost-effectiveness ratio, which is sometimes referred to by the Greek letter λ (lambda). The ICER for B will obviously be much higher than that for A. Clearly these are quite different scenarios, one of which is highly acceptable while the other is not, although they inhabit the same quadrant of the plane. As we move from scenario A to scenario B, we must travel through a point at which decision-makers change their minds, and decide that they are no longer prepared to pay the additional cost for the additional benefit. We can think of this as this maximum acceptable ICER, and we can represent it by the broken diagonal line running through the plane.

Therefore, when working in the two-dimensional world of cost-effectiveness analysis, there are two uncertainties that will be encountered. Firstly, there will be uncertainty concerning the location of the intervention on the cost-effectiveness plane: how much more or less effective and how much more or less costly it is than current treatment. Second, there is uncertainty concerning how much the decision-maker is willing to pay for health gain: the maximum value of λ. Later in this book we shall see that these two uncertainties can be presented together in the form of the question 'What is the probability that this intervention is cost-effective?', a question which effectively divides our cost-effectiveness plane into just two policy spaces—below the maximum acceptable line, and above it (Van Hout *et al.* 1994).

2.3 Incremental versus average cost-effectiveness

When discussing cost-effectiveness in section 2.1.3, we emphasized that the main interest was in the incremental cost-effectiveness ratio, defined as the difference in costs between two alternatives divided by the difference in effects. What do we mean by alternatives, and how do we establish whether or not it is appropriate to make an incremental comparison between a given pair of treatments? To clarify this, suppose that we were considering first-line treatment for people newly diagnosed with type 2 diabetes. In recent years, as a result of convincing evidence on effectiveness and cost-effectiveness, it has become standard practice in many countries to use the oral medication metformin as first-line therapy. In Figure 2.2, metformin is represented by point A, and in this example giving metformin to the population of interest (let us say 200 patients) is assumed to increase survival by a total of 250 life-years and increase cost by £500k compared with basic diet and exercise advice but no medication, shown as point C at the origin. Therefore the resulting incremental cost-effectiveness ratio is £500k/250 life-years, or £2000 per life-year gained (some evaluations have found that metformin is so cost-effective that it can even be cost-saving (Clarke *et al.* 2001)).

Now let us assume that a new class of drug, which is considerably more expensive than metformin but is also more effective at controlling blood glucose, is launched on the market. If given to the same target population, this new drug would increase survival compared with basic diet and exercise advice by a total of 300 life-years at a total cost of £2.5 million, shown by point B on Figure 2.2. Therefore, compared with diet and exercise, this new drug would have a cost-effectiveness ratio of £8333 per life-year gained (£2500k/300). On this basis, the manufacturer argues that this new drug should replace metformin as first line therapy.

However, by calculating the cost-effectiveness of the new drug B in this way, we are ignoring alternative treatments, such as metformin. Most of the health gain obtained with the new therapy (250 of the 300 life-years gained) could be obtained using metformin, and so the next best alternative to the new drug is not the diet and exercise option, but metformin therapy. Therefore the relevant comparison is between the new drug alone versus metformin alone, or between the new drug + metformin versus metformin alone. It is not appropriate to ignore the existence of metformin.

Conventionally, cost-effectiveness ratios that have been calculated against a baseline or do-nothing option without reference to any alternatives are referred to as *average* cost-effectiveness ratios, while comparisons with the next best alternative are described as *incremental* cost-effectiveness ratios (Detsky and Naglie 1990; Johannesson 1996). In Figure 2.2, it can be seen that the new drug B has an average cost-effectiveness ratio of £8333 per life-year gained. However, compared with the alternative (metformin), drug B yields just 50 additional life-years at an additional cost of £2 million, and so has a much higher incremental cost-effectiveness ratio of £40,000 per life-year gained.

The importance of differentiating between average and incremental cost-effectiveness ratios is illustrated in Figure 2.3, drawn from a classic article by

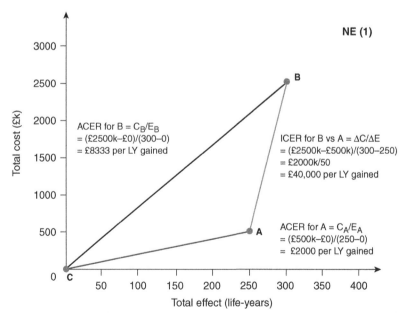

Fig. 2.2 Average and incremental cost-effectiveness: ACER, average cost-effectiveness ratio; ICER, incremental cost-effectiveness ratio; LY, life-year.

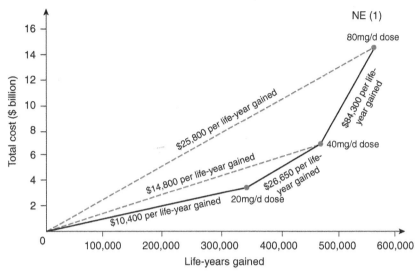

Fig. 2.3 Cost-effectiveness of three different statin doses to reduce cholesterol. Derived from Goldman *et al.* (1991).

Goldman *et al.* (1991) which explored the cost-effectiveness of different policy options involving statin therapy to reduce cholesterol. Note that the baseline or origin here was not strictly a do-nothing option: for example, patients having a myocardial infarction would still incur costs and benefits from treatment they received. This is why the *x*-axis is labelled 'life-years gained', which strictly makes all comparisons incremental. However, the baseline does represent a do-nothing option in the sense that the comparisons were between using statins or not using them, rather than using a next-best cholesterol-lowering therapy, and so cost-effectiveness ratios calculated against the origin here can be described as average cost-effectiveness ratios.

The authors considered policies to target patients with no prior history of heart disease (primary prevention) and patients with a history of heart disease (secondary prevention); they also examined cost-effectiveness in different age-groups, and the cost-effectiveness of different drug doses. Clearly, it would be possible to implement both primary *and* secondary prevention; these are independent policies affecting different patient groups, and so the appropriate approach would not be to calculate the incremental cost-effectiveness of primary versus secondary prevention, but rather to calculate the incremental cost-effectiveness of statins in each relative to the next best alternative for that group of patients. The resulting ICERs could then be compared to see which offered the best value for money. Similarly, policies aimed at different age groups are independent, and a direct incremental calculation of the cost-effectiveness in one age group versus another would not be appropriate. However, different doses of statin are a different matter. Giving a 20 mg/day dose cannot be considered independently of giving the same person a 40 mg/day or 80 mg/day dose; these are mutually exclusive alternatives. As a result, while the average cost-effectiveness of a 40 mg/day dose is $14,800 per life-year gained in this example, the incremental cost-effectiveness compared with 20 mg/day is significantly higher at $26,650, and while the average cost-effectiveness of the 80 mg/day dose is $25,800, the incremental cost-effectiveness compared with 40 mg/day is very much higher at $84,300 per life-year gained. Clearly, as this example shows, it is quite misleading to calculate average cost-effectiveness ratios, as they ignore the alternatives available.

2.4 Mutually exclusive alternatives: dominance and extended dominance

Figure 2.4 shows five mutually exclusive treatment options (V, W, X, Y and Z) plotted on the cost-effectiveness plane. All five treatments cost more than the no-treatment alternative, and all five are more effective than no treatment, so they are all in the north-east quadrant. As they are mutually exclusive, it is appropriate to compare them directly. Bear in mind that at all times we are trying to maximize health gain with the available resources, which here means pushing as far to the right as possible while moving up the vertical axis as little as possible. Therefore we can think of the line running from the origin to option W, and then on to options X and Z, as the **cost-effectiveness frontier**—for any given level of spending and with the available options, health gain will be maximized by choosing one of the treatments on that frontier.

The first point of note is that intervention V is less effective than intervention W, but is also more costly. This is sometimes described as **dominance** or **strong dominance**: one option dominates another on both dimensions of interest—effectiveness and cost. In Figure 2.4, it is evident that all points in the shaded area above and to the left of point W are (strongly) dominated by option W. Therefore option V should be eliminated from any further comparisons between these options.

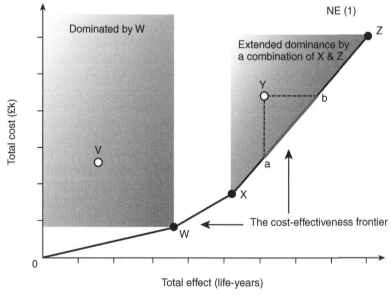

Fig. 2.4 Dominance and extended dominance.

The second point of note in Figure 2.4 concerns intervention Y. It is not strongly dominated by options X or Z, as it is more effective than X and less costly than Z. Indeed, any point in the shaded triangle above the line from X to Z is more effective than X but is also less costly than Z.

What happens if the budget constraint allows us to do more than option X but prevents adoption of alternative Z? Should option Y be considered? Imagine that the line running from X to Z describes what happens as we gradually increase the proportion of patients receiving treatment Z instead of treatment X from 0% to 100%. As we move along this line, it can be seen that there is a portion of the line—the portion marked a to b—which does dominate point Y, i.e. any point between a and b is less costly and more effective than option Y. Therefore it would be better to adopt some combination of X and Z than to adopt option Y. This situation is described as a position of **extended dominance** (the origin of the term is discussed by Cantor (1994)). Note that extended dominance requires two assumptions: (1) the treatment options that need to be combined are perfectly divisible, i.e. they can be produced at any scale, and there is no technical difficulty in providing the treatment to a small fraction of the eligible population; (2) there are constant returns to scale with the same treatment cost per person irrespective of whether 10%, 50%, or 100% of the eligible patients are being treated. In other words, the extended dominance approach set out above depends on an assumption that cost-effectiveness is not affected by the proportion of the eligible patient population receiving that treatment. That may be a reasonable assumption for many interventions, but may not hold for others (for example, screening or diagnostic interventions that require substantial investment in capital equipment).

Table 2.1 shows a worked example where five mutually exclusive treatment options exist (labelled A to E). Option A represents the baseline or no-treatment option, which for simplicity is assumed to have no costs or effects. The other options, labelled B to E, have been arranged in order of increasing total cost (column 1), where total cost and total effect (columns 1 and 2) are calculated in comparison with the no treatment option. Note, however, following the preceding discussion, that we are not interested in the average cost-effectiveness ratio (column 1 divided by column 2) of the options, as these are alternative and mutually exclusive options which need to be compared directly. Instead, we are interested in calculating the incremental costs, effects, and cost-effectiveness of these alternatives relative to the next most effective non-dominated alternative.

In the top part of Table 2.1, we begin by calculating the incremental cost and incremental effect of each option compared with the previous less expensive alternative (B versus A, C versus B, etc.) in columns 4 and 5. From these values, the incremental cost-effectiveness can be calculated, as ΔCost/ΔEffect (column 6). For example, compared with option D, option E costs an additional £15,000 for an additional health gain of 0.5 QALYs, and so has an ICER of £30,000. However, it is immediately obvious that option D is in fact more expensive and less effective than (i.e. is dominated by) the previous less expensive alternative (option C); therefore D can be eliminated.

The central part of Table 2.1 recalculates the ICERs with option D eliminated. The ICER for option E is now calculated in comparison with option C, which has become

Table 2.1 Calculating incremental cost-effectiveness and identifying dominated and extended dominated alternatives

	1	2	3	4	5	6
Option	Total cost	Total QALYs	Comparison	Incremental cost	Incremental QALY	ICER
A	0	0	–	–	–	–
B	£10,000	0.4	B vs. A	£10,000	0.4	£25,000
C	£22,000	0.55	C vs. B	£12,000	0.15	£80,000
D	£25,000	0.5	D vs. C	£ 3,000	–0.05	Dominated
E	£40,000	1	E vs. D	£15,000	0.5	£30,000
After excluding strongly dominated options:						
A	0	0	–	–	–	–
B	£10,000	0.4	B vs. A	£10,000	0.4	£25,000
C	£22,000	0.55	C vs. B	£12,000	0.15	Extended dominated
E	£40,000	1	E vs. C	£18,000	0.45	£40,000
After excluding extendedly dominated options:						
A	0	0	–	–	–	–
B	£10,000	0.4	B vs. A	£10,000	0.4	£25,000
E	£40,000	1	E vs. B	£30,000	0.6	£50,000

the previous less expensive alternative. However, it is now obvious that as we move from option C to option E the ICER falls from £80,000 to £40,000. This indicates that we cannot be on the cost-effectiveness frontier, and so option C must be extended dominated and should also be removed from the comparison. The bottom part of Table 2.1 shows the final situation, now with option E's ICER calculated against option B. Having eliminated all dominated and extended dominated options, the ICER will always rise as we move to the next most costly (and next most effective) option.

Figure 2.5 summarizes this example, immediately making clear the relative positions of these options and illustrating the value of plotting results on the cost-effectiveness plane. The cost-effectiveness frontier runs from A to B to E and its slope increases when moving from the least costly/least effective treatment (A) towards the most costly/most effective treatment (E). Any combination of B and E along the heavily shaded portion of the line will be more cost-effective than the extended dominated option C. As Figure 2.5 shows, failing to remove dominated and extended

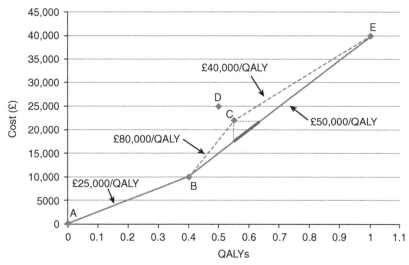

Fig. 2.5 Graphic illustration of Table 2.1.

dominated options before the final ICERs are calculated will result in comparisons with irrelevant alternatives and misleading conclusions about cost-effectiveness.

2.5 Using cost-effectiveness to maximize health gain

Let us now assume that the methods set out in the previous section have been followed to calculate the incremental cost-effectiveness of a whole series of independent programmes under consideration by a newly established health promotion agency. Note that we are now moving from a comparison of mutually exclusive options to the consideration of a set of independent programmes, for each of which incremental costs and effects have already been calculated against the next best alternative. The distinction between mutually exclusive options and sets of independent programmes is further explored with worked examples by Karlsson and Johannesson (1996).

Table 2.2 summarizes the results of this initial exercise. A total of 12 possible independent interventions have been identified, and for each of them the ICER has been calculated against the next best alternative, in addition to the total incremental costs and total incremental health gains that would result from giving these treatments to all eligible patients in the population of interest. The total annual cost of providing all 12 interventions is £10.5 million, a total of 698 additional QALYs are obtained for this expenditure, and their ICERs range from £4706 per QALY gained to £92,500 per QALY gained.

The agency is then informed that its annual budget will be capped at £10 million. Therefore in order to maximize the health gains possible within its budget, it ranks all the possible interventions it can undertake by cost per QALY, and establishes that to stay within budget it can afford all the interventions except numbers 11 and 12, which are the least cost-effective, i.e. have the highest ICERs. That leaves it in the position where, by spending a total of £9.71 million, it can afford to provide 10 interventions

Table 2.2 Using cost-effectiveness to maximize health gain: step 1

Intervention	Incremental cost (£k)	Incremental effectiveness (QALYs)	ICER (cost per QALY) (£)
1	1300	165	7879
2	600	28	21,429
3	750	110	6818
4	750	13	57,692
5	2200	75	29,333
6	400	85	4706
7	800	18	44,444
8	1200	65	18,462
9	1500	96	15,625
10	210	32	6563
11	420	7	60,000
12	370	4	92,500
Total	10,500	698	

which together will yield a total of 687 QALYs gained. Table 2.3 shows the same information as Table 2.2, but with the interventions ordered by cost-effectiveness, with the two least cost-effective interventions dropped, and with the cumulative cost and cumulative QALYs gained calculated as each intervention is added.

Figure 2.6(a) shows the same information as Table 2.3, plotting the cumulative costs and health gains as each intervention is added to form the cost-effectiveness frontier for the agency. Recall that this is now a frontier constructed from a set of independent programmes, and not the frontier identified in Figure 2.4 to compare mutually exclusive options.

Shortly after implementing these interventions, the agency is instructed to implement an entirely new intervention, but within its existing budget. When implemented, this new intervention will cost £1.6 million annually and gain 122 QALYs, giving an incremental cost-effectiveness of £13,115 per QALY gained. Fortunately, this is better than several existing interventions, and Table 2.4 shows the position once the new programme has been adopted.

The new intervention comes fifth when ranked by cost-effectiveness, and the two least-effective interventions (7 and 4) are pushed above the budget constraint and have to be dropped to release enough resources to pay for the new intervention. Most importantly, however, despite dropping these interventions, the total QALYs gained by the agency's programme of interventions have increased from 687 to 778, while expenditure remains within the existing budget constraint of £10 million.

Figure 2.6(b) again shows this information in the form of a cost-effectiveness frontier, which has now been pushed out so that more health gain is obtained with the

Table 2.3 Using cost-effectiveness to maximize health gain: step 2

Intervention	Incremental cost (£k)	Incremental effectiveness (QALYs)	ICER (cost per QALY) (£)	Cumulative cost (£k)	Cumulative effectiveness (QALYs)
6	400	85	4706	400	85
10	210	32	6563	610	117
3	750	110	6818	1360	227
1	1300	165	7879	2660	392
9	1500	96	15,625	4160	488
8	1200	65	18,462	5360	553
2	600	28	21,429	5960	581
5	2200	75	29,333	8160	656
7	800	18	44,444	8960	674
4	750	13	57,692	9710	687
Total	9710	687			

same resources. The area between the two frontiers represents the gain in health as a result of adopting the new intervention.

Clearly, there will be many complicating factors in practice, not least the far from simple task of extracting money from existing interventions to pay for new ones! In fact this is one of the key points raised by critics of the cost-effectiveness approach, who argue that typically it does not identify the opportunity cost of adopting a new intervention, i.e. the health gain from existing activities that may be displaced and so may lead to inappropriate resource allocation decisions and uncontrolled expenditure growth rather than maximization of health gain from the existing budget (Gafni and Birch 1993; Sendi *et al.* 2002). However, the worked example does illustrate how the cost-effectiveness approach can inform the priority that a new intervention should be given and, equally importantly, helps to identify what activities should be dropped if required to fund a cost-effective new treatment within the existing budget.

2.6 **What is the maximum acceptable incremental cost-effectiveness ratio**

As we shall see in this book, a great deal of effort in recent years has been directed at ways of defining, handling, and reducing uncertainty in our estimates of incremental cost-effectiveness. In contrast, comparatively little attention has been paid to the uncertainty around the maximum value of the incremental cost-effectiveness ratio, a neglect memorably described in one critical article as 'the silence of the lambda' (Gafni and Birch 2006). There are at least four ways of approaching this question: a rule of thumb (which may be more or less arbitrary), a league table approach, a revealed

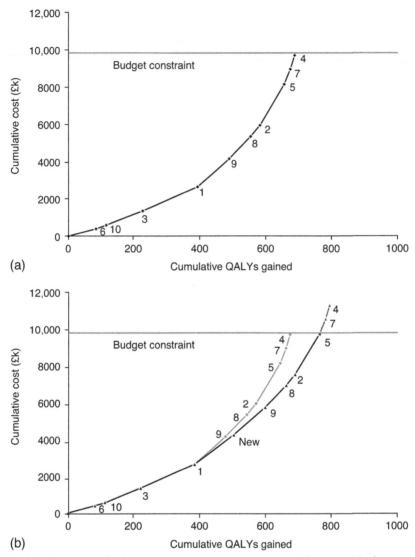

Fig. 2.6 Using cost-effectiveness to maximize health gain: (a) before and (b) after introduction of new intervention.

preference approach, and a stated preference approach. For a fuller discussion, see Weinstein (1995).

2.6.1 Rule-based approaches

One of the earliest attempts to set rules for cost-effectiveness threshold values was made by Kaplan and Bush (1982). Based on their knowledge of the US health system and existing cost-effectiveness literature, they claimed that three categories of

Table 2.4 Using cost-effectiveness to maximize health gain: step 3

Intervention	Incremental cost (£k)	Incremental effectiveness (QALYs)	ICER (cost per QALY) (£)	Cumulative cost (£k)	Cumulative effectiveness (QALYs)
6	400	85	4706	400	85
10	210	32	6563	610	117
3	750	110	6818	1360	227
1	1300	165	7879	2660	392
New	1600	122	13,115	4260	514
9	1500	96	15,625	5760	610
8	1200	65	18,462	6960	675
2	600	28	21,429	7560	703
5	2200	75	29,333	9760	778
7	800	18	44,444	10,560	796
4	750	13	57,692	11,310	809
Total	9760	778			

the cost-utility or 'cost per well-year' ratio could be defined: those less than $20,000, considered cost-effective by current standards; those between $20,000 and $100,000, considered possibly controversial but justifiable based on many current examples; and those greater than $100,000, considered questionable compared with other health care expenditures. Based on simple consumer price index and exchange rate calculations, these figures would correspond approximately to $52,000 and $260,000 in 2009 US dollars, and to £27,000 and £137,000 in 2009 UK pounds.

Curiously, Laupacis *et al.* (1992) adopted identical cut-off points of CAN$20,000 per QALY gained, up to which level they considered that there would be strong grounds for adoption, and CAN$100,000 per QALY gained, above which they considered that evidence for adoption was weak. However, as they were working in 1990 Canadian dollars, their thresholds were rather different: again based on simplified calculations, their figures correspond to approximately $28,100 and $141,000 in 2009 US dollars, and to approximately £15,600 and £78,900 in 2009 UK pounds. One contemporary commentary referred to this as 'cross border shopping with 10-year-old dollars' (Naylor *et al.* 1993).

Kaplan and Bush did not claim that their thresholds were empirically based, but did suggest that their guidelines 'emerge from several previous analyses' (Kaplan and Bush 1982, p.74). Similarly, Laupacis and colleagues made no empirical claims regarding their guidelines, referring to them as 'arbitrary limits' (Laupacis *et al.* 1992, p.476), based partly on a review of previous economic evaluations and guidelines, and partly on what seemed to be routinely, partly, or not provided at that time in the Canadian health care system. Despite this lack of analytical foundation, these threshold values gained widespread currency, and in a review of published cost-effectiveness evidence Neumann *et al.* (2000) found that 34% of the 228 articles they examined quoted a cost-effectiveness threshold value, with a median value squarely within these ranges at $50,000 per QALY gained.

Attempts to trace the genealogy of this $50,000 per QALY figure have suggested that it may originate in an estimate of the amount that the US Medicare programme was prepared to spend on dialysis for patients with endstage renal disease (Hirth *et al.* 2000). One peculiarity of this figure is that it does not seem to have changed much over time despite price changes and economic growth (Ubel *et al.* 2003). More recently, Braithwaite *et al.* (2008) adopted a different perspective, asking whether a $50,000 per QALY rule would be consistent with societal preferences in the USA. They attempted to define a lower bound based on society's willingness to devote a larger share of national income to the health sector over the period from 1950 to 2003, and an upper bound from the willingness or unwillingness of non-elderly adults to buy health insurance voluntarily, even when not constrained by income. This approach suggested that plausible lower and upper bounds for a cost-effectiveness decision rule were $183,000 per life-year and $264,000 per life-year, respectively, or approximately $109,000 to $297,000 per QALY saved. All their base-case and sensitivity analyses results were substantially higher than $50,000 per QALY.

Another rule-based approach to setting cost-effectiveness threshold values has been set out by the National Institute for Health and Clinical Excellence (NICE), which was established in 1999 as part of the publicly funded UK National Health Service (NHS) with the objective of giving advice to health professionals on the highest attainable standards of care for NHS patients in England and Wales (Rawlins 1999). The NICE threshold values have been influential not least because cost-effectiveness analysis plays an important role in guidance issued by NICE on whether or not the NHS should adopt new technologies (or continue existing ones). NICE has never stated any explicit ceiling, citing a lack of empirical evidence, a reluctance to give cost-effectiveness absolute priority over other objectives such as equity, and a desire to encourage price competition amongst suppliers (Rawlins and Culyer 2004). However, in 2004 the Chair and Deputy Chair of NICE sketched a decision framework indicating the relationship in NICE deliberations between the probability of accepting a technology and its cost per QALY. This is shown in Figure 2.7.

Figure 2.7 shows a curve with two inflection points, A and B. Up to inflection point A, with a cost per QALY gained in the range £5000–£15,000, it is highly unlikely that a technology would be rejected on cost-effectiveness grounds. However, once that cost-effectiveness figure had risen to inflection point B, or approximately £25,000–£35,000, it is unlikely that the technology would be accepted, unless there were other compelling reasons for doing so (Rawlins and Culyer 2004).

More recently this general approach has been restated as follows:

> NICE has never identified an ICER above which interventions should not be recommended and below which they should. However, in general, interventions with an ICER of less than £20,000 per QALY gained are considered to be cost effective. [...] Above a most plausible ICER of £20,000 per QALY gained, judgements about the acceptability of the intervention as an effective use of NHS resources will specifically take account of

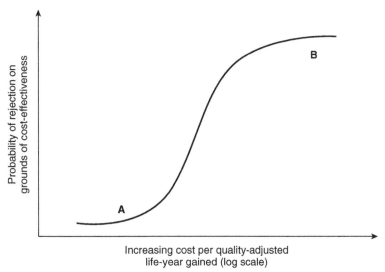

Fig. 2.7 Relation between probability of a technology being rejected by NICE as cost-ineffective and its incremental cost-effectiveness ratio. Reproduced from Rawlins and Culyer (2004), with permission from the BMJ Publishing Group Ltd.

> [additional] factors. [...] Above a most plausible ICER of £30,000 per QALY gained, advisory bodies will need to make an increasingly stronger case for supporting the intervention as an effective use of NHS resources with respect to the[se] factors. (NICE 2008b, p.18)

NICE indicated that these additional factors comprise the degree of certainty around the estimated cost-effectiveness ratio, the possibility that changes in quality of life (as measured) may not fully capture the health gain, and whether the technology has other innovative benefits that are not adequately captured in the measurement of health gain (NICE 2008b, p.19). The extent to which NICE's actual decisions relate to these stated thresholds is considered in section 2.6.3.

Finally, an alternative rule-based approach has been proposed in which the maximum willingness to pay for a QALY is related to the country's gross domestic product (GDP) per capita. Williams (2004) advanced one line of reasoning in support of this, arguing that each person has an entitlement to a 'fair share' of the country's wealth and that this can be approximated by average national product per person.

The World Health Organization (WHO) has advocated a similar approach, which goes further by suggesting as a rule of thumb that interventions with a cost-effectiveness ratio less than the country's GDP can be considered very cost-effective, those with a cost-effectiveness ratio of between one and three times GDP can be considered cost-effective, and those with a ratio greater than three times GDP should be considered not cost-effective (Tan-Torres *et al.* 2003). Thus, for the poorest countries of Africa for example, interventions costing less than $1695 per disability adjusted life-year (DALY) averted (in 2005 international dollars calculated using purchasing power parities (see Chapter 6 for details)) would be considered very cost-effective, and those costing up to $5086 per DALY averted would be considered cost-effective. DALYs are discussed in Chapter 5. By contrast, in Western Europe (including the UK) treatments would be considered very cost-effective up to a ratio of $30,439 per DALY and cost-effective up to a ratio of $91,318 per DALY (equivalent to £18,900 and £56,600 per DALY). The WHO approach is based on a discussion in the report of the Commission on Macroeconomics and Health to the WHO (WHO 2001, p.31), which in turn cites previous literature on the value of a life (e.g. Cutler and Richardson 1997; Murphy and Topel 2006) suggesting that a year of life is valued at around three times annual earnings. If that is the case, the WHO report argues that it must be worth spending up to three times per capita annual income, or 'conservatively' the same amount as per capita annual income, to gain one QALY or to avert one DALY. Decision rules in low- and middle-income countries are discussed in detail by Shillcutt *et al.* (2009).

The flaws in the Williams approach, despite the appeal to 'common sense', are that a similar claim for a 'fair share' could in principle be made for education or any other good or service, undermining the approach as a method of prioritization, and it also fails to take into account either society's willingness to pay for health gains or the ability of any particular system to afford new interventions assessed using these criteria (McCabe *et al.* 2008). The WHO approach avoids the 'fair share' problem and has a clearer, if indirect, link to society's willingness to pay for health gains via the value of life literature, but also fails to address the ability of any particular system to afford new interventions that might be deemed cost-effective using these criteria.

2.6.2 The league table approach

Another way of trying to identify the maximum willingness to pay for health gain is by means of cost-effectiveness league tables (Mason *et al.* 1993). If we had full information on the ICERs of all available interventions, it would be possible to rank them by ICER, calculate the cumulative cost of adopting them in turn from the treatment with the lowest ICER up to the treatment with the highest ICER, identify the point at which the budget constraint was reached, and then note the ICER of the last treatment that is adopted before the budget runs out. Having done this, the decision-maker could then set an explicit maximum acceptable ICER, and any future intervention with an ICER below this maximum could be adopted within the budget constraint and still produce health gain.

A hypothetical example of this was previously seen in Tables 2.2 and 2.3. In that example, having ranked all interventions by ICER, it became clear that the hypothetical agency reached its budget constraint at intervention 4, with an ICER of £57,692 per QALY, and could not adopt the interventions with ICERs higher than this. Therefore the maximum acceptable ICER in that situation is £57,692 per QALY.

Of course in practice it is unlikely that full information on all interventions will be available, and it must also be noted that league tables constructed from many different sources may be quite unreliable, for example because estimates were obtained using different methodologies or assumptions or were performed in different countries at varying times (Drummond *et al.* 1993; Gerard and Mooney 1993; Petrou *et al.* 1993). However, compared with early efforts in this field, significant progress has been made in constructing detailed and quite comprehensive tabulations of cost-effectiveness studies. For example, by early 2010, the Cost-Effectiveness Analysis (CEA) Registry maintained by the Center for the Evaluation of Value and Risk in Health at Tufts University/New England Medical Center had incorporated data on more than 2000 studies (https://research.tufts-nemc.org/cear/Default.aspx) with detailed information on methodology and results. As a result specific questions can be explored from the literature while including only studies meeting specific quality criteria. For example, in 2008 the Registry was used to demonstrate that the distributions of ICERs for preventive measures and for treatment interventions in the published literature were very similar, in contrast with the widespread supposition that prevention offers much better value for money and should be prioritized (Cohen *et al.* 2008).

2.6.3 **Revealed preference**

An alternative approach to finding the amount that decision-makers or society are willing to pay for improvements in health is to systematically examine the preferences of decision-makers as revealed in the decisions they have made. For example, until May 2005 the Standing Medical Advisory Committee (SMAC) was a statutory body providing advice to the Minister of Health in England and Wales on services provided by the NHS. In 1997, when asked to produce guidelines on the use of statins as cholesterol-lowering therapy, it recommended that the priority was to treat patients with a history of myocardial infarction or angina (secondary prevention) rather than patients with no prior history of coronary heart disease but a high risk of developing it (primary prevention).

Available contemporary evidence on the cost-effectiveness of statin therapy in different patient groups (Jonsson *et al.* 1996; Pharoah and Hollingworth 1996; Caro *et al.* 1997) could be used to infer the point at which the SMAC recommendations switched from 'treat' to 'do not treat'. These studies suggest that secondary prevention had an ICER between £5000 and £10,000 per life-year gained, and that primary prevention at the risk cut-off level they specified had an ICER of anywhere between £20,000 and £60,000 per life-year gained, depending on the study. Therefore revealed preference would suggest that the decision-makers (in this case SMAC) had a maximum acceptable ICER between £20,000 and £60,000, although the SMAC report made no reference to cost-effectiveness evidence or the uncertainty surrounding it when framing its recommendations.

Devlin and Parkin (2004) published a study examining whether the actions of NICE as revealed by their decisions were in line with the stated thresholds or 'inflection points'. They fitted various model specifications to data on the cost per QALY and other characteristics of the technology being appraised from the first 51 observable yes/no decisions that NICE made in its first 3 years of operation, and concluded that the threshold for rejecting technologies seemed to be in the range £35,000–£48,000 per QALY, considerably above the stated range. However, in a later exercise surveying 117 technologies that had been the subject of NICE guidance up to April 2005, Raftery (2006) concluded that none had been approved with a cost per QALY gained greater than £39,000.

Similar methods have been used to look at other decision-making bodies. For example, in Australia, George *et al.* (2001) examined 355 recommendations made by the Pharmaceutical Benefits Advisory Committee (PBAC), which has a mandatory role in determining whether new pharmaceuticals should receive public reimbursement. For the 26 submissions made to PBAC over the period 1991–1996 for which cost-effectiveness data were available, they found that none were rejected at a cost per life-year gained of less than Au$39,800 (Australian dollars in 1998–99 prices), equivalent to UK£14,700, while none were accepted at a cost per life-year gained of more than Au$75,300 (UK£27,900).

An alternative to looking at national decision-making bodies is to look at more microlevel clinical decisions. Williams *et al.* (2006) demonstrated this approach by looking at a sample of women treated for breast cancer and comparing the actual clinical decisions concerning who was selected for different adjuvant therapies with the predicted cost-effectiveness of treatment derived from a prognostic model. Using the prognostic model, women could be rank-ordered by the predicted cost-effectiveness of treating each person. It was then possible to observe the cost-effectiveness ratio at the point at which the current budget for adjuvant therapy for breast cancer would have been exhausted if the women had been treated in strict order of cost-effectiveness. This could be interpreted as a 'revealed' ceiling, in the sense that the budget allocated to adjuvant breast cancer therapy would not permit anyone to be treated beyond that point, even if available resources were allocated strictly on the basis of cost-effectiveness. Figure 2.8 shows some illustrative results from this exercise.

The bars and left axis show the frequency distribution of the predicted or modelled cost-effectiveness of providing adjuvant treatment to each of 1058 women with breast cancer compared with not treating them. The line and right axis show the cumulative percentage of women, starting from the left with the 5% of women who could have been treated for less than £2500 per QALY gained, and rising to 100%; note that for the 30% of women in the two bars furthest right, treatment either cost more than £75,000 per QALY gained or would have increased costs and reduced quality-adjusted survival, mainly because of treatment-related side effects.

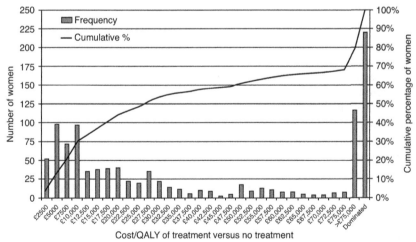

Fig. 2.8 Frequency distribution of cost-effectiveness of adjuvant treatment of 1058 women with breast cancer. Derived from data reported by Williams *et al.* (2006).

From Figure 2.8 it is easy to see that a budget allowing up to 30% of women to be treated would suggest a ceiling ratio of around £10,000 per QALY gained, while a budget allowing up to 50% of women to be treated would suggest an upper cost-effectiveness value of approximately £25,000 per QALY. In practice, around 26% of women had been treated over the whole period covered by the data, although this proportion had been rising over time and the current protocol suggests that around 36% should be treated. Nevertheless, these results suggest that the threshold values being used by NICE may be above those in use in routine clinical practice, at least in this clinical area.

Yet another way of trying to look at the current willingness to pay for health gain by some form of revealed preference is a study by Martin *et al.* (2008) which looked at variations between 295 English Primary Care Trusts in their health expenditure in different disease areas, and their health outcomes in these disease areas measured in terms of deaths from causes amenable to health care. Their results suggested that, at the margin, the cost of a life-year saved from expenditure on existing cancer services was about £13,100, and about £8000 for circulatory disease. Adjusting for quality of life would suggest that these equate to £19,000 and £12,000 per QALY gained. In both cases cost-effectiveness remained well below the threshold values being used by NICE when deciding what new interventions to approve (NICE 2008a).

2.6.4 **Stated preference**

An alternative to revealed preference methods is to use a stated preference (SP) technique to obtain estimates of the value respondents place on a good, service, or effect. These techniques usually fall into two broad categories: choice modelling (CM) and contingent valuation (CV). Choice modelling methods typically aim to reveal the preferences people have for specific characteristics or attributes, for example the waiting time for a surgical procedure or the reassurance provided by better diagnostic information. Contingent valuation (CV) methods usually aim to obtain valuations for a good or service as a whole, for example an entire surgical procedure including the process and the outcomes. Details of these methods are available elsewhere; Bateman *et al.* (2002) provide a manual for the methods across a range of areas, and a companion volume to this book deals with the application of these methods in cost-benefit analyses of health care interventions (McIntosh *et al.* 2010).

The use of stated preference methods to estimate the maximum willingness to pay for a QALY has been quite limited; some studies have drawn widely on literature in areas other than health interventions, while others have relied on less formal survey methods. For example, Hirth *et al.* (2000) conducted a systematic review of all value-of-life estimates published in the English language between 1969 and 1997, and then classified them into contingent valuation studies, human capital studies, revealed preference studies based on willingness to take riskier jobs for higher rewards, and other revealed preference studies. They found eight contingent valuation studies, and having made a quality-of-life adjustment to the results, found that the median valuation of a QALY was $161,305 in 1997 US dollars, well above the maximum willingness to pay for health interventions implied by rule-based approaches. However, there was tremendous variation between studies around this median value, and the studies were not concerned with health interventions but with other areas such as transport.

Another study (Nadler *et al.* 2006) did focus on health interventions, but was effectively a straight survey rather than a contingent valuation exercise. These authors asked 139 academic medical oncologists at two American hospitals to provide estimates for the cost, effectiveness, and perceived value for money of an actual cancer drug, and also asked respondents to state how large a gain in life expectancy would be required to justify a hypothetical cancer drug costing $70,000 per year. Based on the results, they calculated that the implied cost-effectiveness threshold, i.e. the point up to which oncologists considered a treatment offered good value for money, was approximately $300,000 per QALY, well above the $50,000 per QALY figure most frequently quoted.

The importance of the cost-effectiveness threshold value to the work of NICE in England and Wales has led to a number of research projects being commissioned. In one such study, Mason *et al.* (2009) reviewed existing studies that used contingent valuation methods to look at willingness to pay for road safety improvements resulting in a reduced risk of death. They then adjusted these results for quality of life and for age-related variations in attitudes to risk, and used discounting to vary the assumption that all future years have equal value. Their results are presented in Table 2.5.

The results suggested that the willingness to pay for a discounted QALY was around £69,000 if no adjustment was made for variations between age groups in their valuations. If this adjustment is made, and young adults who typically have a lower valuation of reductions in risk than older adults are included, the willingness to pay for a QALY falls to around £31,000. When these 'reckless' younger adults are excluded, the figure

Table 2.5 Estimates of the value of a life-year and a QALY

		Value of a life-year (median)		Value of a QALY (median)	
		Undiscounted (£)	Discounted (£)	Undiscounted (£)	Discounted (£)
1	No adjustment for effect of age on valuation	42,626	54,550	54,091	68,656
2	Adjusting for effect of age on valuation	20,422	26,070	24,219	30,745
3	Adjusting for effect of age on valuation, excluding 'reckless youth'	38,764	55,749	46,504	65,338
4	Focusing only on quality-of-life effects of non-fatal injuries	–		6414–21,519	

Source: Mason *et al.* 2009.

rises again to around £65,000 per QALY. Finally, when the risk of death is excluded from the calculations, so that valuations relate only to the risk of a serious non-fatal accident, the valuation of a QALY falls to somewhere in the range £6,400–£21,500.

In addition to the variations arising from different methods of calculation in this study, it should also be noted that these results are median values, behind which are very wide variations in individual valuations. Therefore it seems clear that contingent valuation studies can be used to obtain estimates of willingness to pay for reductions in mortality and morbidity, but the sample sizes and analytical methods required to obtain reliable and usable estimates for economic evaluation are not yet settled.

2.7 Summary

This chapter has introduced the different types of economic evaluation, noting that cost-utility analysis is currently the preferred framework by many analysts and decision-making agencies. The chapter then demonstrated how cost-effectiveness information can contribute towards the objective of maximizing health gain from available resources, and this was followed by a discussion of different ways to estimate the maximum willingness to pay for health gain. The following chapter (Chapter 3) is the first of three addressing the question of how health gains can be quantified and valued.

References

Anderson, J.P., Bush, J.W., Chen, M., and Dolenc, D. (1986). Policy space areas and properties of benefit-cost utility analysis. *Journal of the American Medical Association*, **255**, 794–95.

Bateman, I., Carson, R.T., Day, B., *et al.* (2002). *Economic Valuation with Stated Preference Techniques: A Manual*. Edward Elgar, Cheltenham.

Black, W.C. (1990). The CE plane: a graphic representation of cost-effectiveness. *Medical Decision Making*, **10**, 212–14.

Braithwaite, R.S., Meltzer, D.O., King, J.T., Leslie, D., and Roberts, M.S. (2008). What does the value of modern medicine say about the $50,000 per quality-adjusted life-year decision rule? *Medical Care*, **46**, 349–56.

Briggs, A.H. and O'Brien, B.J. (2001). The death of cost-minimization analysis? *Health Economics*, **10**, 179–84.

Brouwer, W.B.F., Culyer, A.J., van Exel, N.J.A., and Rutten, F.F.H. (2008). Welfarism vs. extra-welfarism. *Journal of Health Economics*, **27**, 325–38.

Cantor, S.B. (1994). Cost-effectiveness analysis, extended dominance, and ethics: a quantitative assessment. *Medical Decision Making*, **14**, 259–65.

Caro, J., Klittich, W., McGuire, A., *et al.* (1997). The West of Scotland coronary prevention study: economic benefit analysis of primary prevention with pravastatin [see comments]. *British Medical Journal*, **315**, (7122) 1577–1582

Clarke, P.M. (1998). Cost-benefit analysis and mammographic screening: a travel cost approach. *Journal of Health Economics*, **17**, 767–87.

Clarke, P., Gray, A., Adler, A., *et al.* (2001). Cost-effectiveness analysis of intensive blood-glucose control with metformin in overweight patients with type II diabetes (UKPDS No. 51). *Diabetologia*, **44**, 298–304.

Cohen, J.T., Neumann, P.J., and Weinstein, M.C. (2008). Does preventive care save money? Health economics and the presidential candidates. *New England Journal of Medicine*, **358**, 661–3.

Cookson, R., McCabe, C., and Tsuchiya, A. (2008). Public healthcare resource allocation and the Rule of Rescue. *Journal of Medical Ethics*, **34**, 540–4.

Culyer, A.J. (1989). The normative economics of health care finance and provision. *Oxford Review of Economic Policy*, **5**, 34.

Cutler, D.M., and Richardson, E. (1997). Measuring the health of the US population. *Brookings Papers on Economic Activity*, **28**, 217–82.

Detsky, A.S. and Naglie, I.G. (1990). A clinician's guide to cost-effectiveness analysis. *Annals of Internal Medicine*, **113**, 147–54.

Devlin, N. and Parkin, D. (2004). Does NICE have a cost-effectiveness threshold and what other factors influence its decisions? A binary choice analysis. *Health Economics*, **13**, 437–52.

Drummond, M., Torrance, G., and Mason, J. (1993). Cost-effectiveness league tables: more harm than good? *Social Science and Medicine*, **37**, 33–40.

Drummond, M.F., Sculpher, M.J., Torrance, G.W., O'Brien, B.J., and Stoddart, G.L. (2005). *Methods for the Economic Evaluation of Health Care Programmes* (3rd edn). Oxford University Press.

Elixhauser, A. (1993). Health care cost-benefit and cost-effectiveness analysis (CBA/CEA) from 1979 to 1990: a bibliography. *Medical Care*, **31**, JS1–JS141.

Elixhauser, A., Halpern, M., Schmier, J., and Luce, B.R. (1998). Health care CBA and CEA from 1991 to 1996: an updated bibliography. *Medical Care*, **36**, (Suppl) MS1–147.

Ellstrom, M., Ferraz-Nunes, J., Hahlin, M., and Olsson, J.H. (1998). A randomized trial with a cost-consequence analysis after laparoscopic and abdominal hysterectomy. *Obstetrics and Gynecology*, **91**, 30–4.

Gafni, A. and Birch, S. (1993). Guidelines for the adoption of new technologies: a prescription for uncontrolled growth in expenditures and how to avoid the problem [comment]. *Canadian Medical Association Journal*, **148**, 913–17.

Gafni, A. and Birch, S. (2006). Incremental cost-effectiveness ratios (ICERs): the silence of the lambda. *Social Science and Medicine*, **62**, 2091–2100.

Garber, A.M. and Phelps, C.E. (1997). Economic foundations of cost-effectiveness analysis. *Journal of Health Economics*, **16**, 1–31.

George, B., Harris, A., and Mitchell, A. (2001). Cost effectiveness analysis and the consistency of decision making: evidence from pharmaceutical reimbursement in Australia (1991 to 1996). *PharmacoEconomics*, **19**, 1103–9.

Gerard, K. and Mooney, G. (1993). QALY league tables: handle with care. *Health Economics*, **2**, 59–64.

Goldman, L., Weinstein, M.C., Goldman, P.A., and Williams, L.W. (1991). Cost-effectiveness of HMG-CoA reductase inhibition for primary and secondary prevention of coronary heart disease. *Journal of the American Medical Association*, **265**, 1145–51.

Gyrd-Hansen, D. (1997). Is it cost effective to introduce screening programmes for colorectal cancer? Illustrating the principles of optimal resource allocation. *Health Policy*, **41**, 189–99.

Hirth, R.A., Chernew, M.E., Miller, E., Fendrick, A.M., and Weissert, W.G. (2000). Willingness to pay for a quality-adjusted life year: in search of a standard. *Medical Decision Making*, **20**, 332–42.

Johannesson, M. (1996). *Theory and Methods of Economic Evaluation of Health Care*. Kluwer Academic, Boston, MA.

Jonsson, B., Johannesson, M., Kjekshus, J., Olsson, A.G., Pedersen, T.R., and Wedel, H. (1996). Cost-effectiveness of cholesterol lowering. Results from the Scandinavian Simvastatin Survival Study (4S). *European Heart Journal*, **17**, 1001–7.

Kaplan, R.M. and Bush, J.W. (1982). Health-related quality of life measurement for evaluation research and policy analysis. *Health Psychology*, **1**, 61–80.

Karlsson, G. and Johannesson, M. (1996). The decision rules of cost-effectiveness analysis. *PharmacoEconomics*, **9**, (2) 113–120

Laupacis, A., Feeny, D., Detsky, A.S., and Tugwell, P.X. (1992). How attractive does a new technology have to be to warrant adoption and utilization? Tentative guidelines for using clinical and economic evaluations [see comments]. *Canadian Medical Association Journal*, **146**, 473–81.

McCabe, C., Claxton, K., and Culyer, A.J. (2008). The NICE cost-effectiveness threshold. What it is and what that means. *PharmacoEconomics*, **26**, 733–44.

McIntosh, E., Louviere, J.J., Frew, E., and Clarke, P.M. (2010). *Applied Methods of Cost–Benefit Analysis in Health Care*. Oxford University Press.

Martin, S., Rice, N., and Smith, P.C. (2008). Does health care spending improve health outcomes? Evidence-from English programme budgeting data. *Journal of Health Economics*, **27**, 826–42.

Mason, H., Jones-Lee, M., and Donaldson, C. (2009). Modelling the monetary value of a QALY: a new approach based on UK data. *Health Economics*, **18**, 933–50.

Mason, J., Drummond, M., and Torrance, G. (1993). Some guidelines on the use of cost effectiveness league tables [see comments]. *British Medical Journal*, **306**, 570–2.

Murphy, K.M. and Topel, R.H. (2006). The value of health and longevity. *Journal of Political Economy*, **114**, 871–904.

Nadler, E., Eckert, B., and Neumann, P.J. (2006). Do oncologists believe new cancer drugs offer good value? *Oncologist*, **11**, 90–5.

Naylor, C.D., Williams, J.I., Basinski, A., and Goel, V. (1993). Technology assessment and cost-effectiveness analysis: misguided guidelines? *Canadian Medical Association Journal*, **148**, 921.

Neumann, P.J., Sandberg, E.A., Bell, C.M., Stone, P.W., and Chapman, R.H. (2000). Are pharmaceuticals cost-effective? A review of the evidence. *Health Affairs*, **19**, 92–109.

NICE (2008a). *Guide to the Methods of Technology Appraisal*. National Institute for Health and Clinical Excellence, London.

NICE (2008b). *Social Value Judgements: Principles for the Development of NICE Guidance* (2nd edn). National Institute for Health and Clinical Excellence, London.

Pearce, D. and Nash, C. (1981). *The Social Appraisal of Projects: A Text in Cost-Benefit Analysis.* (2nd edn). Macmillan, London.

Petrou, S., Malek, M., and Davey, P.G. (1993). The reliability of cost-utility estimates in cost-per-QALY league tables. *PharmacoEconomics*, **3**, 345–53.

Pharoah, P.D. and Hollingworth, W. (1996). Cost effectiveness of lowering cholesterol concentration with statins in patients with and without pre-existing coronary heart disease: life table method applied to health authority population. *British Medical Journal*, **312**, 1443–8.

Raftery, J. (2006). Review of NICE's recommendations, 1999–2005. *British Medical Journal*, **332**, 1266–8.

Rawlins, M. (1999). In pursuit of quality: the National Institute for Clinical Excellence. *Lancet*, **353**, 1079–82.

Rawlins, M.D. and Culyer, A.J. (2004). National Institute for Clinical Excellence and its value judgments. *British Medical Journal*, **329**, 224–7.

Sendi, P., Gafni, A., and Birch, S. (2002). Opportunity costs and uncertainty in the economic evaluation of health care interventions. *Health Economics*, **11**, 23–31.

Shillcutt, S., Walker, D., Goodman, C., Mills, A., and Street, K. (2009). Cost-effectiveness in low-and middle-income countries: a review of the debates surrounding decision rules. *Pharmacoeconomics*, **27**, 903–17.

Tan-Torres, E., Baltussen, R., and Adams, T. (2003). *Making Choices in Health: WHO Guide to Cost-Effectiveness Analysis*. World Health Organization, Geneva.

Torrance, G.W. (1976). Toward a utility theory foundation for health status index models. *Health Services Research*, **11**, 439–69.

Ubel, P.A., Hirth, R.A., Chernew, M.E., and Fendrick, A.M. (2003). What is the price of life and why doesn't it increase at the rate of inflation? *Archives of Internal Medicine*, **163**, 1637–41.

Van Hout, B., Al, M.J., Gordon, G.S., and Rutten, F.F. (1994). Costs, effects and C/E-ratios alongside a clinical trial. *Health Economics*, **3**, 309–19.

Warner, K.E. and Hutton, R.C. (1980). Cost-Benefit and cost-effectiveness analysis in health-care: growth and composition of the literature. *Medical Care*, **18**, 1069–84.

Weinstein, M.C. (1995). From cost-effectiveness ratios to resource allocation: where to draw the line?. In: *Valuing Health Care: Costs, Benefits and Effectiveness of Pharmaceuticals and Other Medical Technologies* (ed. F.A. Sloan), pp. 77–97. Cambridge University Press.

Weinstein, M.C. and Manning, W.G. (1997). Theoretical issues in cost-effectiveness analysis. *Journal of Health Economics*, **16**, 121–8.

Weinstein, M.C. and Stason, W.B. (1977). Foundations of cost-effectiveness analysis for health and medical practices. *New England Journal of Medicine*, **296**, 716–21.

Weisbrod, B.A. (1971). Costs and benefits of medical research: case study of poliomyelitis. *Journal of Political Economy*, **79**, 527–44.

WHO (2001) *Macroeconomics and Health: Investing in Health for Economic Development. Report of the Commission on Macroeconomics and Health*. World Health Organization, Geneva.

Williams, A. (2004). *What Could be Nicer Than NICE?* Office of Health Economics, London.

Williams, C., Brunskill, S., Altman, D., *et al.* (2006). Cost-effectiveness of using prognostic information to select women with breast cancer for adjuvant systemic therapy. *Health Technology Assessment*, **10**, iii–xi.

Exercise

Interpreting and using cost-effectiveness analysis

Questions

Question 1

Table 2E.1 shows the costs and cost effectiveness of screening programmes for colorectal cancer. The information is based on a Danish study (Gyrd-Hansen 1997). The effectiveness of the programmes is measured in terms of life-years gained, and the cost per life-year figures presented are calculated compared with a 'no screening programme' option. The programmes in Table 2E.1 are mutually exclusive, i.e. only one will be implemented.

Table 2E.1 Costs and cost effectiveness of screening programmes for colorectal cancer

Programme	Costs (£)	Life-years gained (£)	Cost per life-year gained* (£)
Every 2 years; age 55–74	2,900,000	1800	1611
Every 2 years; age 60–74	2,100,000	1400	1500
Every 2 years; age 65–74	1,400,000	1000	1400
Every year; age 50–74	6,700,000	3100	2161
Every year; age 55–74	5,000,000	2600	1923
Every 1.5 years; age 55–74	3,600,000	2100	1714

*Compared with no screening programme.

Since the programmes are mutually exclusive, the appropriate comparison is the incremental cost effectiveness ratio, comparing each option in turn with the next most effective option.

◆ Work out the incremental cost per life-year gained figures, and put in a new table. *Hint*: Incremental rather than average comparisons are required.

◆ Which programme would you recommend implementing? Why?

Question 2

Table 2E.2 shows cost per QALY figures for a number of interventions (this is for illustrative purposes only and the actual figures may not be reliable). Imagine that you must decide how many of these interventions to introduce in a health authority. The interventions are ranked in terms of increasing cost per QALY and are independent, i.e. more than one can be implemented. The interventions in the table are each compared with a 'do nothing' option of no new intervention. Table 2E.2 shows the annual cost of implementing each intervention (this is based on the number of patients in the imaginary health authority that would receive the intervention).

Table 2E.2 Cost and cost per QALY gained for a set of independent interventions

Intervention	Cost per QALY gained* (£)	Annual cost (£)	Cumulative total cost (£)
Hip replacement	1677	20,100,000	
Kidney transplant	6706	168,000	
Breast cancer screening	7397	408,000	
Haemodialysis at home	24,590	590,000	
Beta-interferon	809,900	350,000	

*Compared with no intervention.

♦ Suppose that the health authority has an annual budget constraint of £21 million. Which interventions would they introduce? *Hint*: Work out the cumulative total cost figures.

♦ What is the implied ceiling ratio for acceptable cost-effectiveness?

Answers

Question 1 (Table 2E.3)

Table 2E.3 Costs and cost effectiveness of screening programmes for colorectal cancer

Programme	Incremental costs (£)	Incremental life-years gained	Incremental cost per life-year gained (£)
Every 2 years, age 65–74	1,400,000	1000	1400
Every 2 years, age 60–74	700,000	400	1750
Every 2 years, age 55–74	800,000	400	2000
Every 1.5 years, age 55–74	700,000	300	2333
Every year, age 55–74	1,400,000	500	2800
Every year, age 50–74	1,700,000	500	3400

- First rank the programmes in terms of increasing effectiveness, i.e. by life-years gained.
- Then calculate the incremental costs and incremental effects for each more effective option.
- Divide the incremental costs by the incremental effects to estimate the incremental cost per life-year gained.
- For example, (£2,100,000 – £1,400,000)/(1400–1000) gives an incremental cost per life-year gained of £1750.
- Incremental cost per life-year gained estimates for each option are shown in the final column of Table 2E.3.
- The programme chosen will depend on what the ceiling ratio (cost per life-year gained) is. If the ceiling ratio is £3000 per life-year gained, the annual screening aged 55–74 would be adopted.

Question 2 (Table 2E.4)

Table 2E.4 Cost and cost per QALY gained for a set of independent interventions

Example intervention	Cost per QALY gained* (£)	Annual cost (£)	Cumulative total cost
Hip replacement	1677	20,100,000	20,100,000
Kidney transplant	6706	168,000	20,268,000
Breast cancer screening	7397	408,000	20,676,000
Haemodialysis at home	24,590	590,000	21,266,000
Beta interferon	809,900	350,000	21,616,000

*Compared with no intervention.

- The total cost calculations are shown in the final column of Table 2E.4 and are the sum of the annual costs.
- All programmes up to and including 'Breast screening' would be implemented.
- The implied ceiling ratio is the cost per life-year gained ratio of the last intervention to be implemented, i.e. £7397 per QALY.
- This example highlights the fact that although hip replacement has a low cost per QALY, once the number of patients requiring a hip replacement is taken into account the total cost of hip replacements is very high.

Chapter 3

Life tables and extrapolation

This chapter is the first of three which examine methods of estimating health-related outcomes, and focuses on life expectancy and life-years gained. The chapter reviews life-table methods as a means of estimating life expectancy. It then demonstrates how to use a life table to generate a survival curve, and how to use life tables to calculate changes in life expectancy arising from interventions that reduce mortality. It then considers cause-specific life tables and the issue of competing risk, and concludes with a consideration of using life tables to extrapolate survival benefits.

3.1 Life-table methods

Life-table methods were first developed in the seventeenth century to study patterns of mortality based on church burial records (Graunt 1662). Since then, methods for calculating and manipulating life tables have been developed principally by actuaries and demographers. Health economists may also find life tables useful as they are the principal method of estimating life expectancy from medical interventions.

A life table provides a method of summarizing the mortality experience of a group of individuals. The purpose of this section is not to provide a comprehensive overview of life-table methods, which can be obtained from the references at the end of this chapter, but to show the relevance of this method for quantifying outcomes in economic evaluations. Here we provide an overview of the key concepts used to construct life tables, show how life tables can be used to calculate changes in life expectancy, and then give an example where life tables are used to inform a health economic evaluation. While the main emphasis here is on calculating life expectancies based on estimates of mortality, it is also possible to use life-table methods to quantify other outcomes. However, since the same methods are used, we will not address this issue separately but discuss it at the end of this chapter.

There are two main types of life table. First there is a **cohort life table**, which is constructed based on the mortality experience of a group of individuals (Chaig 1984). While this approach can be used to characterize life expectancies of insects and some animals, human longevity makes this approach difficult to apply as the observation period would have to be sufficiently long to be able to observe the death of all members of the cohort. Instead, **current life tables** are normally constructed using cross-sectional data of observed mortality rates at different ages at a given point in time (Chaig 1984).

Life tables can also be classified according to the intervals over which changes in mortality occur. A **complete life table** displays the various rates for each year of life; while an **abridged life table** deals with greater periods of time, for example 5 year age intervals (Selvin 1996).

Table 3.1 reproduces a part of a complete life table for the first and last twenty years of life (for brevity the portion of the table reporting the experience of individuals between the ages of 20 and 80 years has been omitted). This life table is based on the mortality experience of males in the UK between 2003 and 2005 (this and other life tables can be downloaded from http://www.statistics.gov.uk).

Table 3.1 Part of a complete life table for males, United Kingdom, 2003–05.

Age x	q_x	l_x	d_x	L_x	T_x	e_x
0	0.005683	100000	568	99602	2439752	76.52
1	0.000406	99432	40	99412	2340150	75.95
2	0.000249	99391	25	99379	2240738	74.98
3	0.000207	99367	21	99356	2141360	74.00
4	0.000139	99346	14	99339	2042003	73.02
5	0.000119	99332	12	99326	1942664	72.03
6	0.000134	99320	13	99314	1843338	71.04
7	0.000098	99307	10	99302	1744024	70.05
8	0.000107	99297	11	99292	1644722	69.05
9	0.000110	99287	11	99281	1545430	68.06
10	0.000110	99276	11	99270	1446149	67.07
11	0.000121	99265	12	99259	1346878	66.07
12	0.000158	99253	16	99245	1247620	65.08
13	0.000167	99237	17	99229	1148375	64.09
14	0.000199	99221	20	99211	1049146	63.10
15	0.000255	99201	25	99188	949935	62.12
16	0.000348	99176	35	99158	850747	61.13
17	0.000540	99141	54	99114	751588	60.15
18	0.000685	99088	68	99054	652474	59.19
19	0.000667	99020	66	98987	553421	58.23
20	0.000756	98954	75	98916	454434	57.26
---Age groups 21–79 have been omitted from the table---						
80	0.074002	48246	3570	46461	355518	7.37
81	0.082437	44676	3683	42834	309057	6.92
82	0.089902	40993	3685	39150	266223	6.49
83	0.098441	37307	3673	35471	227073	6.09

(continued)

Table 3.1 (continued) Part of a complete life table for males, United Kingdom, 2003–05.

Age x	q_x	l_x	d_x	L_x	T_x	e_x
84	0.105530	33635	3550	31860	191602	5.70
85	0.114978	30085	3459	28356	159742	5.31
86	0.127949	26626	3407	24923	131386	4.93
87	0.147394	23219	3422	21508	106463	4.59
88	0.160128	19797	3170	18212	84955	4.29
89	0.175957	16627	2926	15164	66743	4.01
90	0.182653	13701	2503	12450	51579	3.76
91	0.198975	11199	2228	10085	39129	3.49
92	0.217279	8971	1949	7996	29044	3.24
93	0.237222	7021	1666	6189	21048	3.00
94	0.247104	5356	1323	4694	14860	2.77
95	0.275402	4032	1111	3477	10166	2.52
96	0.292685	2922	855	2494	6689	2.29
97	0.313100	2067	647	1743	4195	2.03
98	0.336227	1420	477	1181	2452	1.73
99	0.349848	942	330	777	1271	1.35
100	0.389974	613	239	493	493	0.80

Each of the columns of the life table can be defined as follows:

◆ **Age interval (x to $x + 1$)** Each interval in the first column represents a 1 year period except for the last interval (age 100+) which is open ended.

◆ **Proportion dying each year (q_x)** Each row of the second column q_x represents the conditional probability that an individual dies between age x and age $x + 1$.

◆ **Number alive (l_x)** This column reports the exact number of individuals alive at each age. The initial size of the population (l_0), which is termed the **radix**, is normally set at an arbitrary value such as 100,000.

◆ **Deaths (d_x)** This column represents the number of individuals dying within each age interval (i.e. x to $x+1$) and so $d_x = l_x q_x$. For example, in Table 3.1 the probability of dying in the first year of life is $q_0 = 0.005683$ and so d_0 is 568.3.

◆ **Number of years lived (L_x)** Number of years lived by the cohort within the interval x to $x + 1$. Each individual who is alive at $x + 1$ contributes 1 year to L_x, while those who die within this interval contribute only a fraction of a year so that

$$L_x = (l_x - d_x) + a_x d_x \tag{3.1}$$

where a_x is the average time contributed by those who died in the interval x to $x+1$. After the first few age intervals a_x is normally assumed to be 0.5, based on the assumption that individuals die at a similar rate throughout the interval. When this is the case, Hinde (1998) has shown that:

$$L_x = (l_x + l_{x+1})/2 \tag{3.2}$$

◆ **Total time lived (T_x)** The total number of years lived beyond age x, or

$$T_x = L_x + L_{x+1} + L_{x+2} + \dots + L_{100+} \tag{3.3}$$

This quantity is used in the calculation of life expectancy.

◆ **Expectation of life at age x** This represents the average number of additional years at age x and can be calculated by $e_x = T_x / l_x$

Moving beyond definitions, life tables have common features that are worth noting. Firstly, in Table 3.1 $q_0 = 0.005683$ (first row of column 2) is more than an order of magnitude greater than q_1, reflecting hazards during the first year of life. More generally the number of deaths in each age interval continues to fall until the seventh interval and then begins to rise. If we turn to the bottom half of the life table, $q_{80} = 0.074002$, indicating that around 7.4% of males aged 80 years will die before their 81st birthday.

Life expectancies are also reported in Table 3.1. The calculation of these can easily be verified. Firstly, we can calculate the column L_x for each interval from 80 years. For example, $L_{80} = 1/2(l_{80} + l_{81}) = 1/2(48{,}246 + 44{,}676) = 46{,}461$. The total number of years lived ($T_{80} = 355{,}518$) can then be calculated by summing all the remaining rows of this column. The life expectancy of an individual at their 80th birthday is then easily calculated:

$$e_{80} = T_{80}/l_{80} = 355{,}518/48{,}246 = 7.37 \text{ years.}$$

3.2 Survival curves and hazard functions

A life table can be used to generate a survival curve $S(x)$ for the population at any point in time. This represents the probability of surviving beyond a certain age x (i.e. $S(x) = \Pr[X > x]$). We shall discuss the survival curve in more detail in the next chapter. If we consider the life table shown in Table 3.1, l_0 represents the number of males who are born, which is set at 100,000. Of these individuals 48,246 can expect to be alive on their 80th birthday and so $S(80) = 48{,}245/100{,}000 = 0.48$ or, more generally, $S(x) = l_x/l_0$. A survival curve derived from the English 2003–2005 life table is shown in Figure 3.1(a).

The chance of a male living to the age of 60 years is high (around 0.9) and so the survival curve is comparatively flat up until this age. The proportion dying each year from the age of 60 years rapidly increases, so the curve has a much steeper downward slope. In the last part of the survival curve there is an inflection, indicating a slowing rate of increase in the proportion dying each year among the very old (over 90 years).

It also possible to calculate a survival curve that is conditional on having attained a certain age y (i.e. $S'(x) = \Pr[X > x | x \geq y]$). For example, the survival curve for an individual on their 80th birthday could be calculated using $S'(x) = l_x/l_{80}$ and this is shown

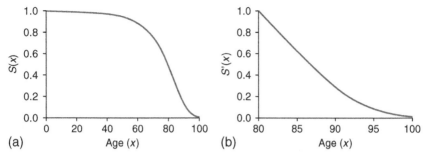

Fig. 3.1 Survival curves derived from the English 2003–2005 life table: (a) from birth; (b) conditional on attaining age 80 years.

in Figure 3.1(b). By definition $S'(80) = 1$ and the probabilities are much higher than those reported in Figure 3.1(a) as they are conditional on living to the age of 80 years. The life expectancy, which is the area under the survival curve, can also be calculated by numerical integration.

Another important concept which determines the shape of $S(x)$ is the **hazard rate** which is sometimes referred to as the force of mortality. The hazard rate is the slope of the survival curve at any point, given the instantaneous chance of an individual dying. In the case of a complete life table, the hazard rate can be represented in several ways, but the most intuitive formula (see Selvin (1996) for its derivation) is based on dividing the number of deaths in each interval by the population at risk at the midpoint of the interval (i.e. $x + 1/2$):

$$h(x+1/2) \approx \frac{d_x}{l_x - 0.5d_x}$$

(3.4)

When mortality rates are low (i.e. $q_x < 0.1$), $h(x+1/2) \approx q_x$. The hazard function underlying the English life table can be calculated using equation (3.4), and this is illustrated in Figure 3.2. In Figure 3.2(b) a natural logarithmic scale is used to highlight changes in the hazard for younger ages. These figures indicate that those aged between 7 and 10 years have the lowest overall risk of mortality.

3.3 Calculation of changes in life expectancy

Life tables are a useful tool for estimating changes in life expectancy from interventions that reduce mortality. In order to estimate a change in life expectancy we must first make an assumption about how the intervention impacts on the hazard. Typically, we assume that the hazard is shifted upwards or downwards by a fixed proportion. For example, if an intervention alters the hazard rate of all-cause mortality (i.e. $h'(x)=rh(x)$, where r represents the hazard ratio), the change in hazard will alter the mortality rate q_x, which in turn changes the rest of the quantities in the life table including e_x.

To work through an example, consider a clinical trial conducted over a period of 5 years in which an intervention significantly reduced the relative risk of mortality of

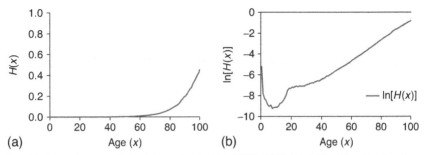

Fig. 3.2 Hazard curves derived from the English 2003–2005 life table: (a) natural scale; (b) logarithmic scale.

older age men by 50% relative to the control group. While reporting relative risk over a defined period is a clinically meaningful outcome, it is less relevant for cost-effectiveness analysis as the outcomes are normally quantified in a metric such as life expectancy.

It is possible to calculate the increased life expectancy accruing from a change in the risk of mortality using a life table and by making assumptions about relative risks with and without the intervention. In this example, we focus on a male who is 80 years of age, but the same techniques can be used to estimate life expectancy for other years. Table 3.2 is divided into two sections, the left-hand side of which is the same life table for England 2003–2005 shown in Table 3.1.

As can be seen, the q_x reported in Table 3.1 is identical to $^{NT}q_x$ on the left-hand side of Table 3.2, but we have rescaled $^{NT}l_x$ so that $^{NT}l_{80}$ is 100,000 (this can easily be done by dividing all values in the column l_x reported in Table 3.1 by the number of persons surviving to their 80th birthday (48,246 individuals) and then multiplying through by 100,000). Rescaling $^{NT}l_x$ has no effect on the estimated life expectancy (see later in this section), but makes it easier to interpret the reported number of survivors and decedents in subsequent intervals as they can be compared with the 100,000 persons alive at 80 years of age.

Firstly, we must calculate the life expectancy if the individual had not received the intervention. The number alive at each age interval can be recalculated as $^{NT}l_{x+1} = {^{NT}l_x} - {^{NT}q_x}{^{NT}l_x}$. For example, the number of individuals surviving to their 81st birthday can easily be calculated as $^{NT}l_{81} = 100,000 - 0.074002 \times 100,000 = 92,600$. The other elements of the life table can then be calculated in the usual way (i.e. $^{NT}L_x$, $^{NT}T_x$, and $^{NT}e_x$). The values for life expectancy without the intervention at various ages in Table 3.2 are identical to those reported in the bottom half of Table 3.1.

Secondly, we need to calculate what effect the intervention has on life expectancy, and this is illustrated in the life table on the right-hand side of Table 3.2. Based on the results of the trial we must make assumptions about the mortality rate in the intervention group. One way of capturing the reduction in risk observed in the trial is to adjust the mortality rate (i.e. $^{T}q_x = 0.5^{NT}q_x$) for age groups 80–84. The mortality rate is left unaltered in the rest of the life table. A life table based on these reduced mortality rates is reported on the right-hand side of Table 3.2. Using this approach the life expectancy $^{T}e_{80}$ for an individual at the age of 80 years who receives the therapy is 8.74 years.

Table 3.2 Using a life table to estimate differences in life expectancy associated with an intervention

Age	Without the intervention					With the intervention				
	NT_{q_x}	NT_{l_x}	NT_{L_x}	NT_{T_x}	NT_{e_x}	T_{q_x}	T_{l_x}	T_{L_x}	T_{T_x}	T_{e_x}
80	0.074002	100000	96300	738352	7.38	0.037001	100000	98150	873895	8.74
81	0.082437	92600	88783	642052	6.93	0.041219	96300	94315	775745	8.06
82	0.089902	84966	81147	553269	6.51	0.044951	92331	90255	681429	7.38
83	0.098441	77327	73521	472122	6.11	0.049221	88180	86010	591174	6.70
84	0.10553	69715	66037	398601	5.72	0.052765	83840	81628	505164	6.03
85	0.114978	62358	58773	332564	5.33	0.114978	79416	74851	423536	5.33
86	0.127949	55188	51658	273791	4.96	0.127949	70285	65789	348685	4.96
87	0.147394	48127	44580	222133	4.62	0.147394	61292	56775	282897	4.62
88	0.160128	41034	37748	177553	4.33	0.160128	52258	48074	226122	4.33
89	0.175957	34463	31431	139805	4.06	0.175957	43890	40029	178048	4.06
90	0.182653	28399	25805	108374	3.82	0.182653	36167	32864	138019	3.82
91	0.198975	23212	20903	82568	3.56	0.198975	29561	26620	105155	3.56
92	0.217279	18593	16573	61666	3.32	0.217279	23679	21107	78534	3.32

(continued)

Table 3.2 (continued) Using a life table to estimate differences in life expectancy associated with an intervention

Age	Without the intervention					With the intervention				
	$^{NT}q_x$	$^{NT}l_x$	$^{NT}L_x$	$^{NT}T_x$	$^{NT}e_x$	$^{T}q_x$	$^{T}l_x$	$^{T}L_x$	$^{T}T_x$	$^{T}e_x$
93	0.237222	14553	12827	45093	3.10	0.237222	18534	16336	57428	3.10
94	0.247104	11101	9729	32265	2.91	0.247104	14138	12391	41092	2.91
95	0.275402	8358	7207	22536	2.70	0.275402	10644	9178	28701	2.70
96	0.292685	6056	5170	15329	2.53	0.292685	7713	6584	19523	2.53
97	0.313100	4283	3613	10159	2.37	0.313100	5455	4601	12939	2.37
98	0.336227	2942	2448	6546	2.22	0.336227	3747	3117	8337	2.22
99	0.349848	1953	1611	4099	2.10	0.349848	2487	2052	5220	2.10
100	0.389974	1270	2487	2487	1.96	0.389974	1617	3168	3168	1.96

Hence the increase in life-expectancy due to the intervention is 8.74 − 7.38 = 1.36 years.

It is important to note that the overall increase in life expectancy is due to a combination of two factors: the reduction in mortality observed during the 5 years of the trial and the ongoing effects of having a larger number of people alive in the intervention arm at the end of the trial. The relative importance of these two factors can be appreciated visually from Figure 3.3 which compares the number of survivors at each age for a hypothetical cohort of the general population with the number of survivors in the group receiving the intervention between the ages of 80 and 85 years. The grey shaded area represents the additional number of survivors in the intervention group at each age.

Within the period of the trial, the risk reduction leads to increasing divergence in the proportion surviving in each group. At the end of the trial, which we assume occurs at a person's 85th birthday, there are around 79,400 people alive in the intervention group compared with around 62,400 in the control group. The within-trial difference in survival contributes 0.45 years, or about a third of the overall difference in life expectancy. The rest of the difference in life expectancy is simply due to having more people (around 17,000) in the intervention group alive at the end of the trial. As it would seem unlikely that these people die immediately after the trial is completed, we can expect more people to be alive in the intervention group in the period following the trial, and this difference needs to be taken into account in the calculation of overall life expectancy. For the extrapolation represented in Figure 3.3 we have assumed that the mortality of both groups is governed by the life-table experience of the general population for all years beyond the trial. Based on this assumption, the contribution to overall life expectancy from the period of extrapolation is 0.91 years, or about twice as much as that observed within the trial.

The assumption that, beyond the trial, both the intervention group and the control group are based on the same life table is just one of a range of assumptions that can be adopted for the extrapolation. We could also assume that the therapy continues to

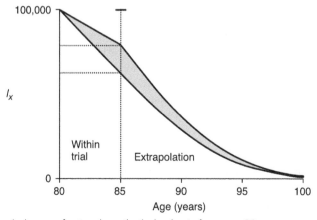

Fig. 3.3 Survival curves for two hypothetical cohorts from age 80 years.

have a protective effect on the intervention even after the trial concludes. There is evidence for what has been termed a **legacy effect** with some classes of drugs such as statins (Ford *et al.* 2007). Alternatively, it is also possible that the side effects of treatment may increase mortality risks after the trial. For example, radiotherapy reduces deaths from breast cancer in the short term, but there is evidence that it increases the risk of mortality from vascular disease in the longer term (Gagliardia *et al.* 1998). Positive or negative effects of an intervention can be taken into account in the extrapolation by adjusting the mortality rates.

Figure 3.3 highlights the importance of extrapolating outcomes over a lifetime. The change in life expectancy observed within the trial may be a fraction of the overall benefits of the therapy, and this is likely to impart a bias to cost-effectiveness analysis if steps are not taken to capture the full health effects. Based on the results presented in Figure 3.3 this bias can be substantial, as the cost-effectiveness ratio would be three times higher if it was based on the observed survival difference within the trial than if it was based on estimates which also take into account extrapolated effects, even assuming that the therapy has no legacy effects.

3.4 **Multiple-cause life tables**

So far we have examined life tables that are based on all-cause mortality. In practice death can be attributed to a range of specific causes. The principle cause of death is recorded on a death certificate in most developed countries, and is coded according to a common disease classification system which can be used to construct multiple-cause life tables. The most frequently used classification systems are the 9th and 10th revisions of International Classification of Diseases, commonly known as ICD9 and ICD10, respectively. Medical interventions normally reduce the risk of one or a limited range of causes. For example, treatments for hypertension have been shown to significantly reduce the risk of cardiovascular mortality, but not the risks of mortality due to other causes such as cancer (Patel *et al.* 2007). Multiple-cause life tables are a way of quantifying outcomes when there is more than one mutually exclusive cause of death. These life tables can estimate the potential gains from the elimination of a cause of death and are also useful in calculating the benefits of interventions that reduce the risk of a particular cause of death.

Table 3.3 provides an example of a multiple-cause life table. Before examining it in detail, we must first explain the abridged life table. The first row quantifies the risk of mortality in the first year of life, but the remaining rows cover longer periods of time (in most cases 5 years). If we denote the width of an age group in years by n, the various values required to obtain estimates of life expectancy are as follows:

- **Deaths during the period** ($_nd_x$) The number of deaths occurring between ages x and $x + n$ years, i.e. $_nd_x = l_{x+n} - l_x$.
- **Proportion dying during the period** ($_nq_x$) The proportion of those people reaching their xth birthday who reach their $(x + n)$th birthday, i.e. $_nq_x = {}_nd_x/l_x$.
- **Number of person-years lived during the period** ($_nL_x$) The number of years lived between exact ages x and $x + n$.

A number of assumptions can be made in order to calculate $_nL_x$. The simplest is that deaths are evenly distributed within each interval. If this is the case then person-years lived is given by

$$_nL_x = (n/2)(l_x + l_{x+n}) \tag{3.5}$$

This equation, which is simply a generalization of equation (3.2), can be a poor approximation, especially within the first year of life (i.e. the first age group) where deaths are more likely occur towards the beginning of the interval. Adjustments can be made using by setting a_x to less than 0.5 in equation (3.1).

Table 3.3 shows such an abridged life table, constructed from US Decennial Life Tables 1989–1991 for white females, which divides the conditional probability of mortality ($_nq_x$) into that due to major cardiovascular diseases (defined as ICD9 390–448), denoted as $^{CVD}_nq_x$, and all other causes ($^{oc}_nq_x$). These three quantities are reported in the columns on the left-hand side of the table and are used to calculate the number of people alive and the number of person-years lived. A potential application of this life table is calculation of the potential increase in life expectancy if a type of disease is removed as a cause of death (see right-hand side of Table 3.3). As the calculations suggest, life expectancy at birth could rise from 79.45 to 86.06 years in the absence of cardiovascular deaths.

One issue that arises when death is divided into multiple causes in this type of life table is **competing risk**. As Pintilie (2006) notes, competing risk can arise 'when an individual can experience more than one type of event and the occurrence of one type of event hinders the occurrence of other types of events'. Competing risks affect life tables, as those who die from a specific cause have no chance of dying from other causes during the remainder of the interval and so $^{CVD}_nq_x$ is not independent of $^{oc}_nq_x$. In practice this will mean that as soon as one cause is eliminated the probabilities of dying of other causes increase (Mackenbach et al. 1995). Several methods have been proposed (Chiang 1991; Selvin 1996) to correct for competing risks when calculating life tables.

3.5 Using life tables in practice

One cost-effectiveness study that used life-table methods to estimate outcomes is that of Pharoah and Hollingworth (1996), who evaluated cholesterol-lowering therapy using life tables to estimate the expected life years gained by use of statins in people with and without pre-existing coronary heart disease. To adjust for the higher risk in people with pre-existing heart disease, Pharoah and Hollingworth proposed a method for scaling q_x that takes into account the relative risk of those with and without the disease and its prevalence within the existing population:

$$\theta = \frac{r}{pr + (1-p)} \tag{3.6}$$

where r is the hazard ratio of those with and without the disease and p is prevalence of the disease in the population. The **scale-up factor** θ ranges between r and 1. For rare diseases p will be close to zero and so θ will be approximately equal to r. As a disease becomes

Table 3.3 Abridged multiple cause life-table for the USA: White females

Age group	q_x^{CVD}	q_x^{OC}	q_x^{AC}	$^{CE}l_x$	$^{CE}L_x$	$^{CE}e_x$	$^{NC}l_x$	$^{NC}L_x$	$^{NC}e_x$
0–1	0.00016	0.00651	0.00667	100,000	99480	86.06	100000	99467	79.45
1–5	0.00008	0.00139	0.00147	99349	397065	85.62	99333	396981	78.99
5–10	0.00004	0.00085	0.00089	99211	495829	81.74	99187	495699	75.10
10–15	0.00005	0.00088	0.00093	99127	495450	76.80	99099	495300	70.17
15–20	0.00007	0.00207	0.00214	99039	494723	71.87	99007	494542	65.23
20–25	0.00014	0.00237	0.00251	98834	493595	67.01	98795	493360	60.36
25–30	0.00022	0.00246	0.00268	98600	492413	62.17	98547	492091	55.51
30–35	0.00036	0.00314	0.00350	98358	491054	57.31	98283	490593	50.65
35–40	0.00060	0.00417	0.00477	98049	489288	52.49	97939	488598	45.82
40–45	0.00115	0.00607	0.00722	97640	486828	47.69	97472	485726	41.03
45–50	0.00233	0.00966	0.01199	97047	483083	42.97	96768	481171	36.30

(continued)

50–55	0.00442	0.01522	96110	477173	38.36	95608	473699	31.71
55–60	0.00819	0.02319	94647	468149	33.91	93730	461827	27.29
60–65	0.01461	0.0344	92452	454795	29.65	90789	443491	23.09
65–70	0.02513	0.04848	89272	436148	25.62	86339	416694	19.14
70–75	0.04518	0.06922	84944	410846	21.79	79984	378325	15.46
75–80	0.07878	0.09599	79064	377235	18.21	70834	324662	12.11
80–85	0.13840	0.13840	71475	333455	14.87	58454	253141	9.12
85–90	0.22276	0.20313	61583	276559	11.84	42274	166239	6.62
90–95	0.31246	0.29632	49073	206521	9.22	24270	81879	4.69
95–100	0.36422	0.39997	34532	132493	7.13	9495	26373	3.36
100+	0.40000	0.60000	20720	113565	5.48	2239	5571	2.49

Reproduced from National Center for Health Statistics, *US Decennial Life Tables for 1989–91*, Vol II, *State Life Tables No. 33, New York*. Hyattsville, MD, 1998, with permission. Major cardiovascular disease defined as ICD9 390–448.

more common, θ will decline as less scaling up is required because the higher mortality risk associated with the disease is already captured within the existing life table.

Table 3.4 illustrates how to calculate the increase in life expectancy from statin treatment for men with pre-existing coronary heart disease (CHD) aged 50–60 years based on information provided by Pharoah and Hollingworth (1996). Columns 1 and 2 report age-specific mortality rates for the general population for CHD ($^{G}q_{x}^{CHD}$) and all other causes of death ($^{G}q_{x}^{oc}$). By using these rates and some additional information it is possible to use life tables to calculate incremental outcomes using the following steps:

1 **Adjust disease-specific mortality rates of the general population to reflect the risk in the population involved in the evaluation.** To calculate the life expectancy of men with a history of pre-existing CHD the rates for the general population must be adjusted upwards to reflect the higher risk of mortality of those with a history of this disease. To do this, Pharoah and Hollingworth assume that the mortality ratio of those with pre-existing CHD to those without is 3.4 and the prevalence of CHD in this age range is 4.4%. From equation (3.6) the scale-up factor θ is 3.08. The mortality rate of those with pre-existing disease who are not treated can be obtained by multiplying column 1 by θ (i.e. $^{NT}q_{x}^{CHD} = {^{G}q_{x}^{CHD}} \times \theta$).

Table 3.4 A partial life table constructed for men between 50 and 60 years with pre-existing coronary heart disease according to treatment for raised cholesterol

	Mortality rates						No. alive		Person-years lived	
Col. no.	1	2	3	4	5	6	7	8	9	10
	General population		No treatment		Treatment					
Age (x)	$^{G}q_{x}^{CHD}$	$^{G}q_{x}^{oc}$	$^{NT}q_{x}^{CHD}$	$^{NT}q_{x}^{AC}$	$^{T}q_{x}^{CHD}$	$^{T}q_{x}^{AC}$	$^{NT}l_{x}$	$^{T}l_{x}$	$^{NT}L_{x}$	$^{T}L_{x}$
50	0.0008	0.0027	0.0024	0.0051	0.0014	0.0041	1000	1000	997	998
51	0.0009	0.0029	0.0027	0.0056	0.0016	0.0045	995	996	992	994
52	0.0010	0.0032	0.0031	0.0063	0.0018	0.0050	989	991	986	989
53	0.0011	0.0036	0.0035	0.0070	0.0020	0.0056	983	986	980	984
54	0.0013	0.0039	0.0039	0.0079	0.0023	0.0062	976	981	972	978
55	0.0014	0.0043	0.0044	0.0088	0.0026	0.0069	968	975	964	972
56	0.0016	0.0048	0.0050	0.0098	0.0029	0.0077	960	968	955	964
57	0.0018	0.0052	0.0057	0.0109	0.0033	0.0085	951	961	945	957
58	0.0021	0.0058	0.0064	0.0122	0.0037	0.0095	940	953	935	948
59	0.0024	0.0064	0.0072	0.0136	0.0042	0.0105	929	944	923	939
60	–	–	–	–	–	–	916	934		

Adapted from Pharoah and Hollingworth (1996).
Mortality from cardiovascular disease includes codes 401-405, 410-414, 430-438 of ICD9.

2 **Estimate the mortality rates of the population if they received treatment.** Pharoah and Hollingworth assume that statins reduce cardiovascular mortality by 42%, so the mortality rate for the treated group is $^{T}q_x^{CHD} = {}^{NT}q_x^{CHD} \times 0.58$ (i.e. 1–0.42).

3 **Calculate the all-cause mortality rates for those with and without treatment.** The all-cause mortality rates for those with a history of CHD without treatment is simply column 3 plus column 2 (i.e. $^{NT}q_x^{AC} = {}^{NT}q_x^{CHD} + {}^{G}q_x^{OC}$). Similarly, the mortality rate of the treated group is $^{T}q_x^{AC} = {}^{T}q_x^{CHD} + {}^{G}q_x^{OC}$.

4 **Calculate the number alive at each age.** We set the radix l_{50} to 1000, and then the number of persons alive without treatment ($^{NT}l_x$) and with treatment ($^{T}l_x$) can be calculated using the all-cause mortality rates reported in columns 4 and 6, respectively.

5 **Calculate the person-years lived.** If we assume a constant mortality rate within each age group, equation (3.2) can be used to estimate person-years lived for the no-treatment group ($^{NT}L_x$) and the treatment group ($^{T}L_x$).

6 **Estimate life expectancy.** A partial estimate of life expectancy can be made by summing person-years lived between the age 50–60 years and dividing by 1000. On this basis, the life expectancy for the treatment group is 9.72 years compared with 9.65 years for those without treatment.

Pharoah and Hollingworth (1996) used this approach to estimate the benefits of using statin therapy to lower cholesterol for a range of subgroups including men and women with and without CHD. Their overall estimates of average cost-effectiveness for patients with pre-existing CHD and a cholesterol concentration >5.4 mmol/l was £32,000 per life-year. This estimate is considerably higher than more recent estimates based on the Heart Protection Study (Mihaylova *et al.* 2006), which showed the cost-effectiveness of statin therapy to be as low as £2,500 per life year and in some cases cost-saving.

While the improvements in cost-effectiveness are in part due to reductions in the price of statins following the introduction of generic medications, there are also probable differences in the quantification of benefits. Pharoah and Hollingworth (1996) appear only to calculate the difference in life expectancy using a life table from ages 50 to 60 years, and do not extrapolate the observed survival difference over remaining lifetimes. As Figure 3.3 illustrated, this approach is likely to underestimate the benefits even if there is no continuing benefit from therapy and so bias the cost-effectiveness ratio upwards.

3.6 **Extrapolating life expectancy**

How can we use life tables to extrapolate outcomes from clinical studies such as randomized controlled trials (RCTs)? One advantage of using life tables is that they are available for almost all countries (Lopez *et al.* 2001), so they can assist in generalizing results. In this section we outline the steps required to construct a life table using clinical and other information. As its main focus is on the specific issues pertaining to trials, it should be read in conjunction with more general guidelines on the development of decision analytic models such as those of the ISPOR panel (Weinstein *et al.* 2003).

1 **Define the patient group under evaluation.** When an economic evaluation is being conducted alongside a clinical trial, it is important to consider first whether the patients in the trial are representative of patients in the population where the intervention will be applied. In many cases selection or eligibility criteria or differences in standards of care will mean that the patients involved in a clinical study may have different characteristics and different outcomes to patients with the same disease who would be seen in routine clinical practice. Does this matter? The answer to this question depends on the aim of the economic analysis. If the purpose is to conduct a CEA of the population enrolled in the trial, the answer is 'No', but such an analysis is likely to be limited in scope, as often the selection criteria mean that only a proportion of patients with that disease have been included in the clinical study. Hence the findings of the CEA may not pertain to those patients excluded from the trial.

Examples where particular selection criteria may impact on a CEA include clinical trials of therapies to reduce cardiovascular disease, which often have selection criteria that exclude patients who have cancer or other life-threatening illnesses. Such criteria will tend to reduce the observed mortality from non-cardiovascular causes, especially within the first few years of the trial. This may increase the risk reductions associated with effective therapy, as those patients who benefit from a reduction in cardiovascular disease can be expected to live longer as they have less chance of dying of a non-cardiovascular cause such as cancer. This phenomenon, which is another example of competing risks, only becomes an issue if the CEA is being used to evaluate therapies that will also be available to patients with life-threatening illnesses. The higher competing risk tends to reduce the benefit for these patients, and so a CEA that only takes into account the risks observed in the trial population may produce different results than if the whole population was considered.

2 **Construct a life table for the population under evaluation.** The construction of a life table requires information on disease-specific hazards by age and sex for the population under evaluation. Most medical interventions are not applied to the whole population but to specific subpopulations, and impact on the mortality of a specific disease. For example, suppose that we are interested in the cost-effectiveness of breast cancer screening in women aged 40–50 years. This would require information on the age-related mortality from breast cancer and from all other diseases from a cause-elimination life table. Such a life table may require some modification to adjust for either the risk of cancer mortality or the competing risk from all other diseases. For example, it is known that women with variations of the *BRCA1* gene are at an increased risk of breast cancer, and so if the screening programme was applied to this subpopulation, a life table for the general population would have to be manipulated to reflect this increase in risk. Similarly, improvements in treatments of cardiovascular disease may reduce the mortality associated with other causes of death, which will also have an effect on outcomes.

3 **Construct a life table for the population with and without the intervention.** In order to estimate incremental benefits it is necessary to calculate life tables for patients with and without the intervention. Here clinical trials are useful in isolating the effect of an intervention on relative risk. For example, if a randomized trial showed that women aged 40–50 years who were regularly screened for breast cancer had a 30% lower mortality from breast cancer, this could be used to adjust the life table for those receiving the intervention to reflect these lower risks. Assumptions regarding whether there are any continuing benefits of the intervention would also need to be made.

4 **Calculation and reporting results.** By using life tables, the effects of the intervention on life expectancy can easily be calculated with the methods outlined in this chapter. When reporting results, although medical journals do not have established reporting requirements for such life-table analyses, it would seem prudent to separate life expectancy differences observed within a trial from those extrapolated over the patient's remaining life time. It is also useful to report undiscounted life expectancies as well as discounted life expectancies which assume that future benefits have a lower net present value and apply a positive discount rate.

3.7 Summary

Life-table methods for estimating health-related outcomes in terms of life expectancy and life years gained have been described in this chapter. These methods are particularly useful when an estimate of the likely effect of an intervention on life expectancy has to be made from summary data. When individual patient information is available, other techniques become possible and these are considered in Chapter 4.

References

Chaig, C.L. (1984). *The Life Table and its Applications*. Krieger, Malabar, FL.

Chiang, C.L. (1991). Competing risks in mortality analysis. *Annual Review of Public Health*, **12**, 281–307.

Ford, I., Murray, H., Packard, C.J., Shepherd, J., Macfarlane, P.W., Cobbe, S.M. (2007). Long-term follow-up of the West of Scotland Coronary Prevention Study. *New England Journal of Medicine*, **357**, 1477–86.

Gagliardia, G., Lax, I., Söderström, S., Gyenes, G., Rutqvist, L.E. (1998). Prediction of excess risk of long-term cardiac mortality after radiotherapy of stage I breast cancer. *Radiotherapy and Oncology*, **46**, 63–71.

Graunt, J. (1662). *Natural and Political Observations, Mentioned in a Following Index and Made Upon the Bills Of Mortality London*. Facsimile available online at: http://www.edstephan.org/Graunt/bills.html

Guillaume, W., Mouchart, M., Duchêne, J. (eds) (2002). *The Life Table: Modelling Survival and Death (European Studies of Population)*. Kluwer, Dordrecht.

Hinde, A. (1998). *Demographic Methods*. Arnold, New York.

Lopez, A.D., Salomon, J., Ahmad, O., Murray, C.J.L., and Mafat, D. (2001). *Life Tables for 191 Countries: Data, Methods and Results. GPE Discussion Paper Series No. 9*. World Health Organization, New York.

Mackenbach, J.P., Kunst, A.E., Lautenbach, H., Bijlsma, F., and Oei, Y.B. (1995). Competing causes of death: an analysis using multiple cause of death data from the Netherlands. *American Journal of Epidemiology*, **141**, 466–75.

Mihaylova, B., Briggs, A., Armitage, J., Parish, S., Gray, A., Collins, R. (2006). Lifetime cost effectiveness of simvastatin in a range of risk groups and age groups derived from a randomised trial of 20,536 people. *British Medical Journal*, **333**, 1145.

Office of National Statistics (2009). *England, Interim Life Tables, 1980–82 to 2006–08*. Stationery Office, London (available online at: http://www.statistics.gov.uk).

Patel, A., MacMahon, S., Chalmers, J., *et al.* (2007). Effects of a fixed combination of perindopril and indapamide on macrovascular and microvascular outcomes in patients with type 2 diabetes mellitus (the ADVANCE trial): a randomised controlled trial. *Lancet*, **370**, 829–40.

Pharoah, P.D.P. and Hollingworth, W. (1996). Cost effectiveness analysis of lowering cholesterol concentration with statins in patients with and without pre-existing coronary heart disease: life table methods applied to health authority population. *British Medical Journal*, **312**, 1443–8.

Pintilie, M. (2006). *Competing Risks: A Practice Perspective*. John Wiley, New York.

Selvin, S. (1996). *Statistical Analysis of Epidemiologic Data*. Oxford University Press, New York.

Weinstein, M.C., O'Brien, B., Hornberger, J., *et al.* (2003). Principles of good practice for decision analytic modeling in health-care evaluation: Report of the ISPOR task force on good research practices—modeling studies. *Value in Health*, **6**, 9–17.

Exercise

Analysis of health outcomes

If you go to the website www.herc.ox.ac.uk/books/applied you will find an Excel file *Outcomes2.xlsx* which contains five worksheets. The first sheet, **Life Table**, contains a set of mortality rates that can be used in the construction of a life table. (The remaining sheets will be used in a continuation of this exercise in Chapters 4, 5, and 11). A written step-by-step guide is also provided below.

Using life-table methods

The first worksheet contains all-cause and cerebrovascular disease (stroke) mortality rates for men aged 70 years and over.

(i) Construct a multiple-decrement life table and use this to estimate the increase in life expectancy for men aged 70 years if we could eliminate stroke as a cause of death. Patients who have had a stroke in the past are at an elevated risk of having a fatal stroke compared with the general population. A new drug is being developed to reduce the risk of cerebrovascular mortality in these patients. Preliminary trial data suggest that this drug can reduce cerebrovascular mortality by 30%. The prevalence of cerebrovascular disease in the population is 5% between 65 and 74 years and 10% in the 75+ age group. Assume that patients who have had a stroke have twice the rate of cerebrovascular mortality as the general population.

(ii) What is the gain in life expectancy from using the drug on a male patient aged 72 years?

(iii) What is the gain in life expectancy if we apply a discount rate of 3.5% per year to health benefits?

Step-by-step guide

Using life-table methods

Click on the first worksheet **Life Table**. The first work sheet contains all-cause mortality rates under the column heading **qxAC** and cerebrovascular disease (stroke) mortality rates (**qxCB**) for men aged 70 years and over.

(i) *Construct a multiple-decrement life table and use this to estimate the increase in life expectancy for men aged 70 years if we could eliminate stroke as a cause of death.*

♦ Copy the data from the all-cause mortality column **qxAC** to the first column of the multiple-decrement life table.

♦ Copy data in **qxCB** to the second column.

- The column **IxAC** represents the number of people still alive at each birthday.
- Place an initial value in the first cell of **IxAC** (it is best to use a round number such as 1000—this is already entered for you) to represent the number of people alive at their 70th birthday.
- Calculate the number of people alive at each subsequent birthday using the mortality rate in column **qxAC**. For example, the number of people alive at their 71st birthday is 957 (formula: =H17–F17*H17).
- Copy this formula down to the rest of column **IxAC.**
- The column **Ix(AC-CB)** represents the number of people still alive at each birthday if stroke were eliminated as a cause of death.
- The value of 1000 in the first cell in this column represents the number of people alive at their 70th birthday (this is already entered for you).
- This time all-cause mortality rate is reduced since stroke is eliminated as a cause of death, so recalculate the number of people alive at each birthday with the reduced mortality rate. Now 960 people should be alive at their 71st birthday (formula: =I17–(F17–G17)*I17).
- The column **LxAC** represents the number of person-years lived between age x years and age $x + 1$ years.
- For the first cell in **LxAC** average the first two cells in column **IxAC** (i.e. number of persons alive at their 70th and 71st birthdays).
- Copy this down the rest of column **LxAC.**
- The column **Lx(AC-CB)** represents the number of person-years lived between age x years and age $x + 1$ years when stroke is eliminated as a cause of death.
- Calculate number of person-years lived again, using **Ix(AC-CB)** instead of **IxAC** for all cells in **Lx(AC-CB)**.
- Sum **LxAC** (cells J17:J55) and place this value at the bottom on the column next to **Total Lx.**
- Do the same for **Lx(AC-CB)**
- Calculate the life expectancy for all-cause mortality by dividing the total person-years lived by the number of persons alive at age 70 (starting cohort) and place it in the column next to the cell **Life Expectancy.**
- Do the same when stroke is eliminated as a cause.
- Calculate the difference.

Patients who have had a stroke in the past are at an elevated risk of having a fatal stroke compared with the general population. A new drug is being developed to reduce the risk of cerebrovascular mortality in these patients. Preliminary trial data suggest that this drug can reduce cerebrovascular mortality by 30%. The prevalence of cerebrovasuclar disease in the population is 5% between 65 and 74 years and 10% in the 75+ age group. Assume that patients who have had a stroke have twice the rate of cerebrovascular mortality as the general population.

(ii) *What is the gain in life expectancy from using the drug on a male patient aged 72 years?*

This exercise is similar to the example from Pharoah and Hollingworth (1996) described in section 3.5. Firstly, we need to calculate the life expectancy of patients who are *not* treated with the new drug.

- ◆ Again, copy the data from the all-cause mortality column **qxAC** and the cerebrovascular disease mortality (**qxCB**) to the first and second columns of the life table.
- ◆ Under the third column **Prevalence** place the value 0.05 for ages 70–74 years and 0.10 for ages 75 years and above.
- ◆ The fourth column **s** is for calculating the degree by which the cerebrovascular mortality rate must be scaled up for patients who have had a stroke (i.e. these patients are at an elevated risk compared with the general population).
- ◆ Use equation 3.6 to scale up, where *r* is mortality ratio (2 in this example) and *p* is prevalence of the disease, to calculate *s* for each age.
- ◆ Multiply *s* by cerebrovascular disease mortality rate (**qxCB**) to create a new column **qxCB1**.
- ◆ Calculate the number of people surviving (**lx**) in a similar manner to part (i). However, this time we must subtract from **qxAC** the stroke mortality rate in the general population **qxCB** and replace it with the stroke mortality rate for this population **qxCB1** (e.g. the second cell in column **lx** will have the formula =J69–(E69–F69+I69)*J69.
- ◆ Calculate **Lx**.
- ◆ Obtain **Tx** by summing **Lx** over the age range 72–108 years (cells K71:K107).
- ◆ Calculate **ex** (life expectancy) for a patient aged 72 years by dividing **Tx** by **lx** for a patient aged 72 years.

Now we need to calculate the life expectancy of the group receiving the drug. Go to cell **M69**.

The drug reduces mortality by 30%; hence **qxcb2** (e.g. the first cell, M69) will have the formula =I69*0.7. That is, we need to reduce **qxCB1** (CB is the disease mortality rate of those who have previously had a stroke) by 30%.

- ◆ Calculate **lx** again (NB: start with 1000). In cell N70, the formula should be: =N69–(E69–F69+M69)*N69.
- ◆ Calculate **Lx** for the treatment group.
- ◆ Obtain **Tx** for the treatment group by summing **Lx** over the age range 72–108 years (cells O71:O107).
- ◆ Calculate **ex** (life expectancy) for a patient aged 72 years in the treatment group by dividing **Tx** by **lx** for a patient aged 72 years.
- ◆ Calculate the difference in life expectancy by subtracting the life expectancy (**ex**) in the no-treatment group from the life expectancy in the treatment group (**ex**).

(iii) *What is the gain in life expectancy for a male aged 72 years if we apply a discount rate of 3.5% per year to health benefits?*

The formula for discounting is $1/(1 + r)^n$ where r is the rate of interest (3.5%) and n is the number of years into the future. (Tip: For the first cell (**R71**), use the formula: =K71*(1/(1.035)^Q71) and copy this down for the rest.)

Reminder glossary of terms

q_x	mortality rate
q_xAC	all-cause mortality rate
q_xCB	mortality rate for cerebrovascular disease
I_xAC	number of people still alive at each birthday
I_x(AC-CB)	number of people still alive at each birthday if stroke was eliminated as a cause of death
L_xAC	number of person-years lived between ages x and x + 1 years
l_x	number of people experiencing their x th birthday
L_x	number of person-years lived between ages x and x + 1
e_x	life expectancy
T_x	sum of all L_x (total person-years lived between ages x and x + 1)

A completed version of this exercise is available from the website www.herc.ox.ac.uk/books/applied in the Excel file *Outcomes2 solutions.xlsx*

Chapter 4

Modelling outcomes using patient-level data

Chapter 3 focused on life-table methods as a way of measuring life expectancy differences in economic evaluations. However, the use of published life-table methods may have limitations, especially when considering particular populations which may have very different risks from the general population. In these cases, there are a host of techniques referred to as **survival analysis** which enable risks to be estimated from patient-level data.

This chapter provides an introduction to the survival analysis techniques that health economists can use in estimating patient outcomes. The initial focus of the chapter is on using survival analysis to estimate changes in life expectancy associated with an intervention. We primarily use survival analysis to estimate gains in life expectancy, but the methods can be applied to other outcomes (for example, occurrence of stroke). We also consider how survival analysis can be integrated with quality-of-life measures to measure quality-adjusted survival. Different ways of measuring and valuing quality of life are considered in detail in Chapter 5.

4.1 Overview of survival analysis

Survival analysis typically involves observing one or more outcomes in a population of interest over a period of time. The outcome, which is often referred to as an **event** or **endpoint** could be death, a non-fatal outcome such as a major clinical event (e.g. myocardial infarction), the occurrence of an adverse event, or even the date of first non-compliance with a therapy.

4.1.1 Key features of survival data

A key feature of survival data is censoring, which occurs whenever the event of interest is not observed within the follow-up period. This does not mean that the event will not occur some time in the future, just that it has not occurred while the individual was observed. This could be for a variety of reasons. For example, a subject may withdraw from a study before its conclusion because they move from the area where it is conducted. Alternatively, as most studies involve observing patients for a finite period, the end of the follow-up period may be the reason for censoring. Finally, for non-fatal events, dying from an unrelated cause could censor outcomes. For example, if the event of interest is a cardiovascular event, death from cancer would censor the patient as they are no longer at risk of the event of interest.

The most common case of censoring is referred to as **right censoring**. This occurs whenever the observation of interest occurs after the observation period. For a study where the individuals are observed for a fixed period, all those who have not experienced the event at the end of the study will in effect be right censored. An alternative form of censoring is **left censoring**, which occurs when there is a period of time when individuals are at risk prior to the observation period.

A key feature of most survival analysis methods is that they assume that the censoring process is **non-informative**, meaning that there is no dependence between the time to the event of interest and the process that is causing the censoring. However, if the duration of observation is related to the severity of a patient's disease, for example if patients with more advanced illness are withdrawn early from the study, the censoring is likely to be informative and other techniques are required (Siannis *et al.* 2005)

4.1.2 Key concepts in survival analysis

Here we will only provide definitions for the essential elements of survival analysis that are used in this chapter. These are derived in a more rigorous fashion elsewhere (Collett 2003; Machin *et al.* 2006; Cleves *et al.* 2008), and it would be useful for those unfamiliar with the methods of survival analysis to consult one of these sources.

At the core of survival analysis is the notion of survivor and hazard functions, which we define in turn. Let T be a non-negative random variable indicating the time of the event of interest, which is often referred to as a failure. As Cleves *et al.* (2008) note, the survivor function is defined as:

$$S(t) = \Pr(T > t)$$

where $S(t)$ is the probability of surviving beyond time t. We first encountered this function in Chapter 3, except that there the survivor function was defined in terms of surviving beyond a certain age x rather than a period of time t.

By definition $S(t) = 1$ when $t = 0$ and declines monotonically as t increases. The hazard function $h(t)$ is the instantaneous rate of failure, and can range from zero (when no event occurs) to infinity (when all events occur simultaneously). It can be defined in the limit as the probability that a failure occurs with a defined interval, given that the individual has survived to the beginning of the interval:

$$h(t) = \lim_{\Delta t \to 0} \frac{\Pr(t + \Delta t > T > t \mid T > t)}{\Delta t}$$

Finally, there is the cumulative hazard function, which measures the accumulated hazard up to time t:

$$H(t) \int_0^t h(u) du$$

It can also be shown that all these functions are related, so that $H(t) = -\ln[S(t)]$ or alternatively $S(t) = \exp[-H(t)]$. More details can be found in Chapter 2 of Cleves *et al.* (2008).

4.1.3 Overview of typical survival data

In this section we examine the various techniques that can be employed to measure outcomes in the context of a clinical trial involving survival data. To start, consider an 'ideal study', where all patients could be followed until the outcome of interest has occurred. While this level of patient monitoring is unlikely to occur in practice, it provides us with a 'gold standard' against which we can compare the ability of various survival analysis methods to capture health economic outcomes such as improvement in life expectancy between treatment groups.

Let us consider a randomized controlled trial of an intervention in which 200 patients are evenly divided between the intervention and control groups. The primary outcome of the trial is all-cause mortality. Figure 4.1(a) illustrates the overall survival times for the intervention and control groups in such a study (this figure plots survival time data that are contained in the file SURVIVAL_DATA which is in both Excel and STATA format and can be downloaded from www.herc.ox.ac.uk/books/applied). As all patients are observed continuously for a period of up to 40 years, there is no censoring.

Information is also collected on a secondary outcome, which we term an event, that is known to raise the risk of subsequent mortality. The type of event will depend on the nature of the clinical study under examination. For example, if we were evaluating a therapy for diabetes this could be a major diabetes-related complication. Alternatively, if the trial involved a therapy to prevent cancer this event could be recurrence of a tumour. The survivor function for the event is shown in Figure 4.1(b). We initially focus on mortality alone as the outcome of interest, but return to a discussion on applying survival analysis to non-fatal events in section 4.2.4.

Our first task is to estimate the life expectancy of each group from these survival curves. As there is no censoring, this can be done by calculating the area under the both survivor functions. So for example, consider the survivor function associated with the control group. The time to death of the first five and last five patients are listed in Table 4.1.

The area is easily calculated numerically. If the first patient dies 0.027 years into the follow-up period, the area under the first step of the survival curve is 0.027 (width) × 1 (height) = 0.027. The width of each of the remaining steps can easily be calculated in the same way: for example, the width for the second patient is 0.279 − 0.027 = 0.253. The life expectancy is simply the cumulative area across all 100 patients, which in this case is 13.743 years. The life expectancy of 18.166 years for the intervention group can be calculated in a similar fashion.

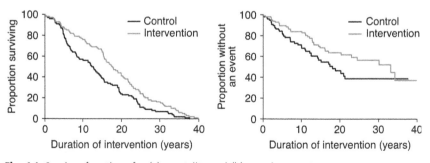

Fig. 4.1 Survivor functions for (a) mortality and (b) a major event.

Table 4.1 Illustration of how to calculate the area under a survivor function

Patient no.	Time to death	Width	% alive	Area	Cumulative area
1	0.027	0.027	1.00	0.027	0.027
2	0.279	0.253	0.99	0.250	0.277
3	0.676	0.397	0.98	0.389	0.666
4	1.191	0.515	0.97	0.499	1.165
5	2.472	1.281	0.96	1.230	2.395
--------------Patients 6–95 have been omitted from the table--------------					
96	33.212	0.960	0.05	0.048	13.656
97	33.657	0.444	0.04	0.018	13.674
98	33.716	0.059	0.03	0.002	13.675
99	36.514	2.799	0.02	0.056	13.731
100	37.689	1.174	0.01	0.012	13.743

4.1.4 Introducing the problem of censoring

Now let us assume that the trial is conducted in a real-world setting in which some patients drop out or are lost during follow-up. Furthermore, the period of follow-up normally ends before outcomes are known for all patients. This is particularly likely when the outcome is mortality, as it may take many years for all patients to die. For example, Table 4.1 indicates that the last patient in the control group lives for over 37 years after entering the study.

To introduce censoring into our dataset we have randomly applied durations of follow-up for each of the 200 patients. Figure 4.2 plots the time that each patient is under observation in the control group. The black lines represent the survival times of patients who have died, while the grey lines represent the duration of follow-up for patients who are censored. We observed the time of death for 58 of the 100 patients in the control group. The remaining 42 are censored; 29 of these are censored in the 15th and final year of observation, while an additional 13 patients are censored in earlier years of the study.

4.2 Quantifying outcomes using survival analysis

4.2.1 Characteristics of the patients

It is also useful to examine the characteristics of patients in the two groups at the start and end of follow-up (i.e. those patients who are alive and censored in the final year of follow-up). Table 4.2 lists the summary statistics for age, sex, and number of events in the intervention and control groups. At the commencement of the study the groups are balanced in the sense that there are equal numbers of men and women in the intervention and control groups and no significant differences in the mean age. By the end of the

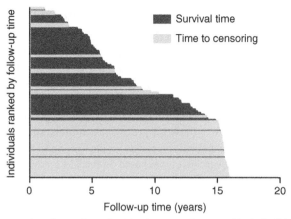

Fig. 4.2 Follow-up time for each patient in the control group: black, individuals whose survival times are determined; grey, individuals who are censored.

study there are substantial differences between the groups: the control group is around 5 years younger than the intervention group and has a larger proportion of females.

Differences in the composition of the intervention and control groups at the end of follow-up may have important implications for estimating outcomes, especially when we are interested in extrapolation. If we know that the intervention group is older and has a lower proportion of females, we would expect these characteristics to increase the hazard mortality in this group over their remaining lifetimes. However, if the intervention group has experienced a lower number of events, this may significantly reduce the hazard for some individuals. They may also benefit from a past treatment which continues to reduce the hazard of a primary outcome such as death. This effect, which is known as the **legacy effect** (Chalmers and Cooper 2008), was noted in Chapter 3 in relation to life-table methods and may also be important when extrapolating outcomes. However, before we examine survival analysis methods to adjust for each of these factors, it is useful to provide a general framework for measuring outcomes involving patient-level data.

Table 4.2 Summary of individual characteristics by allocation group

Characteristic	Participant summary variables			
	At randomization		At end of the study*	
	Control (*n* = 100)	Intervention (*n* = 100)	Control (*n* = 25)	Intervention (*n* = 38)
Males (%)	50	50	40	52
Mean age (SD) (years)	61.9 (11.9)	61.6 (11.4)	65.06 (8.7)	70.46 (10.4)
No. of events	–	–	23	12

*Estimated from patients who do not die and have at least 15 years of follow-up data.

4.2.2 **Estimating outcomes during the study follow-up**

Different strategies are required when estimating outcomes for the period of follow-up and for post-trial extrapolation. During the period when the clinical trial is running, we observe the outcomes in both groups, but we must account for censoring due to loss to follow-up or the early withdrawal of patients. Here non-parametric methods, such as the Kaplan–Meier (KM) or product limit method (Collett 2003), can be applied to the observed data and form the basis of calculations of outcomes such as differences in life expectancy between groups. To understand how the method accounts for censoring, it is helpful to provide an illustration of how it can be calculated manually. In practice survival curves based on the KM method are automatically generated by most statistical analysis packages such as STATA or SAS.

A key feature of the KM method is that probability of survival to time t changes only at times when events occur (in this case death). This method involves multiplying a series of probabilities that are calculated for each interval to represent the proportion of patients for which failure does not occur and then dividing by the number of patients alive at the start of the interval. As Machin *et al.* (2006) indicate, this can be represented by

$$S(t) = (1 - \frac{d_1}{n_1})(1 - \frac{d_2}{n_2})...(1 - \frac{d_t}{n_t})$$

or

$$S(t) = \prod_t (1 - \frac{d_t}{n_t})$$

Table 4.3 illustrates how this formula can be applied to calculate $S(t)$ for the control group of our sample dataset. At time zero there are 100 people at risk, as by definition $S(t) = 1$. The first death occurs at time 0.027, so the first conditional probability of survival is $(1 - d_1/n_1)$ or $1 - 1/100 = 0.99$. Then $S(t)$ on the first step of the KM can be calculated as 1.000×0.990, or 0.990. When $t = 0.099$ the next person is censored from the data, and as there are no events during this interval the conditional probability of survival is $1 - 0/99 = 1$, and so $S(t)$ does not change. This procedure can be used to calculate the entire survivor function: for example, after 2.607 years three patients have been censored and seven have died so the estimated $S(t) = 0.939$. Continuing the procedure for all patients, the follow-up time for the 100th patient is 15.902 and by that time $S(t) = 0.325$. The same KM curve would be generated automatically using the STATA command **sts list**.

Life expectancy can then be calculated as the area under $S(t)$ for the entire duration of follow-up using the methods outlined in section 4.2.1. Alternatively, using STATA, the life expectancy of the control group can be estimated automatically using the command **stci, rmean** (StataCorp 2009). Applying either of these approaches gives a life expectancy for the control group of 10.61 years compared with 13.03 years for the intervention group, indicating an incremental gain in life expectancy of 2.42 years.

Capturing uncertainty around these measures is relatively straightforward. STATA routinely reports confidence intervals for estimates of average survival. For example, the 95% confidence interval for life expectancy in the control group is 9.55 to

Table 4.3 Illustration of the product limit method for calculating the survivor function

T	Deaths	Censored	No. at risk	$1 - d_t/n_t$	S(t)
0.000	0	0	100	1.000	1.000
0.027	1	0	99	0.990	0.990
0.099	0	1	98	1.000	0.990
0.279	1	0	97	0.990	0.980
0.676	1	0	96	0.990	0.970
1.158	0	1	95	1.000	0.970
1.191	1	0	94	0.989	0.960
1.931	0	1	93	1.000	0.960
1.994	0	1	92	1.000	0.960
2.472	1	0	91	0.989	0.949
2.607	1	0	90	0.989	0.939

---------Data on the remaining 90 individuals has been omitted from this table--------

11.67 years, and for the intervention group is 12.08 to 13.99 years. Since the confidence intervals do not overlap, the incremental gain in life expectancy must be significant, but unfortunately the confidence intervals of the difference are not routinely reported. One way of estimating uncertainty around the gain in life expectancy is to use bootstrapping, a resampling method that is considered in detail in Chapters 7 and 11. Using this approach (see www.herc.ox.ac.uk/books/applied which contains a do file (SURVIVAL. do) illustrating how to implement this in STATA) we obtain a 95% confidence interval around the increase in life expectancy due to the intervention of 0.38 to 4.32.

The KM method is just one approach to estimating survival during the follow-up period of the study. Another useful technique is the **Cox proportional hazards model** (Cox 1972) which is one of the most widely employed techniques in survival analysis. The Cox model, as it is commonly known, is a semi-parametric method which assumes that any covariate has a proportional effect on the hazard in that it multiplicatively shifts the baseline hazard function upwards or downwards (for a detailed overview see Cleves *et al.* 2008). Hence the hazard rate for the ith individual in the data is

$$h(t \mid x_i) = h_0(t)\exp(x_i\beta_x)$$

where $h_0(t)$ is known as the **baseline hazard** and the β_x are regression coefficients indicating the effect of each covariate x_i. The baseline hazard is the hazard when all $x_i = 0$, as the relative hazard is equal to one. Many statisticians involved with clinical studies are primarily interested in the relative effect of a factor (or a treatment) on risk, and consider it a key virtue of the Cox model that $h_0(t)$ has no parametric form and is therefore completely flexible. However, from a health economist's perspective this is also the model's key limitation, as it does not permit extrapolation beyond the period of follow-up without imposing additional assumptions.

Despite these limitations, there are several reasons why health economists may want to use Cox models when quantifying outcomes. Firstly, it provides an easy way of estimating the benefits of an intervention in terms of its impact on relative risk during the follow-up period. Second, it provides a way of adjusting for covariates if the trial or study from which we obtain patient-level data is not representative of the population that is the focus of the economic evaluation. For example, if we are interested in whether an intervention is cost-effective for women and the clinical study involves both men and women, then we could apply the method to adjust for the hazards that the different subgroups face. Finally, a Cox model could be used to construct life tables on the assumption that the mortality experience of older individuals in the data can be used to estimate the hazard of younger individuals. Such an approach involves using age rather than study follow-up time as the underlying time at risk. As a baseline hazard can now be obtained across a range of ages it can be used to extrapolate outcomes. Clarke *et al.* (2009) give an example of where this approach has been used to estimate the effect that a quality-of-life rating can have on life expectancy.

To illustrate the use of a Cox model we apply it to the full example dataset and include an indicator variable for the allocation group (i.e. *Intervention* is set equal to one for those receiving the treatment and zero otherwise). In addition, we have estimated a model that also includes *Age* in years and *Male* which is again defined using a zero–one indicator variable. Table 4.4 reports the hazard ratios for each of these covariates of the Cox models. Those in the intervention group are at a considerably lower level of risk (i.e. around 50%) than the control group in both the *Therapy only* and the *Full model* which also adjusts for age and sex. If we turn to the interpretation of other covariates, each year of age increases an individual's risk by around 8%; and being male increases risk by 48%, but this is not statistically significant at the 5% level ($P = 0.066$).

Table 4.4 Hazard ratio (95% CI) for covariates of the Cox regression models

	Therapy only model	Full model
Intervention	0.473 (0.309,0.723)	0.461 (0.301, 0.709)
Age	–	1.084 (1.061,1.108)
Male	–	1.480 (0.975, 2.248)

It is important to test if the proportional hazards assumption holds for the Cox model and other parametric models of this form (see section 4.2.3). There are many alternative methods for undertaking diagnostic tests. One such test is based on Schoenfeld residuals and can be routinely estimated using the STATA command **estat phtest** (StataCorp 2009). When applied to the sample dataset the following output is produced:

Test of proportional-hazards assumption

Time: Time

	rho	chi2	df	Prob>chi2
therapy	−0.07941	0.58	1	0.4448
age	0.07682	0.54	1	0.4615
male	0.05932	0.34	1	0.5625
global test		1.41	3	0.7032

Applying this test to the current data indicates there is no evidence that the specification violates the proportional hazards assumption. The combined test statistic, which is distributed χ^2 with three degrees of freedom of 1.41, is well below the cut-off value and there is no evidence of violations in individual variables.

While violation of the proportional hazards assumption is not an issue in the current application, there will be times when these diagnostic tests indicate that one or more covariates are not having a proportional effect on the baseline hazard. What can be done when this problem arises? As these are mis-specification tests, the way to overcome this violation is to re-specify the model. This could take a number of directions: (i) consider whether any important covariates have been omitted from the model; (ii) stratification or transformation of the variables that are having a non-proportional effect; (iii) use of time-varying covariates to allow a factor to have different effects on the hazard at different times.

4.2.3 Parametric models

The final class of survival analysis models we consider are parametric proportional hazard models. Like the Cox model, these models have covariates, but they also assign parameters to represent the baseline hazard $h_0(t)$. A number of functional forms are commonly employed, the simplest of which is the exponential regression which assumes that baseline hazard is constant, i.e. $h_0(t) = \exp(\alpha)$ This effectively means that the model is memoryless. Two other common forms are (Hougaard 2000):

- the *Weibull* regression $h_0(t) = pt^{p-1}\exp(a)$
- the *Gompertz* regression $h_0(t) = \exp(\alpha)\exp(\gamma t)$

Weibull regression allows quite a flexible specification of the hazard: when $p > 1$ the hazard is continually increasing with time, and when $p < 1$ a decreasing hazard is obtained. When $p = 1$ the exponential model is obtained. Similarly, in the Gompertz regression model if $\gamma > 0$ the hazard is increasing, if $\gamma < 0$ it is decreasing, and if $\gamma = 0$ the model again reduces to the exponential model (Cleves 2008).

The choice between these parametric models will depend on the application. Gompertz regression was originally developed for predicting human mortality (Gompertz 1825), and is often used to model survival and life expectancy. Weibull regression has been widely used for other outcomes, such as major complications of

Table 4.5 Coefficients and hazard ratios of three parametric survival analysis models

	Model coefficient (standard error)			Hazard ratio (95% CI)		
	Exponential	Weibull	Gompertz	Exponential	Weibull	Gompertz
Intervention	−0.684 (0.216)	−0.750 (0.217)	−0.776 (0.218)	0.504 (0.330, 0.772)	0.472 (0.308, 0.723)	0.460 (0.301, 0.705)
Age	0.0683 (0.010)	0.077 (0.011)	0.081 (0.011)	1.071 (1.049, 1.092)	1.080 (1.057, 1.103)	1.084 (1.061, 1.108)
Male	0.331 (0.211)	0.392 (0.213)	0.411 (0.213)	1.393 (0.920, 2.109)	1.480 (0.975, 2.248)	1.509 (0.993, 2.293)
Constant	−7.32 (0.729)	−8.946 (0.885)	−8.921 (0.854)			
ρ		1.441 (0.13)				
γ			0.112 (0.025)			
LLF	−190.277	−183.250	−180.221			
AIC	388.554	376.499	370.443			

diabetes (Clarke *et al.* 2004) or the failure of different hip prostheses (Briggs *et al.* 2004). As both models contain the exponential as a nested model, it is easy to test whether the underlying hazard is constant. Likelihood-based tests such as the Akaike information criterion (AIC) can also be used to choose between alternative models.

Table 4.5 reports the coefficients of the exponential, Weibull, and Gompertz models. The left-hand side of the table reports the coefficients and standard errors, and the right-hand side reports the hazard ratios and 95% confidence intervals (CI). The hazard ratios can easily be calculated by taking the exponential of each of the coefficients: for example, the relative effect of the intervention in the exponential model of 0.504 is exp(–0.684). The hazard ratios are similar across each type of parametric model, and those of the Cox model are reported in Table 4.4. Both the Weibull and the Gompertz models have an additional parameter which determines the shape of the hazard. Both indicate an increasing hazard, and in the Weibull model, ρ has an additional interpretation: 1.441 is between 1 and 2, and so it indicates that the hazard is increasing at a decreasing rate.

It is easy to calculate the AIC for each of the models in STATA (StataCorp 2009):

$$AIC = -2LLF + 2(K + C)$$

where LLF is the logarithm of the likelihood function, K is the number of model covariates, and C is the number of distributional parameters. Applying this formula to the exponential model gives

$$AIC_{exp} = -2 \times (-190.277) + 2(3 + 1) = 388.554$$

If this criterion is used to choose between the three models, the Gompertz regression would be selected as it has the lowest AIC (370.443).

Using these equations it is possible to estimate the survivor functions for each individual in the example dataset using the following formulae (Cleves *et al.* 2008):

$$\text{exponential: } S(t|x_k) = \exp(-\exp(\beta_0 + x_k\beta_x)t)$$

$$\text{Weibull: } S(t|x_k) = \exp(-\exp(\beta_0 + x_k\beta_x)t^p)$$

$$\text{Gompertz: } S(t|x_k) = \exp(-\frac{1}{\gamma}\exp(\beta_0 + x_k\beta_x)(\exp(\gamma t) - 1))$$

where β_0 is the regression constant, β_x is a vector of coefficients for the k explanatory variables. For example, the first individual in the sample is a male aged 51 years who receives the intervention. Using the exponential formula the probability that the individual will live to 52 can be calculated as:

$$S(1) = \exp(-\exp(-7.32 - 0.684 + 51 \times 0.0683 + 0.0331) \times 1) = 0.985$$

The proportion surviving at other times and for the other parametric models can be derived similarly.

Figure 4.3 plots the survivor functions for each of the parametric forms for the 49 years until the individual reaches the age of 100 years (the calculations underlying this figure are contained in the downloadable spreadsheet parametric_survival_analysis.xls). Figure 4.3 also contains an empirical survivor function for a male of the same age derived from the complete English Life Tables 2003–2005 similar to that used in

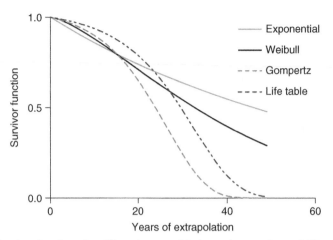

Fig. 4.3 Survivor functions for different parametric forms for a male aged 51 years.

Chapter 3 (Office of National Statistics England 2009). Such a comparison is useful as it gives an indication of how the mortality experience of the population under study differs from the general population, and thereby provides a useful reality check.

It is evident from Figure 4.3 that the Gompertz model has a very similar shape to the survivor function derived from the population life table, except that there is much higher mortality in the sample dataset than in the general population. The other parametric forms have quite different shapes. While the hazards associated with the Weibull and exponential models are initially higher relative to the Gompertz model, from the age of around 75 years there is a greater probability of survival. The probability of survival at 100 years of age is around 0.48 for the exponential model and 0.29 for the Weibull model, which is implausibly high given that fewer than 1% of males in the general population who were alive at 51 years survive to this age. This again suggests that the Gompertz is likely to be the most appropriate parametric form, and so we shall use it for the extrapolation.

While it is possible to derive life expectancies directly from some parametric forms such as Weibull, which has well defined moments, this is not possible using other distributions such as Gompertz (Hougaard 2000, p.68). Alternatively, life expectancies can be estimated through methods of numerical integration such as the trapezoidal rule (Atkinson 1989):

$$\int_{t_0}^{t_1} S(t) \approx (t_1 - t_0) \frac{S(t_0) + S(t_1)}{2}$$

where t_0 and t_1 are two time points that span the interval being numerically integrated. Applying this method to successive 1 year intervals, the life expectancies for the 51-year-old male based on the three models are 64.7 years, 38.3 years, and 23.0 years for the exponential, Weibull, and Gompertz models, respectively. This compares with the male life expectancy of 28.3 years from the English life table.

4.2.4 **Modelling and extrapolating outcomes**

The final stage is to employ survival analysis methods to quantify the outcomes of an intervention. Several approaches could be adopted. First, one could estimate the within-trial benefits using a non-parametric approach such as the KM or Cox model. However, if there is a significant difference in outcomes observed with the trial, such as a greater number of survivors in the intervention group, it will be important to extrapolate beyond the follow-up period in order to fully account for the benefits.

There are two alternative approaches that could be adopted. First, one could employ a pure modelling approach, which would involve using a parametric survival analysis method, such as the Gompertz model, to estimate a survivor function which would then be used to estimate all the benefits. The idea here is that the trial data are simply a way of informing a more general model (Sculpher *et al.* 2006). An alternative is to combine trial-based outcomes with model-based extrapolation. This would involve estimating the within-trial benefits non-parametrically and the benefits beyond the trial parametrically from a model that is fitted to the available data. We shall consider each of these approaches in turn.

One way of implementing the modelled approach is to estimate survivor functions and then apply these to the population that is the focus of the economic evaluation. Where patient-level data are available an overall survivor function could be calculated using

$$\hat{S}(t) = \sum_{i=l}^{n} S_i(t) / n$$

where n is the number of patients. By way of example, we apply this approach to estimate separate survivor functions for the treatment and control groups of the sample survival analysis dataset (although these estimated functions could be applied to other populations). Figure 4.4 uses the estimated Gompertz model to plot survivor functions for the treatment and control groups based on the model reported in Table 4.5. We also plot the non-parametric survivor functions derived using the KM method (see section 4.2.1) in the same figure.

There are some differences between the non-parametric and parametric survivor functions, but the two approaches generally produce similar results. Estimates of life

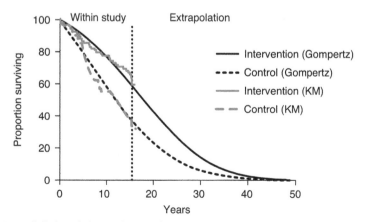

Fig. 4.4 Modelled and observed survival.

expectancy obtained from the Gompertz model using numerical integration during the period of follow-up (i.e. within first 16 years) are 10.69 and 13.00 years, very close to those reported in section 4.2.1 which were derived using KM (10.61 and 13.03 years).

When the Gompertz model is used to extrapolate survivor function until all patients have died (i.e. over the 50 year period), the life expectancies for the control and intervention groups are 13.51 years and 18.55 years, respectively. One can compare this with the actual estimates reported in section 4.1.3 from the original (uncensored) data. The comparable estimates for the control and intervention groups were 13.74 years and 18.17 years, respectively. This suggests that the Gompertz model fitted to only 15 years of follow-up data provides useful estimates of the benefits of treatment if it were continued for a period of 50 years.

The second approach is to extrapolate only for those individuals who are censored as a way of filling in information about survival beyond the period they are observed within the study. Again, the estimated Gompertz regression model could be used to undertake this, but the age of each individual needs to be increased to reflect the time that they are observed in the study. It is also important to make a decision about the nature of the treatment effect beyond the end of the study. Some assumptions are possible:

◆ the intervention group continues to experience the lower hazard observed during the study

◆ the intervention group reverts to the hazard of the control group

◆ the hazard in the control group is reduced to that of the treatment group.

It is comparatively easy to implement these assumptions by switching the intervention indicator variable on (or off) when extrapolating. It is also possible to assume that the intervention continues to have only a partial effect over time. The choice between these assumptions will depend on the evaluation, but the most conservative is the second assumption that there are no ongoing treatment effects. Figure 4.5 illustrates how different assumptions impact on outcomes.

The life expectancy for those individuals alive at the end of follow-up in the intervention group is 11.15 years without treatment effects and 15.75 years with treatment

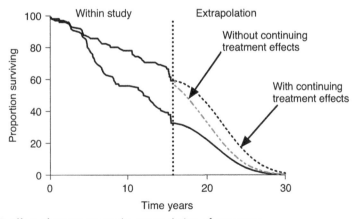

Fig. 4.5 Effect of treatment on the extrapolation of outcomes.

effects included. However, these differences only impact on the period of extrapolation, and the impact on overall incremental life expectancy is more modest (increasing it by around 20%).

4.2.5 Applying survival analysis to other outcomes

The same survival analysis techniques can be used to model other outcomes such as time to first event. Two issues need to be taken into account when modelling these outcomes. First, although we have seen above that the Gompertz distribution represents overall mortality quite well, it may not be appropriate for other outcomes. Specification and diagnostic testing are always required to determine a preferred model. Secondly, in studies where there is a high rate of mortality (or mortality is stratified into different causes), **competing risks** are likely to be an issue (Hougaard 2000). This is the case with the sample dataset as 92 patients died during follow-up. There are now a variety of different estimators for dealing with competing risk (Pintilie 2006), some of which have recently been implemented in statistical software packages such as STATA (StataCorp 2009).

4.3 Combining quantity and quality of life

In Chapter 5 we consider in more detail the other dimension to health outcomes—the measurement and valuation of quality of life. Ideally, changes in both life expectancy and quality of life will be brought together in a metric such as the quality-adjusted life-year (QALY) in which quality associated with each year of life is quantified on a 0 to 1 scale (which is often referred to as utility). The purpose of this section is to discuss ways of combining survival data with quality-of-life data, using either individual or population-level data.

If survival times and the health-related quality of life over time are known for all the patients in a study (i.e. none are censored), standard techniques for dealing with continuous data can be used. The sample mean and standard deviation of the QALYs for the patients in each treatment and control arm of a study could be calculated and used to provide an estimate of the mean treatment difference in QALYs, together with an appropriate CI.

If the data for some patients are censored, a standard survival analysis using QALYs for each individual as an endpoint rather than the actual survival time may seem appropriate. However, the problem of informative drop-out or censoring is a particular problem when trying to measure QALYs. This can arise when patients with low quality of life drop out early from a study (Billingham *et al.* 1999).

Even if this is not the case, patients with poor quality of life will receive a lower weighting than patients with good quality of life, and therefore will accumulate QALYs at a slower rate. Thus they are likely to be censored earlier on the QALY timescale than those with good quality of life. This will bias KM estimates and other standard survival analysis techniques.

Two options are available for a valid analysis: the subject-based approach and the population-based approach. We will consider each of these in turn.

4.3.1 Subject-based approach

Billingham and Abrams (2002) suggest that one approach to combining survival analysis with quality of life is to set the censoring date for the analysis to the smallest censored survival time value, thus restricting the analysis to a period during which all subjects have full follow-up and eliminating censoring. This is only feasible if the smallest censored value is quite large; otherwise, a considerable number of events may be lost, reducing the statistical power of the analysis.

An alternative approach is to use either extrapolation or imputation to fill in event and QALY histories from the point when patients are censored. An example of this approach is the UKPDS Outcomes Model (Clarke *et al.* 2004), a computer simulation model developed using patient-level information from the UK Prospective Diabetes Study. The Outcomes Model involves probabilistic discrete-time computer simulation and is based on an integrated system of parametric proportional hazards risk equations. The current version of the model includes both macrovascular complications (e.g. myocardial infarction, other ischaemic heart disease, congestive heart failure, stroke) and selected microvascular complications (e.g. blindness). The model is based on a combination of Weibull and Gompertz parametric survival models estimated from an average of 10 years of follow-up data on 3642 patients. Figure 4.6 shows each of the equations with hazard or odds ratios for each risk factor, and also shows event-related dependencies in the form of arrows linking equations.

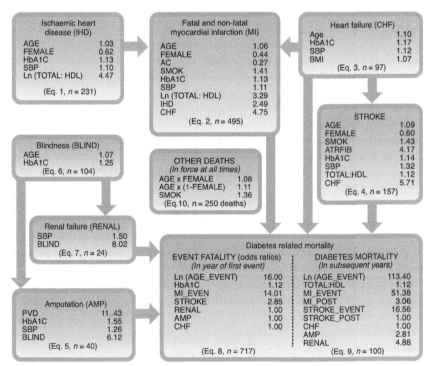

Fig. 4.6 Summary of model equations showing event-related dependencies and hazard/odds ratio for each risk factor. Reproduced from Clarke *et al.* (2004), with kind permission from Springer Science+Business Media.

For example, looking at the top right-hand corner of Figure 4.6, the risk of heart failure increases by 10% with each year of age, and by 17% for each 1% increase in haemoglobin (HbA1c). It also increases with systolic blood pressure (SBP) and body mass index (BMI). The arrows indicate that patients who have a history of heart failure are at a significantly higher risk of subsequent stroke and myocardial infarction.

In order to implement this approach, the impact of each type of event on quality of life or utility is also required. Clarke *et al.* (2002) report an example of this approach, in which quality of life data from a large randomized trial (measured using the EQ-5D, which is described in Chapter 5) was analysed in relation to the prior occurrence of a set of diabetes-related complications. Because of the presence of significant numbers of patients in a state of full health, conventional linear regression was arguably inappropriate, and hence the study adopted a Tobit model with upper censoring at 1.

The results indicated that, for example, a non-fatal myocardial infarction was associated with a decrement of 0.055 in subsequent utility, stroke was associated with a 0.164 decrement, and amputation with a 0.28 decrement. As with event-based costing, which is discussed in Chapter 7, this approach has the advantage of isolating the specific effects of the clinical events of interest, and is also amenable to most forms of extrapolation modelling which are normally based on predicting time to and frequency of such events.

The simulation model shown in Figure 4.6 can be used to predict the timing of events and mortality based on patient characteristics, and utility decrements can then be applied to obtain a profile of QALYs over time. In this way the model can be used to extrapolate outcomes for patients in studies from the point at which they are censored. An example of such a simulation is given in Figure 4.7, which shows the predicted QALYs of patients with type 2 diabetes managed by intensive blood glucose

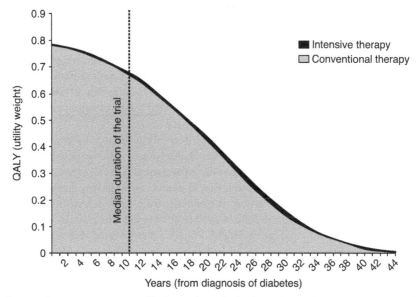

Fig. 4.7 The average QALY profile for patients in the intensive and conventional arms of the UKPDS study.

control compared with those managed less intensively. While this extrapolation is based on the assumption that the direct effects of therapy do not continue beyond the study, it is nevertheless apparent that a substantial proportion of the incremental benefit is attained beyond the median follow-up time of around 10 years. Based on this simulation model, Clarke *et al.* (2005) report QALYs of 16.35 in the conventional group versus 16.62 in the intensively treated group, a gain of 0.27 QALYs from the intervention.

4.3.2 **Population-based approach**

The alternative to the subject-based approach is the population- or group-based approach, which involves estimating survival and quality of life separately and combining them at a group level (Glasziou *et al.* 1998). As Billingham and Abrams (2002) note, the population approach can be represented by:

$$QALY(T) = \int_0^T Q(t)S(t)$$

where $Q(t)$ is the average utility (or quality-of-life score) of the survivors at any given point in time represented by $S(t)$, which is then integrated between zero and a fixed time T. Hence the quality-adjusted survival curve is formed by plotting against time t the product of the mean quality-of-life score of patients alive at time t and the probability of surviving to time t. $S(t)$ can be estimated using standard methods such as the life-table method, KM estimates, or parametric models (for further discussion, see Billingham *et al.* (1999)). It should be noted that this approach is basically very similar to the approach to deal with censored costs that will be covered in Chapter 7.

4.4 **Measuring outcomes in practice**

Changes in life expectancy are a commonly used outcome measure in economic evaluation. In this final section, we briefly review some real-world estimates of the impact of different interventions on life expectancy. Table 4.6 shows selected examples of estimates of the gain in life expectancy for various interventions reported by Wright and Weinstein (1998) in an article arguing that gains in life expectancy from a medical intervention can only be categorized as large or small if they are compared with gains from other interventions aimed at the same target population.

Gains in life expectancy from preventive interventions in populations of average risk generally ranged from a few days to slightly more than a year. For example, regular mammography is reported to increase life expectancy by 0.067 years (or around 24 days). This relatively low average is due to breast cancer having a relatively low prevalence in the population, and so the benefits from early detection have to be spread across a large number of individuals being screened. The gains in life expectancy from preventing or treating disease in persons at elevated risk are generally greater. Interventions that treat established disease vary, with gains in life expectancy ranging from a few months (for coronary thombolysis and revascularization to treat heart disease) to as long as 9 years (for chemotherapy to treat advanced testicular cancer). However, the point that Wright and Weinstein (1998) were making was not that

Table 4.6 The reported effect of selected interventions on life expectancy

Disease and intervention	Target population	Gain in life expectancy (years)
Prevention		
10 years of 2-yearly mammography	50-year-old women	0.067
Measles vaccine	Infants	0.008
Quitting cigarette smoking	35-year-old smokers	2.6
Treatment		
Revascularization to treat heart disease	Men with coronary disease	0.08–1.17
Heart transplant	Patients with endstage cardiac failure	2.5–8.25
Chemotherapy to treat advanced testicular cancer	Men with advanced testicular cancer	8.9

Adapted from Wright and Weinstein (1998).

absolute gains vary widely, but that a gain in life expectancy of a month from a preventive intervention targeted at populations at average risk and a gain of a year from a preventive intervention targeted at populations at elevated risk could both be considered large. It should also be noted that interventions that produce a comparatively small gain in life expectancy when averaged across the population, for example immunization to prevent infectious disease, may still be very cost-effective. For example, Balestra and Littenberg (1993) estimated that a tetanus booster at age 65 years increases life expectancy by 0.000003 years (approximately 2 minutes) at a cost-effectiveness ratio of $4527 per life year gained.

4.5 Summary

This chapter has described survival analysis methods for estimating health-related outcomes when patient-level data are available, but information on the outcomes of some individuals is not available. These methods were applied to a hypothetical dataset, and a range of methods to estimate outcome such as life expectancy were then derived. The issue of how to combine survival analysis with quality-of-life data was then considered. The final section considered some published empirical estimates of the improvements in life expectancy that have been attributed to various interventions.

References

Atkinson, K.A. (1989). *An Introduction to Numerical Analysis* (2nd edn). John Wiley, New York.

Balestra, D.J. and Littenberg, B. (1993). Should adult tetanus immunization be given as a single vaccination at age 65? A cost-effectiveness analysis. *Journal of General Internal Medicine*, **8**, 405–12.

Billingham, L.J. and Abrams, K.R. (2002). Simultaneous analysis of quality of life and survival data. *Statistical Methods in Medical Research*, **11**, 25–48.

Billingham, L.J., Abrams, K.R., and Jones, D.R. (1999). Methods for the analysis of quality-of-life and survival data in health technology assessment. *Health Technology Assessment*, **3**, 1–152.

Briggs, A.H., Sculpher, M.J., Dawson, J., Fitzpatrick, R., Murray, D., and Malchau, H. (2004). The use of probabilistic decision models in technology assessment: the case of total hip replacement. *Applied Health Economics and Health Policy*, **3**, 78–9.

Clarke, P.M., Gray, A.M., Holman, R. (2002). Estimating utility values for health states of type 2 diabetic patients using the EQ-5D. *Medical Decision Making*, **22**, 340–349.

Clarke, P.M., Gray, A.M., Briggs, A., *et al.* (2004). A model to estimate the lifetime health outcomes of patients with Type 2 diabetes: the United Kingdom Prospective Diabetes Study (UKPDS 68) Outcomes Model. *Diabetologia*, **47**, 1747–59.

Clarke, P.M., Gray, A.M., Briggs, A., Stevens, R., Matthews, D., Holman, R. on behalf of the UK Prospective Diabetes Study (UKPDS). (2005). Cost utility analyses of intensive blood-glucose and tight blood-pressure control in Type 2 diabetes. *Diabetologia*, **48**, 866–877.

Clarke, P.M., Hayes, A.J., Glasziou, P.G., Scott, R., Simes, J., and Keech, A.C. (2009). Using the EQ-5D index score as a predictor of outcomes in patients with type 2 diabetes. *Medical Care*, **47**, 61–8.

Cleves, M., Gutierrez, R., Gould, W., and Marchenko, Y. (2008). *An Introduction to Survival Analysis Using STATA* (2nd edn). Stata Press, College Station, TX.

Chalmers, J. and Cooper, M.E. (2008). UKPDS and the legacy effect. *New England Journal of Medicine*, **359**, 1618–20.

Collett, D.(2003). *Modelling Survival Data in Medical Research* (2nd edn). Chapman & Hall, London.

Cox, D.R. (1972). Regression models and life tables. *Journal of the Royal Statistical Society, Series B*, **34**, 187–220.

Glasziou, P.P., Cole, B.F., Gelber, R.D., Hilden, J., and Simes, R.J. (1998). Quality adjusted survival analysis with repeated quality of life measures. *Statistics in Medicine*, **17**, 1215–29.

Gompertz, B. (1825). On the nature of the function expressive of the law of human mortality, and on a new mode of determining the value of life contingencies. *Philosophical Transactions of the Royal Society of London*, **115**, 513–83.

Hougaard, P. (2000). *Analysis of Multivariate Survival Data*. Springer-Verlag, New York.

Machin, D., Cheung, Y.B., and Parmar, M.K. (2006). *Survival Analysis: A Practical Approach* (2nd edn). JohnWiley, New York.

Office of National Statistics England (2009). *Interim Life Tables, 1980–82 to 2006–08*. Stationery Office, London (available online at: http://www.statistics.gov.uk/StatBase/Product.asp?vlnk = 14459).

Pintilie, M. (2006). *Competing Risks: A Practical Perspective*. JohnWiley, New York.

Sculpher, M.J., Claxton, K., Drummond, M., and McCabe, C. (2006). Whither trial-based economic evaluation for health care decision making. *Health Economics*, **15**, 677–87.

Siannis, F., Copas, J., and Lu, G. (2005). Sensitivity analysis for informative censoring in parametric survival models. *Biostatistics*, **6**, 77–91.

StataCorp (2009). *STATA: Release 11. Statistical Software*. StataCorp, College Station, TX.

Wright, J.C. and Weinstein, M.C. (1998). Gains in life expectancy from medical interventions standardizing data on outcomes. *New England Journal of Medicine*, **339**, 380–6.

Exercise

Using survival analysis

If you go to the website www.herc.ox.ac.uk/books/applied you will find an Excel file **Outcomes2.xlsx** which contains five worksheets. The first sheet, **Life Table**, containing a set of mortality rates that can be used in the construction of a life table, was used in the Exercise for Chapter 3. The second sheet, **Survival Times**, contains information on the survival times of patients in the Control Group and Treatment Group of our exercise study, and the questions below relate to this worksheet. (The remaining sheets will be used in a continuation of this exercise in Chapters 5 and 11.)

The second worksheet, **Survival times**, contains survival data on patients in the Control Group and Treatment Group of our exercise study.

(i) Use the product limit method to estimate life expectancy of patients in the Control and Treatment groups.

(ii) Extrapolate from year 5 of the study to obtain an estimate of the proportion in each group surviving at 10 years, and compare this with the actual survival proportion.

(iii) Estimate the discounted life expectancy using an annual discount rate of 3.5%.

Step-by-step guide

The second worksheet **Survival Times** contains survival data on the two groups of patients that are also used in the Costs and the Presenting Results exercises: a Control group and a Treatment group, each containing 100 patients followed for up to 20 years.

(i) Use the product limit method to estimate the life expectancy of patients in each group

The product limit method must be applied to each group of patients. The number at risk for each period of time has already been calculated.

For the Control group patients:

♦ Use the product limit formula to calculate the survival probability for each period of time.

♦ At time zero all patients are alive. Hence the proportion surviving is 100% (place 1 in cell E113).

♦ At 0.724 years one patient has died. Calculate the proportion surviving by applying the product limit formula: = E113*(1–B114/D113).

♦ Copy this formula down column E.

- To estimate life expectancy we must calculate the area under each step of the survival curve.

- Calculate the width of the first step. All patients are alive for the first 0.724 years so the formula for the width of the first rectangle is: = A114–A113.

- Multiply the width by the height, which is the proportion surviving, to estimate life expectancy for each period and place in column **LE**.

- Sum column **LE** to estimate total life expectancy.

Repeat the above steps to calculate life expectancy of the Treatment group patients.

(ii) Part (ii) of the exercise asks you to undertake some simple extrapolation. In this case we have follow-up data up to 20 years, but assume that the study finished after 5 years. Extrapolate to obtain an estimate of the proportion in each group surviving out to 10 years, and then compare your results with the actual proportion surviving to 10 years in each group.

Use the exponential approximation formula. For the Control group you will be using information up to the last point before 5 years, which you will find in row 125: = EXP(10*LN(E125)/A125). For the Treatment group the last point before 5 years is in row 119: = EXP(10*LN(N119)/J119).

Your results should indicate a predicted survival at 10 years of 0.734 in the Control group and 0.868 in the Treatment group; these compare with the actual survival rates at 10 years of 0.715 and 0.841, respectively. This suggests that the exponential assumption in this estimate may overestimate actual survival, at least over this period.

(iii) Estimate the discounted life expectancy.

To do this, paste the survival time data in cells A113–A213 of the **Survival times** sheet to cells A239–A339, making sure that you paste the values rather than the formulae (use paste special). In the column adjacent to this, insert the discounting formula using a discount rate of 3.5%. This will be = 1/((1.035)^INT(A239)). Then go to cell D239 and insert the formula to calculate the life expectancy that has to be discounted. Remember that this is going to be the added life expectancy in each period, not the whole within-trial life expectancy. For example, in cell D239 the formula will be: = (A240-A239)*B239*E113 (i.e. the added life expectancy in that period compared with the previous period times the discount factor times the survival probability).

Repeat these steps for the Treatment group patients, and then sum columns D and I to obtain and compare discounted life expectancy for the two groups.

A completed version of this exercise is available from the website www.herc.ox.ac.uk/books/applied in the Excel file ***Outcomes2 solutions.xlsx***

Chapter 5

Measuring, valuing, and analysing health outcomes

Chapter 4 introduced survival analysis techniques and demonstrated how these could be combined with quality-of-life data to estimate quality-adjusted survival. We now take a closer look at the different types of outcome measures likely to be used in cost-effectiveness and cost-utility analyses, including event-free time, disease-specific measures, and quality- or disability-adjusted life-years. This chapter then considers different instruments for collecting outcome information, including disease-specific instruments, generic quality-of-life instruments such as the SF-36 and SF-12, study- or disease-specific standard gamble and time trade-off exercises, and generic utility-based instruments including the EQ-5D and the Health Utility Index (HUI). The chapter demonstrates the use of scoring tariffs and ways of presenting results, including descriptive information from questionnaire responses. It also considers different methods of mapping between instruments, such as from the SF-36 or SF-12 to utility-based measures of outcome, and concludes by briefly considering possible alternatives to the QALY approach, including DALYs and capabilities.

5.1 Introduction

One of the best-known definitions of health is offered by the World Health Organization in its founding Constitution: 'A state of complete physical, mental and social well-being, and not merely the absence of disease and infirmity' (World Health Organization 1948). This usefully conveys that health has different dimensions or domains (eg physical, mental), and that care is required in deciding what to include or exclude. In practice, the WHO definition has been very hard to use in any measurable way, but the issues of scope and dimension which it raises are very clearly reflected in the many thousands of different instruments that have been developed to measure different aspects of health. It should also be noted that these instruments sometimes claim to be measuring health, or health status, or health-related quality of life, or quality of life, and the use or alleged misuse of these terms has generated a good deal of heat. Here we follow other analysts (Brazier *et al.* 2007) in arguing that the precise terminology is much less important than agreeing exactly what should be included in the outcome component of an economic evaluation: disease-specific symptoms, more all-encompassing measures of health, or very broad measures of social well-being.

It is also important to stress at the outset the distinction between **measurement** and **valuation**. Many researchers working in this field are primarily concerned with **measuring** symptoms, disease progression, or quality of life, and the instruments used to do this are generally referred to by economists as **non-preference-based measures**. However, economists are typically interested in moving beyond measurement to assess what **value** individuals place on symptoms or quality-of-life states. The parallel is with resource use on the cost side of the cost-effectiveness equation, where we are not interested simply in quantifying the volume of resources used *per se*, but in estimating the value of these resources measured by their cost. How resources are valued is dealt with in Chapter 6; **preference-based measures** and different methods of valuing health outcomes are discussed in this chapter.

5.2 Non-preference-based measures of health status

Some non-preference-based instruments are highly specific and are designed to measure specific symptoms in specific diseases, while others are much broader and aim to capture many different aspects or domains of health status.

5.2.1 Disease- and symptom-specific measures

The American Urological Association (AUA) Symptom Index is a good example of a widely used disease-specific instrument which elicits information on the frequency of urinary symptoms related to benign prostatic hyperplasia (Barry *et al.* 1992). It contains seven questions covering symptoms of frequency, nocturia, weak urinary stream, hesitancy, intermittence, incomplete emptying, and urgency; each is scored from 0 to 5, where 0 means 'never' and 5 means 'almost always', and the scores across the seven questions are then summed. Total scores can then be used to make a clinical assessment (for example, to determine whether a patient's symptoms are sufficiently severe to warrant medical or surgical intervention), but they can also be used to make comparisons over time or between groups of patients, either on the continuous scale 0–35, or in clinically defined categories of symptom severity where 0–7 is classified as mild, 8–19 as moderate and 20–35 as severe.

5.2.2 Disease-specific measures

Clearly, the AUA Symptom Index can only be used in a particular group of patients, and moreover is entirely focused on a set of disease-related symptoms rather than the more general health status of these patients. Other instruments are also disease specific but are not confined to measuring symptoms. For example, the EORTC QLQ-C30 questionnaire developed by the European Organization for Research and Treatment of Cancer, while also disease specific in that it is designed to assess quality of life in cancer patients, can be used across a range of different cancers and measures not only symptoms but also emotional, physical, and role functioning (Aaronson *et al.* 1993).

The QLQ-C30 is a 30-item self-reporting questionnaire, with questions grouped into five functional subscales covering role, physical, cognitive, emotional, and social functioning, three multi-item symptom scales covering fatigue, pain, and nausea and vomiting, individual questions concerning common symptoms in cancer patients such as insomnia or loss of appetite, one item assessing perceived financial impact, and one global or general quality-of-life question. Every subscale and single-item measure is scored from 0 to 100, and these are then reported separately for each subscale or single item.

Another example of a disease-specific instrument aiming to measure several dimensions of quality of life is the Diabetes Quality of Life (DQOL) questionnaire, developed by the Diabetes Control and Complications Trial (DCCT) Research Group for use in a large trial of treatment of type 1 diabetes (DCCT Research Group 1988). The original DQOL contained 46 questions, each scored on a five-point scale and then grouped into four subscales intended to measure life satisfaction, diabetes impact, worries about diabetes, and social/vocational concerns. The scores for each subscale were reported separately along with a total score.

5.2.3 Non-disease-specific measures

The SF-36 is the most widely used and best-known example of a generic or non-disease-specific measure of general health; it is not restricted to any particular disease or condition, and is intended to measure quality of life in all major domains. It was developed as a general measure of health outcomes during the Medical Outcomes Study (MOS), an investigation of whether variations in patient outcomes could be explained by differences in systems of health care and clinician characteristics (Tarlov *et al.* 1989). A 116-item questionnaire was initially developed for the MOS to measure physical, mental, and general health aspects of quality of life, from which a shortened version ('short form' or SF) was produced with 36 questions, hence SF-36 (Ware and Sherbourne 1992).

The 36 questions in the SF-36 are grouped into eight different domains or dimensions, with a varying number of questions in each domain, and within each dimension responses are scored and then transformed onto a 0–100 scale. Table 5.1 summarizes the eight dimensions and their content, and also gives the mean scores for each domain from a large population survey conducted as part of the Health Survey for England in 1996 (Health Survey 1998).

The eight dimension scores of the SF-36 are intended to be presented separately and should not be compared directly across dimensions or summed. However, it is possible to combine SF-36 responses into two summary scores of physical and mental health; these are usually described as the physical component summary (PCS) and the mental component summary (MCS), and were developed partly to reduce the number of statistical comparisons involved in the SF-36 and therefore reduce the likelihood that significant differences would be detected simply as a result of play of chance (Ware *et al.* 1995). A shorter version of the SF-36 with just 12 items has also been developed (SF-12), from which it is also possible to generate PCS and MCS scores (Ware *et al.* 1996).

5.2.4 Limitations of non-preference-based measures for economic evaluation

The non-preference-based health status instruments described above are very different in design and purpose. They can be valuable for their descriptive properties and

Table 5.1 Dimensions and content description for the SF-36, and mean scores from an English population survey

Dimension	No. of items	Summary of content	Mean score (SE)
Physical functioning	10	Extent to which health limits physical activities such as self-care, walking, climbing stairs, bending, lifting, and moderate and vigorous exercise	81 (0.21)
Role limitations – physical	4	Extent to which physical health interferes with work or other daily activities, including accomplishing less than wanted, limitations in the kind of activities, or difficulty in performing activities	80 (0.28)
Bodily pain	2	Intensity of pain and effect of pain on normal work, both inside and outside the home	77 (0.21)
General health	5	Personal evaluation of health, including current health, health outlook, and resistance to illness	69 (0.17)
Vitality	4	Feeling energetic and full of life versus feeling tired and worn out	63 (0.16)
Social functioning	2	Extent to which physical health or emotional problems interfere with normal social activities	85 (0.19)
Role limitations – emotional	3	Extent to which emotional problems interfere with work or other daily activities, including decreased time spent on activities, accomplishing less, and not working as carefully as usual	84 (0.25)
Mental health	5	General mental health, including depression, anxiety, behavioural-emotional control, general positive affect	75 (0.14)

Data from Brazier *et al.* (1999) with permission.

clinical relevance, but their direct usefulness as outcome measures in economic evaluations is limited for a variety of reasons:

- ◆ **Lack of comparability** Because they use different items and domains, and are not linked to any underlying valuation of the health states they describe, it is impossible to make direct comparisons between them. A decision-maker trying to decide whether to expand urology or oncology services would have no way of knowing whether an intervention that improves the AUA Symptom Index by 15 points was a better investment than one which greatly reduces nausea and vomiting measured on that subscale of the EORTC QLQ-C30 instrument.

- ◆ **Difficulty in trading-off across profiles** They are frequently presented in the form of a profile or series of scores over different domains. However, it would not be clear how to interpret a change in health status which was manifested in an improvement in one domain of, for example, the DQOL or SF-36, and a simultaneous deterioration in another: for example, an intervention that reduced pain but also led to some increase in nausea.

◆ **Assumptions concerning weighting of domains** Some non-preference-based instruments, such as the DQOL, permit a single score to be calculated across different domains, but they typically do so by giving equal weight to each dimension and then summing them. For example, the DQOL derives a total score by assuming that each subscale has equal importance and summing across the four subscales. In practice many patients, members of the public, or decision-makers might not agree with this weighting.

◆ **Assumptions concerning weighting of questions** The same issues arise even within a single domain, where several different questions are typically given equal weight. For example, the EORTC QLQ-C30 gives equal weight in the physical functioning domain to one question asking 'Do you have any trouble taking a long walk?' and another asking 'Do you need help with eating, dressing, washing yourself, or using the toilet?'. If asked, many people might not consider these to be equally important.

◆ **Equal-interval assumption** Many non-preference-based instruments give equal weight in their scoring system to each interval in the question response scale. For example, in the EORTC QLQ-C30's question '(During the past week) have you had pain?', moving from level 1 (Not at all) to level 2 (A little) is considered equal to moving from level 3 (Quite a bit) to level 4 (Very much). If asked, many people might not consider these to be equivalent in importance.

◆ **Aggregation over time** For the purposes of economic evaluation, where outcome has to be represented by a single number in a cost-effectiveness ratio, it may be important to construct a profile of quality of life over time. For instance, a surgical procedure may create more short-term pain and discomfort than an alternative medical treatment, but produce better long-term results. However, non-preference-based instruments do not readily lend themselves to this form of aggregation, which may again raise issues of trade-off and weighting.

◆ **Time preference** Related to the preceding point, individuals may have different attitudes to immediate versus longer-term health effects, but non-preference-based instruments typically give equal weighting to a given health state or health change irrespective of its timing.

◆ **Death** As noted previously, economic evaluation is typically concerned with estimating a profile of quality of life over time, represented by a single number. Ideally, this would include information on survival as well as quality of life, as both may well be affected by an intervention. The measures considered above do not include any measure of mortality and cannot readily be combined with survival information to form a composite measure.

In summary, non-preference-based health status measures, whether disease specific or generic, are not suitable as outcome measures in economic evaluation. Instead, economists require a measure that combines quality and quantity of life, and that also incorporates the valuations that individuals place on particular states of health.

The outcome metric that is currently favoured as meeting these requirements and facilitating the widest possible comparison between alternative uses of health resources is the **quality-adjusted life-year**, which is described in the next section.

5.3 Quality-adjusted life-years

The quality-adjusted life-year (QALY) is a composite measure of quality of life and quantity of life. The concept was clearly set out by Torrance *et al.* (1972), who referred to a 'utility maximization model' in which 'health days' are computed and summed over the time period of interest. But the first use of the phrase 'quality-adjusted life-years' appears to be in 1976, when Zeckhauser and Shepard (1976) stated: 'We shall employ a hypothetical utility function in our analyses. The unit of output will be quality-adjusted life years, to be referred to by the acronym QALY'. In the same year Weinstein and Stason (1976) used QALYs to try to quantify the impact of various hypertension interventions, and they have been increasingly widely used ever since. The concept and background methodology are dealt with in detail elsewhere (Torrance 1986; Johannesson 1996).

QALYs are a measure of outcome which typically assigns to each period of time a weight corresponding to the health-related quality of life during that period. Normally the weight 1 corresponds to full health and the weight 0 corresponds to a health state equivalent to dead.

Figure 5.1 provides a graphical representation of the QALY approach, in which the life courses of two hypothetical individuals are plotted, with quality of life on the y-axis and time or survival on the x-axis. In this figure, both patients start with similar level of quality of life of 0.83 on a 0–1 scale. After approximately 1.5 years one patient has a complication (C^1) which reduces her quality of life, and this is followed by three

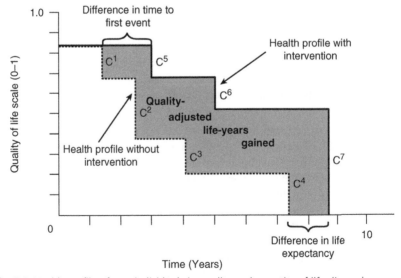

Fig. 5.1 Health profile of two individuals in quality and quantity of life dimensions.

further complications (C^2, C^3, C^4) which adversely affect quality of life, with the final one being fatal after approximately 7.5 years. The second patient does not experience any complications until year 3 (C^5), has one further non-fatal complication (C^6), and then experiences a fatal complication just before year 9 (C^7).

It can be seen that it would be possible to measure the difference between these two hypothetical patients in several different ways: by time to first event or complication-free time (a common measure in clinical trials), by time to death, or by number of complications. In this instance any of these would show some benefit to the patient receiving the intervention. However, all these are partial measures of the differences observed, and measuring the effect of the intervention using any single one of these metrics could be seriously misleading. In contrast, the area under each of the two curves or profiles does capture survival as well as the timing and number of non-fatal events and their health impact, and therefore the difference represented by the shaded area is a measure of QALYs gained.

5.4 Valuing health states

While appealing in principle, it is clear from Figure 5.1 that the most important challenge is to find a reliable way of quantifying the quality of life associated with any particular health state. There are two elements to this: describing the health state, which as discussed earlier could be either a disease-specific description or a generic description intended to cover many different diseases, and placing a valuation on the health state. As noted in Chapter 2, these weights or valuations are related to utility theory and are frequently referred to as **utilities** or **utility values**.

Obtaining utility values almost invariably involves some process by which individuals are given descriptions of a number of health states and then directly or indirectly express their preferences for these states. It is relatively simple to measure **ordinal preferences** by asking respondents to rank-order different health states. However, these give no information on strength of preference and a simple ranking suffers from the equal-interval assumption discussed in section 5.2.4; as a result they are not suitable for economic evaluation. Instead, analysts make use of **cardinal preference** measurement. Three main methods have been used to obtain cardinal measures of health state preferences: the **rating scale**, the **time trade-off**, and the **standard gamble**. Further details of these can be found in Torrance (1986) or in textbooks such as Brazier *et al.* (2007).

5.4.1 The rating scale (RS) method

Rating scales are sometimes referred to as visual analogue scales (VASs) or thermometers. The scale is represented by a line with defined endpoints stretching from the best or most preferred health state to the worst or least preferred. The respondent is then asked to consider a health state that is described for them, or to consider their own health, and indicate where on the line they would locate this health state. If several health states are being considered, they are located on the line in order of preference, and the distance or interval between the points chosen to represent health states is intended to correspond to differences in strength of preference. A well-known example of a rating scale is the EQ-5D visual analogue scale (Figure 5.2).

As Figure 5.2 shows, the EQ-5D VAS is a thermometer-like scale running from 0 to 100 and calibrated in intervals of 1, 5, and 10, with the ends of the line anchored at 'Worst imaginable health state' and 'Best imaginable health state'. In this example, respondents are being asked to use the scale to indicate their own health state, and so no description is required, but it would be quite possible to ask respondents to indicate their preference for a health state described to them.

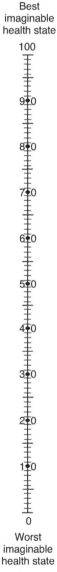

To help people say how good or bad a health state is, we have drawn a scale (rather like a thermometer) on which the best state you can imagine is marked 100 and the worst state you can imagine is marked 0.

We would like you to indicate on this scale how good or bad your own health is today, in your opinion. Please do this by drawing a line from the box below to whichever point on the scale indicates how good or bad your health state is today.

**Your own
health state
today**

Fig. 5.2 The EQ-5D Visual Analogue Scale. © 1990 EuroQol GroupEQ-5D™ is a trade mark of the EuroQol Group. Reproduced with permission.

An essential attribute of instruments such as this intended for use in economic evaluation is that they permit comparison between individuals or groups, and therefore there should not be scope for differences in the interpretation of the health states defined at either end of the scale. In this particular example, there is some ambiguity. For example, 'best imaginable' might not mean the same to someone in advanced old age or with a permanent physical disability as it would to a healthy young adult; equally, 'worst imaginable' could mean death to some respondents but a health state worse than death to others. The ambiguity at the top of the EQ-5D VAS is not easy to avoid and analysts normally have to assume that 'best imaginable' is the same as full health. However, at the bottom of the scale it is possible to ask respondents to indicate where they would place being dead. If this is done, the scale can then be transformed so that death always takes the value 0 and any states worse than death are accorded a negative valuation.

Rating scales are relatively simple to administer. However, respondents sometimes draw more than one line on the EQ-5D VAS, perhaps having misinterpreted the instruction referring to 'how good or bad your health state is today'. There is also a tendency for respondents to avoid using the ends of the scale (end-aversion bias), to make particular use of the 5 or 10 unit calibration marks, and to space out multiple health state valuations evenly.

Another important feature of the rating scale is that it does not explicitly require respondents to make any choices or trade-offs when indicating their preferences, and it has been argued that this weakens its foundations in decision theory and limits the usefulness of the responses. If there is no 'cost' in indicating that a preference is strong or weak, respondents will tend to overstate their preferences. While this view has been contested (Parkin and Devlin 2006, 2007; Brazier and McCabe 2007), analysts have tended to view the information provided by rating scales as inferior to information from choice-based techniques, notably the standard gamble and the time trade-off.

5.4.2 The standard gamble (SG) method

The standard gamble method is generally considered to have the strongest theoretical foundations of choice-based valuation methods, as it can be traced to the theory of rational decision-making under uncertainty set out by von Neumann and Morgenstern (1944). They developed a famous set of axioms, which if satisfied might define an individual acting in a way that would maximize their expected utility. These axioms were as follows.

- **Completeness** An individual has well-defined preferences and can decide between two alternatives.
- **Transitivity** An individual deciding according to the completeness axiom also decides consistently: for example, if A is preferred to B and B is preferred to C, then A will be preferred to C.
- **Independence** The preference order of two choices under uncertainty (gambles) when mixed with a third choice maintains the same preference order as when the two are mixed independently.
- **Continuity** When there are three choices A, B and C, and the individual prefers A to B and B to C, there is some combination of the 'best' and 'worst' choices A and C where the individual will be indifferent between that combination and a certain intermediate outcome B.

Figure 5.3 shows three examples of the standard gamble method for valuing a health state, with the primary difference being in the ordering of the states from best to worst. In Figure 5.3(a) we are interested in valuing a chronic health state that is preferred to death (i.e. it is intermediate between full health and death), in Figure 5.3(b) the chronic health state is considered worse than death (i.e. death is intermediate between full health and the chronic health state), and in Figure 5.3(b) a temporary health state j is ordered as worst with another temporary health state i as the intermediate outcome.

It can immediately be seen that the situation conforms closely to the continuity axiom. The individual is confronted with three health states, and has to choose between alternative 1, which involves some probability P of the best outcome but also some risk of the worst outcome, and alternative 2, which involves the certainty of the intermediate outcome.

For example, state i in Figure 5.3(a) might be someone with Parkinson's disease, and the choice might be between the certainty of continuing with the disease or opting to undergo a neurosurgical procedure which could restore the person to full health but could also kill them. Probability P is varied in this example until the respondent is indifferent between the two alternatives, and P at that indifference point is the valuation placed on health state i, on a scale of 0–1 where 0 = death and 1 = full health. Pursuing the Parkinson's disease example, the worse the patient perceives the chronic health state of having the disease, the greater the risk of death they are prepared to accept for the possibility of being restored to full health.

In Figure 5.3(b) the only difference is that the chronic state is worse than death. Hence the respondent must choose between, for example, alternative 2 which might be thought of as a serious disease with a prognosis of imminent death unless treated, and alternative 1, in which a choice exists between a treatment that may cure the patient completely but may leave them in chronic state i. In this case, once the point of indifference is located, the preference for health state i would be given by $-P/(1-P)$. For example, if the respondent was indifferent between alternative 2 and a 60% probability of full health or a 40% probability of being left in chronic health state i, the value placed on state i would be $-0.6/(1-0.6) = -1.5$. However, if the respondent was very unwilling to run the risk of finishing in health state i they might not be indifferent between the alternatives unless there was a 95% probability of full health or a 5% probability of being left in chronic health state i. In this case the value being placed on state i would be $-0.95/(1-0.95) = -19$. As these lower values could be very large (in fact they are unbounded), it has become conventional to avoid giving them too much weight by simply taking the preference for health state i as $-P$, thus ensuring that it will not be larger than -1.

In Figure 5.3(c) the respondent must choose between alternative 1, which has a probability of being in full health or of being in a temporary poor health state j, or alternative 2, which is the certainty of a less bad temporary health state i. In this case, the valuation placed on state i will be given by $P + (1-P)j$.

Other versions of these standard gamble exercises have been developed, some using different visual aids and devices to help respondents arrive at their point of indifference. However, this has raised the cost of using the method, as face-to-face interviews will typically be required to take respondents through the exercises. Responses may also be

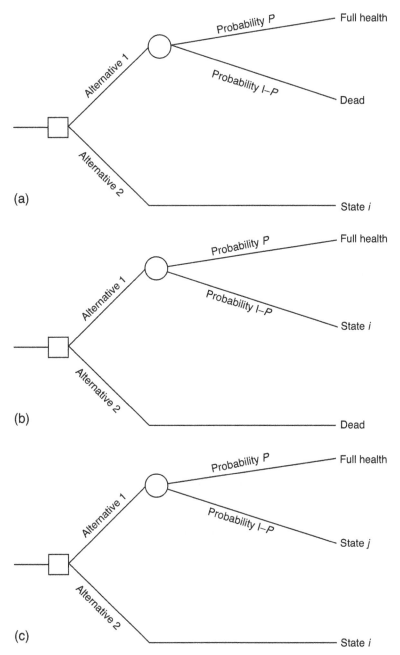

Fig. 5.3 The standard gamble: (a) a chronic health state preferred to death; (b) a chronic health state considered worse than death; (c) a temporary health state.

affected by the attitudes to risk held by different individuals, and by the difficulties many people have in fully understanding probabilities, especially when they are close to 1 or zero. Hence, although the standard gamble method is sometimes considered to be the gold standard of valuation methods, it is not perfect either theoretically or practically, which has prompted a search for alternatives including the time trade-off method.

5.4.3 The time trade-off (TTO) method

The time trade-off method was developed by Torrance and colleagues in the early 1970s (Torrance *et al.* 1972; Torrance 1976) as a simpler alternative to the standard gamble and with health state valuation specifically in mind. Like the SG it involves finding a point of indifference between alternatives, but there are only two outcomes and no uncertainty or probability is involved.

Figure 5.4 shows three examples of the time trade-off method for valuing a health state, corresponding to the SG examples given in Figure 5.3: a chronic health state that is preferred to death (Figure 5.4(a)), a chronic health state considered worse than death (Figure 5.4(b)), and a temporary health state (Figure 5.4(c)).

In Figure 5.4(a) the choice is between being in health state i for time T, or being in full health for a shorter period of time X. Time X is varied until the respondent is indifferent between the two alternatives—clearly the more time the respondent is willing to give up to be out of health state i the worse it must be—and the valuation of state i is then obtained as X/T.

In Figure 5.4(b) the chronic state being valued is worse than death. Here the respondent is given a choice between immediate death (alternative 2) and time X in full health followed by time T in health state i which is worse than death. Again, time X is varied until the respondent is indifferent between the alternatives. (In some representations of Figure 5.4(b), alternative 1 begins at level i and reverts to full health at time X, i.e. the sequence is switched.) As with the SG method, this method of valuing health states worse than death is unbounded and could produce large negative numbers which could have a disproportionate effect on mean values. A simple expedient to deal with this, suggested by Torrance *et al.* (1982), is to set the state given the worst valuation equal to -1.0.

In Figure 5.4(c) a temporary health state is being valued. The choice is between spending time X in health state j and then moving to a state of full health, or spending a longer period T in a less bad temporary health state i, again followed by a move to full health. The valuation of health state i will then be $1 - (1 - hj)X/T$, or, if j is set to zero, as $1 - X/T$.

As with the SG method, a range of graphical devices and decision aids have been developed to help respondents identify their point of indifference in the TTO. Many of these have to be used in a face-to-face interview, but as the TTO is simpler than the SG, it has also been possible to administer it postally or on-line.

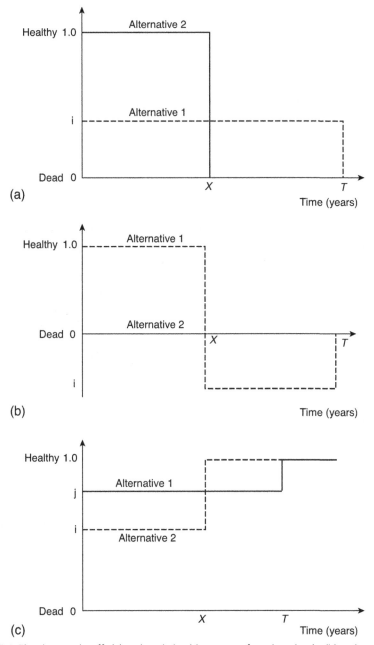

Fig. 5.4 The time trade-off: (a) a chronic health state preferred to death; (b) a chronic health state considered worse than death; (c) a temporary health state.

5.4.4 **Comparison of valuation methods in practice**

A number of studies have compared the results obtained from the RS, SG, and TTO valuation methods, either indirectly or directly. Tengs and Lin (Lin 2003) conducted an indirect comparison, in which 20 articles were identified by means of a systematic review that reported 53 quality-of-life weights for stroke. Regression analysis was then performed to estimate the effect on the estimates of stroke severity, elicitation method, respondent characteristics, and the bounds placed on the scale used. They found that severity of stroke and the bounds of the scale were significant predictors of the quality-of-life valuation, but that the elicitation method used and the respondent characteristics had no significant effect.

Hallan *et al.* (1999) conducted a direct comparison by asking a sample of 158 people to value the health consequences of a minor stroke or a major stroke, using the RS, SG, and TTO methods. Table 5.2 summarizes the results. Although the sample is small and the study is limited in terms of the summary statistics reported (median values), the results clearly show that, as expected, the RS produced substantially lower valuations than either of the choice-based methods, and that the TTO tended to produce slightly lower valuations than the SG.

Similar results have been obtained in other direct comparisons. For example, in a study of quality of life associated with mild and severe menopausal symptoms, Daly *et al.* (1993) found that the mean valuation of mild symptoms was 0.65 (95% CI 0.61, 0.69) using the RS, but was 0.85 (95% CI 0.80, 0.90) using the TTO. The mean valuation for severe symptoms was 0.30 (95% CI 0.26, 0.34) using the RS compared with 0.64 (95% CI 0.57, 0.71) using the TTO.

The large differences typically observed between RS and TTO or SG valuations, and the fact that the TTO and SG methods are choice based and therefore have stronger foundations in decision theory, have led most standard texts and guidelines for technology appraisal to recommend choice-based valuation methods (Gold *et al.* 1996; Drummond *et al.* 2005; Brazier *et al.* 2007; NICE 2008). However, as discussed below, the many remaining theoretical and practical issues in this area have also encouraged analysts to continue looking for alternative valuation methods.

Table 5.2 Utility values of a minor or a major stroke using different valuation methods

Health state	Method	Utility (median)
Minor stroke	Rating scale	0.71
	Time trade-off	0.88
	Standard gamble	0.91
Major stroke	Rating scale	0.31
	Time trade-off	0.51
	Standard gamble	0.61

Source: Data from Hallan *et al.* (1999).

5.5 **Whose preferences: patients, 'experts', general population?**

Controversies over health state valuation are not confined to the valuation method; there are also several strands of opinion concerning who should provide valuations. In principle, valuations could be provided by patients who have had first-hand experience of the health state in question, or by experts such as clinicians with relevant scientific or clinical expertise, or by members of the public.

The arguments in favour of obtaining valuations from patients are primarily that they have insight born of experience (Nord *et al.* 1999), and that potentially they have the most to gain from treatment innovations and the most to lose if treatments are not funded. In addition, as they have direct experience, it is not necessary to create descriptions of that health state, which may be inaccurate or partial (Nord *et al.* 1999). However, there are many states for which patients may be unable to provide valuations, including dementia, severe mental disorders, perinatal or infant health states, and terminal disease states. There is also evidence that, in time, patients may adapt to or reach an accommodation with their health state (Cassileth *et al.* 1984), which may be realistic but could also reflect reduced expectations and hence understatement of the health state's impact.

A major argument deployed in favour of obtaining valuations from the general public is that, as tax or insurance payers, they bear the cost of health care decisions and so are entitled to have some say on the valuations placed on health outcomes (Hadorn 1991). It could also be argued that members of the general public are all potential patients. Asking the public also corresponds more closely to a Rawlsian approach to distributive justice, which strives to blind individuals to self-interest by asking them to make fair choices from behind a hypothetical 'veil of ignorance' (Rawls 1971). However, the fact remains that most members of the public will have no first-hand experience of particular health states, and may project fears or prejudices onto their valuations, or simply struggle to understand detailed descriptions.

While the influence of these countervailing arguments on actual valuations is not clear, there is good evidence that the valuations made by population samples and patients frequently vary quite substantially. For example, Boyd *et al.* (1990) elicited utility values for colostomy following surgery for carcinoma of the rectum, and compared results from five groups of individuals: one group of patients with colostomies, a second patient group with rectal cancer but without colostomies, a group of physicians and surgeons specializing in the area, and two groups of healthy subjects. Utilities were elicited using the standard gamble, category rating, and a treatment choice questionnaire, and Table 5.3 summarizes some of the results.

It was evident that the groups differed substantially in the utilities they assigned to colostomy, with patients with colostomies and physicians giving significantly higher utilities than did healthy volunteers or patients who did not have colostomies. The reasons for these differences were not clear, although the researchers suggested that direct knowledge of the health condition seemed to be the main explanatory factor.

Similar discrepancies have been found in other studies, although the direction of difference is not always consistent. For example, Baron *et al.* (2003) found that members

Table 5.3 Utilities for a colostomy from different groups

	N	Utility value elicited using:	
		Standard gamble	Category rating
Patients with colostomy	40	91.5 (10.0)	80.9 (14.9)
Physicians	40	90.8 (6.5)	71.9 (18.1)
Healthy volunteers A	30	85.1 (9.3)	63.2 (21.4)
Healthy volunteers B	29	80.3 (11.7)	52.7 (24.5)
Patients without colostomy	11	80.4 (11.8)	48.6 (31.8)
P value for intergroup difference		<0.0001	<0.00001

Reproduced from Boyd *et al.* (1990). Reprinted by permission of SAGE Publications.

of the public rated a series of common health problems such as acne and arthritis more severely than people who had the disorders. However, Pyne *et al.* (2009) found that patients with depression reported significantly lower preference scores for depression health states than the general population, indicating that they considered depression to be worse than did people with no direct experience of it.

While further work is clearly required to understand these differences, current practice has moved towards the use of valuations obtained from the general public (Brauer *et al.* 2006), an approach endorsed by recent guidelines in the UK and USA which explicitly recommend that population valuations are used (Gold *et al.* 1996; NICE 2008).

5.6 Multi-attribute utility systems (MAUS)

Devising descriptions for particular states and then eliciting valuations of them using appropriate methods is not straightforward and from a decision-making perspective may be unsatisfactory, as differences in utility between interventions or health states could be at least partly attributable to specific details of the descriptions used or the participating sample. An alternative approach which avoids these problems is to adopt a two-step valuation method, in which patients use a generic descriptive system to describe the health state in which they perceive themselves to be, and then valuations derived from the general public are placed on these health states. Ideally, these generic descriptive systems should be able to register all commonly encountered features or domains of health status, and are sometimes referred to as multi-attribute utility systems (MAUS) or multi-attribute health status classification systems. At least six such systems have been developed, of which three in particular are quite widely used: the EQ-5D, the Health Utilities Index, and the Short Form SF-6D (others include the 15D from Finland (Sintonen 2001), the Assessment of Quality of Life (AQoL) from Australia (Hawthorne *et al.* 1999), and the Quality of Wellbeing (QWB) instrument (Kaplan and Anderson 1988).

5.6.1 **The EQ-5D**

The EQ-5D was developed by the EuroQol Group in the 1980s and has become one of the most widely used instruments of its type (EuroQol Group 1990). The full question-naire includes a visual analogue scale, as shown in section 5.4.1, but the multi-attribute heart of the instrument is a set of five questions, each of which has three response levels, giving a total of 243 ($3 \times 3 \times 3 \times 3 \times 3$) possible health states (Table 5.4). Therefore it is possible to describe any response with a 1, 2, or 3 for each question, and

Table 5.4 The EQ-5D classification system

By placing a tick in one box in each group below, please indicate which statements best describe your own health state today.

Mobility	
I have no problems in walking about	❏
I have some problems in walking about	❏
I am confined to bed	❏
Self-care	
I have no problems with self-care	❏
I have some problems washing and dressing myself	❏
I am unable to wash or dress myself	❏
Usual activities *(e.g. work, study, housework, family, or leisure activities)*	
I have no problems with performing my usual activities	❏
I have some problems with performing my usual activities	❏
I am unable to perform my usual activities	❏
Pain/discomfort	
I have no pain or discomfort	❏
I have moderate pain or discomfort	❏
I have extreme pain or discomfort	❏
Anxiety/depression	
I am not anxious or depressed	❏
I am moderately anxious or depressed	❏
I am extremely anxious or depressed	❏

© 1990 EuroQol GroupEQ-5D™ is a trade mark of the EuroQol Group. Reproduced with permission.

so 11121 would signify 'no problems in walking about, no problems with self-care, no problems with performing usual activities, moderate pain or discomfort, not anxious or depressed', while 22322 would represent 'some problems in walking about, some problems washing or dressing, unable to perform usual activities, moderate pain or discomfort, moderately anxious or depressed'.

The EQ-5D is available in approximately 100 different official language versions and was designed to be self-completed by patients or respondents, but it can also be administered in face-to-face interview, telephone interview, online or by touch-screen, or by a proxy such as a relative or carer. Once a respondent has described their health state by answering the five questions in Table 5.4, the second stage of the procedure is to attach a valuation or utility value to that health state. This was first done by selecting a representative sample of the 243 possible health states, and then asking a large population sample of 3337 British adults to value each of these states using a time trade-off procedure. A regression equation was then derived, from which it is possible to predict or estimate a valuation or 'tariff' for all 243 health states (Dolan *et al.* 1995). The coefficients for the equation are shown in Table 5.5.

Each coefficient can be interpreted as a decrement from a full health state of 1.000. For example, consider the two health states mentioned earlier, 11121 and 22322. A person in health state 11121 would incur a decrement of 0.081 for a downward move in any dimension plus a decrement of 0.123 for being in moderate pain, and so would have a utility of 0.796. A person in health state 22322 would incur a decrement of 0.081 for a downward move in any dimension plus a decrement of 0.069 for some problems in walking about, a decrement of 0.104 for some problems washing or dressing, a decrement of 0.094 for being unable to perform usual activities, a decrement of 0.123 for being in moderate pain or discomfort, a decrement of 0.071 for being moderately anxious or depressed, and a decrement of 0.269 for being at level 3 in any of the dimensions, and so would have a utility of 0.189. The worst possible health state (33333) has a utility value of –0.594.

This UK tariff was the first and to date the most widely used set of valuations for EQ-5D health states. However, valuation sets or tariffs have also been derived using the time trade-off method for a number of other countries, including Denmark, Germany, Japan, Spain, and the USA (Shaw *et al.* 2005). An alternative model of UK valuations, based on differences in valuations between the worst state and all other states, has also been published (Dolan and Roberts 2002).

Although analysts using the EQ-5D frequently proceed directly to report summary results in the form of mean tariff values, it may also be helpful to report descriptive information from the actual health states recorded, for example in the form of proportions recording level 1, 2, or 3 in each question, or the proportions not on level 1 in each question, or possibly even the most commonly reported health states. In a randomized trial comparable data would be reported for two or more groups. For example, a trial examining the consequences of blood glucose self-monitoring in patients with type 2 diabetes found that self-monitoring produced no significant clinical benefits and was associated with a small but significant worsening of quality of life in the patients randomized to it (Simon *et al.* 2008). This was in itself an interesting and important result. However, by looking at the actual responses to each EQ-5D question (Table 5.6), it was possible to drill down into the reasons for this difference. Closer analysis of the distribution of responses across the different levels of each dimension indicated significant increases in the levels of anxiety and depression between baseline and the 12 month follow-up in both the less intensive and more intensive self-monitoring groups compared with usual care.

Table 5.5 Coefficients for the EQ-5D time trade-off tariff

Dimension	Level	Coefficient (decrement)	Illustrative health states:	
			11121	22322
Constant	Any downward move	0.081	−0.081	−0.081
Mobility	2: Some problems	0.069		−0.069
	3: Confined to bed	0.314		
Self–care	2: Some problems	0.104		−0.104
	3: Unable to	0.214		
Usual activities	2: Some problems	0.036		
	3: Unable to perform	0.094		−0.094
Pain/discomfort	2: Moderate	0.123	−0.123	−0.123
	3: Extreme	0.386		
Anxiety/depression	2: Moderate	0.071		−0.071
	3: Extreme	0.236		
N3 constant	Level 3 at least once	0.269		−0.269
			= 1−0.081 −0.123 **= 0.796**	=1−0.081 −0.069 −0.104 −0.094 −0.123 −0.269 **= 0.189**

Reproduced from Dolan *et al*. 1995, with permission.

5.6.2 **The Health Utilities Index**

The Health Utilities Index (HUI) was originally developed in the early 1980s at McMaster University, Ontario, to assess the outcomes of low-birthweight infants (Torrance *et al.* 1982). Two versions are currently in use, HUI2 and HUI3 (Horsman *et al.* 2003). The HUI2 consists of six domains: sensation, mobility, emotion, cognition, self-care, and pain. A seventh domain of fertility can be included if relevant. Each domain has between three and five levels, producing approximately 24,000 possible health states. Quality-of-life valuations were elicited from 293 Canadian parents, using standard gamble and a visual analogue scale (Torrance *et al.* 1996). Whereas the EQ-5D valuation exercise was done using a small sample of health states and then deriving a regression equation to obtain valuations for all remaining states, HUI2 valuations were derived by estimating a utility function for each of the seven domains

Table 5.6 Percentage of EuroQol EQ-5D answers across the dimensions for patients with non-insulin-treated type 2 diabetes receiving standardized usual care, less intensive self-monitoring of blood glucose, or more-intensive self-monitoring (S-M) of blood glucose: complete case analysis

Self-monitoring group:	Mobility			Self-care			Usual activities			Pain			Anxiety		
	1	2	3	1	2	3	1	2	3	1	2	3	1	2	3
Baseline															
Usual care	62	38	0	92	8	0	82	17	1	51	44	5	71	29	0
Less intensive	66	34	0	92	8	0	78	22	0	52	41	7	77	21	2
More intensive	67	33	0	95	5	0	85	14	1	55	42	3	77	23	0
12-month follow-up															
Usual care	66	34	0	90	10	0	77	23	0	53	43	4	82	16	2
Less intensive	61	39	0	90	10	0	78	19	3	55	38	7	72	24	4
More intensive	67	33	0	91	9	0	78	22	0	52	43	5	69	29	2

Source: Simon *et al.* (2008); see supplementary Table C at www.herc.ox.ac.uk/downloads.

or attributes, and then calculating an equation to estimate overall utility as a function of the set of single-attribute utilities. As a result, any health state reported on the questionnaire can be translated into a utility on a scale from 1 (perfect health) to 0 (death). The minimum score on the HUI2, for a state considered worse than death, is –0.03.

The HUI3 has many similarities to the HUI2, but with the sensation domain expanded into three separate attributes of vision, hearing, and speech, and additional response levels added to some domains, resulting in an instrument on which 972,000 possible health states can be recorded. Valuations were elicited from a random sample of 504 members of the Canadian general public using standard gamble and a visual analogue scale and a utility function approach similar to that described for the HUI2 (Feeny *et al.* 2002). The HUI3 is scaled from 1 (perfect health) to 0 (death), and can record states worse than death to a minimum value of –0.36.

5.6.3 **The SF-6D**

The SF-6D took as its starting point the health state classification system used by the SF-36, described in section 5.2.3, and selected from the original 36 items 11 items in six different dimensions—physical functioning, role limitations, social functioning, pain, mental health, and vitality—each with between four and six response levels, thus permitting up to 18,000 different health states. A sample of 249 of these health states was valued using the standard gamble by 611 respondents from a UK general population random sample. Models were then derived to provide utility values for all possible health states (Brazier *et al.* 1998; Brazier *et al.* 2002). With the preferred scoring model, the worst state in the SF-6D has a quality-of-life estimate of 0.296 (Brazier *et al.* 2002, model 10).

As noted in section 5.2.3, a 12-item version of SF-36 has also been developed, and in turn a version of the SF-6D has been derived from the SF-12 using just seven items from the SF-12 health state classification system (Brazier and Roberts 2004) and with valuations derived using the same exercise that provided valuations for the SF-36 version.

5.6.4 **Comparisons between instruments**

Extensive experience has now been accumulated in the use of the HUI, EQ-5D, and SF-6D in different health states and populations and under different conditions of administration. There have also been a substantial number of head-to-head comparisons: Brazier *et al.* (2007) identified at least 24 in the period up to 2005. In general, these comparisons have found that instruments have different characteristics and can produce quite different results. For example, O'Brien *et al.* (2003) examined the correlation between SF-6D utility values and HUI3 utility values when administered to the same sample. The relatively poor correlation between these instruments led the authors to express some doubt as to whether the two sets of utilities were comparable. In a study of health outcomes in 2097 patients with serious spinal disorders, McDonough *et al.* (2005) found that at baseline the EQ-5D, HUI3, and SF-6D gave mean values of 0.39, 0.45, and 0.57 respectively. Rank correlations between these three instruments ranged between 0.67 and 0.72, but there were major differences in the range and distribution of the responses, as shown in Figure 5.5.

These figures display some of the recurring features of these instruments. The EQ-5D has a wider range than other instruments, with valuations down to –0.594. In fact, the UK utility tariff places a valuation of less than zero on over a third (84 of 243) of its potential health states, and Figure 5.5 does show significant numbers of respondents in these lower health states. In contrast, the SF-6D is bounded at the lower end by a minimum score of 0.296, so that those in the lowest SF-6D health state have a utility value a very long way away from those in the lowest health state of the EQ-5D. In fact the SF-6D appears generally to suffer from a floor effect, with significant numbers of respondents often clustered in the lowest health states (Brazier *et al.* 2004).

In contrast, the EQ-5D is often perceived to suffer from a ceiling effect, with substantial proportions of respondents clustered in the full health state. In some population surveys, such as the Medical Expenditure Panel Survey or the Health Survey for England, 40–45% of respondents have reported themselves to be in perfect health on the EQ-5D, even when stating that they have some health problem in response to other questions asked at the same time (Health Survey 1998). This reflects a feature of the EQ-5D scoring algorithm, in which even the smallest move from full health (a one-level drop in one question) equates to a utility decrement of 12–20 percentage points in the UK tariff.

The most important aspect of these differences between instruments is that they could have a significant impact on the estimated cost-effectiveness of interventions, as such evaluations are one of their main uses. For example, Barton *et al.* (2004) found that utility scores for 609 hearing-impaired adults who completed the EQ-5D, HUI3, and SF-6D before and after being provided with a hearing aid showed a mean improvement

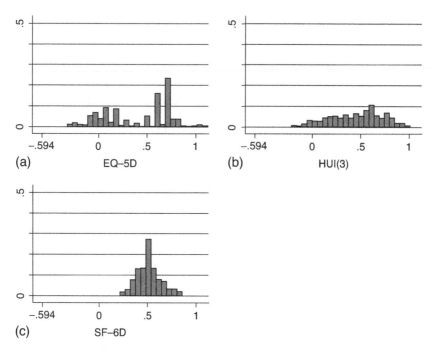

Fig. 5.5 Frequency distributions for EQ-5D, HUI3, and SF-6D at baseline in a sample of 2097 participants in a spine patient outcomes research trial. Reproduced from McDonough *et al.* (2005) with kind permission from Springer Science+Business Media.

of 0.06 in the HUI3, but an improvement of just 0.01 according to the EQ-5D or SF-6D. Such differences might well determine whether or not such an intervention is assessed as cost-effective. In consequence, reimbursement agencies that have to make many comparisons across different economic evaluations have become more prescriptive not only about the valuation methods they wish to see used, but also about the instruments they prefer. For example, in England and Wales NICE now specifically expresses a preference for the EQ-5D (NICE 2008). However, development and comparison work on these and other instruments is certain to continue; for instance, in 2009 the EQ-5D group released a five-level version of the EQ-5D with the same five dimensions or domains but slight changes to the wording of the previous levels and the insertion of intermediate levels between the previous levels 1, 2, and 3 (Herdman *et al.* 2009).

5.6.5 Meaningful differences

Another important issue raised by the observed differences between instruments is how capable they are of registering moderate changes or differences in quality of life. Drummond (2001) has suggested that a difference of 0.03 on the HUI or the 15D instrument on a 0–1 scale is likely to be considered the minimum clinically important difference, although this may differ from an economically important difference. Using data from eight longitudinal studies, Walters and Brazier (2005) estimated the mean change in the EQ-5D and SF-6D that might correspond to a minimally important difference, and found that this was 0.074 for the EQ-5D and 0.041 for the SF-6D, which could be interpreted as similar given that the range of the EQ-5D from minimum to maximum score is approximately twice that of the SF-6D (Walters and Brazier 2005).

A different way of tackling this issue was suggested by Campbell *et al.* (2006), who first used the SF-36 global health questionnaire to divide a group of patients with spinal problems into those who considered their health to have improved or deteriorated over the previous 12 months, and then determined the value of the EQ-5D change that best discriminated between these two groups in terms of sensitivity and specificity. This suggested that a change of 0.069 points was the optimum value, giving a sensitivity of 86% and a specificity of 67%.

The results from Walters and Brazier (2005), Campbell *et al.* (2006), and other studies suggest that instruments such as the HUI, EQ-5D, and SF-6D will be unlikely to provide evidence of significant differences in quality of life of just a few percentage points. Figure 5.6 brings together evidence from six group comparisons of QALYs gained in four trials of moderate size.

It is clear from this figure that only one of these comparisons produced a significant difference in QALYs, and that differences of 3%, 4%, or even 6% were not statistically significant. In short, whereas model-based exercises may produce very small but

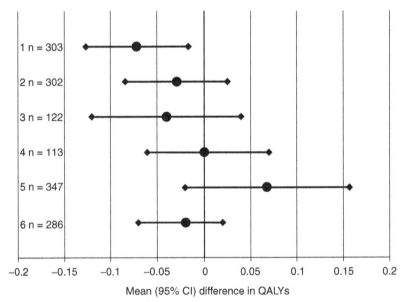

Fig. 5.6 Mean differences in quality of life in six trial-based comparisons: (1) DIGEM trial, more self-monitoring versus usual care (Simon *et al.* 2008); (2) DIGEM trial, less self-monitoring versus usual care (Simon *et al.* 2008); (3) problem-solving trial, problem-solving nurse versus GP care (Kendrick *et al.* 2006); (4) problem-solving trial, generic nurse versus GP care (Kendrick *et al.* 2006); (5) spine stabilization trial (Rivero-Arias *et al.* 2005; (6) physiotherapy treatment versus physiotherapy advice trial (Rivero-Arias *et al.* 2006).

significant differences in QALYs (as we will see in Chapters 8–10), this is less likely to occur in real-life comparisons.

5.7 Mapping between instruments

Despite the growing use of instruments such as the EQ-5D, SF-6D, or HUI, there are many thousands of studies which have recorded outcome information only in the form of non-preference-based instruments, either symptom- or disease-specific or generic. In these circumstances it would clearly be useful to be able to make a reliable translation or mapping from the non-preference-based instrument into health state utilities, so that an outcome or effect can be expressed in terms of QALYs. As a result increasing numbers of such 'mapping' studies have been undertaken.

Mapping studies can be classified into three broad categories: direct elicitation of utility values alongside another instrument; prediction from the health state described on a non-preference-based instrument of a utility level; prediction from the health state described on a non-preference-based instrument of the likely health state on a preference-based instrument.

5.7.1 Direct elicitation of utility values alongside another instrument

The first approach has been to directly elicit utility values alongside a generic instrument such as the SF-12. For example, Lundberg *et al.* (1999) sent a postal questionnaire to 8000 adults asking them to complete the SF-12, a rating scale question, and a time trade-off question, and then used age, gender, and the individual items of the SF-12 as explanatory variables in a linear regression analysis of health-state utilities indicated by the time trade-off question. The results allowed them to suggest a regression equation that could be used when SF-12 data were available to predict a utility level for any health state described by the SF-12. Using a similar approach, Shmueli (1999) used face-to-face interviews with a sample of 2030 adults who rated their own health using the SF-36 and a visual analogue scale, and then used linear and non-linear regression to estimate the association between domains of the SF-36 and VAS scores (Shmueli 1999).

5.7.2 Utility prediction

A second approach is to use data in which respondents have described their health state on a non-preference-based instrument and a preference-based instrument, and then predict the utility value associated with each preference-based instrument response from the response given on the non-preference-based instrument. An early example of this approach is a study by Fryback *et al.* (1997), where the SF-36 and the Quality of Wellbeing index (QWB) instruments were both administered by interview to 1430 people in the Beaver Dam Health Outcomes Study. The domain scales of the SF-36, their squares, and all pairwise cross-products were then used as explanatory variables in stepwise and best-subset regressions to predict the QWB scores. Franks *et al.* (2003) also used this approach to estimate the relationship between SF-12 responses and utility values generated from EQ-5D and HUI3 responses of a convenience sample of 240 patients . They then repeated this approach for the EQ-5D with a much larger sample of 12,998 adults drawn from the 2000 Medical Expenditure Panel Survey (MEPS) (Franks *et al.* 2004).

5.7.3 Item or response prediction

Utility prediction studies of the type mentioned above have typically used ordinary least-squares (OLS) regression or variants. This has simplicity, but does imply that utilities are continuously distributed and so the probability that the utility has a value of 1.0 is small. For example, in the study by Franks and colleagues, 45% of the MEPS sample placed themselves in a full health state when responding to the EQ-5D, but the OLS prediction model had a maximum utility value of 0.97 with no individual at full health (Franks *et al.* 2004). In addition, these methods provide predictions for only one set of utility values, and so separate equations would be required to map the SF-12 to the UK EQ-5D tariff or to the US EQ-5D tariff. The use of OLS in the presence of ceiling effects is also known to produce inconsistent estimates of the coefficients of explanatory variables (Long 1997).

Therefore an alternative is to use the responses to the non-preference-based instrument to estimate probable responses for each question in the preference-based instrument. A utility value can then be calculated based on the set of predicted responses. This approach, sometimes called response mapping or item prediction, was used by Gray *et al.* (2006) to look at the relation between SF-12 responses and EQ-5D responses. They used a sample of 12,967 respondents to MEPS who had completed the SF-12 and the EQ-5D, and then estimated a set of five multinomial logit equations, one for each domain or question of the EQ-5D, to predict the probability of a respondent choosing level 1, 2, or 3. The results, measured in terms of mean estimate, mean squared error, and mean absolute error, were similar to or slightly poorer than the OLS approach, but the approach generates predicted responses by domain as well as an overall utility value, and different tariffs could be attached to the predicted responses without the need for separate models.

The same approach has been used to map from the modified Rankin scale, a widely used neurological outcome instrument, to the EQ-5D (Rivero-Arias *et al.* 2009).

5.7.4 Assessment

Mapping studies are continuing to proliferate, and the literature on new mapping algorithms and methods, and comparisons between approaches, is expanding rapidly. In general, mapping methods seem to have reasonable ability to predict group mean utility scores and to differentiate between groups with or without known existing illness. However, they all seem to predict increasingly poorly as health states become more serious. Reimbursement agencies such as NICE have indicated that they are prepared to consider evidence from mapping studies in the absence of more direct evidence (NICE 2008). However, given the current lack of consensus on the most reliable method and apparent differences in results, it would probably be prudent to use more than one method if relying on such evidence. Finally, it is worth stating that all forms of mapping are 'second best', and the existence of a range of techniques should not be taken as an argument for relying on mapping instead of obtaining direct preference-based measurements in prospectively designed studies.

5.8 Alternatives: disability-adjusted life-years, capabilities

Despite their differences, the EQ-5D, HUI, and SF-6D are all intended to provide a way of making quality-of-life adjustments to survival in order to generate estimates of QALYs. However, some alternative metrics have gained currency in recent years, including disability-adjusted life-years (DALYs) and measures of capability.

5.8.1 DALYs

DALYs were originally developed by the World Bank and the World Health Organization (WHO) as part of a major programme of work to estimate the global burden of disease attributable to different diseases and injuries, and first appeared in the landmark 1993 World Bank Report *Investing in Health* (World Bank 1993; Murray 1994; Murray *et al.* 1994).

The DALY is a health outcome measure which has two main components: the duration of a lifetime lost due to premature death (years of life lost (YLL)), and the reduction in quality of life due to a disability (years of life with a disability (YLD)).

The primary scale is 0–1, with 0 = perfect health with no disability and 1 = dead. The duration of a lifetime lost due to premature mortality is calculated by comparing actual age at death with a standard expectation of life, which was chosen to match the highest national life expectancy observed (in Japan). Thus standard life expectancy was set at 82.5 years for females and 80 years for males.

Calculation of the reduction in quality of life due to a disability was originally based on a simple six-level classification system, with weights allocated by a group of experts. Thus Class 2, 'Limited ability to perform most activities in two of the following areas: recreation, education, procreation or occupation', was given a weight of 0.400, so that each year in that state would lose 0.40 of a DALY, whereas each year in Class 6, 'Needs assistance with activities of daily living such as eating, personal hygiene, or toilet use', would lose 0.920 of a DALY. Subsequently the basis of the weighting system was revised, with a person trade-off system used to derive weights for 22 indicator conditions (Murray 1996).

A simplified illustration of the concept is shown in Figure 5.7. A hypothetical male has a traffic accident at age 20 which results in permanent disability, comparable to Class 2 described in the previous paragraph, and so from that point on has a disability weight of 0.4. He eventually dies at the age of 60.

Forty years with this level of disability would result in a loss of $40 \times 0.40 = 16$ DALYs, and death at age 60 is 20 years short of the standard male life expectancy of 80 and hence results in another 20 DALYs lost, giving a total of 36 DALYs lost. It should be noted that, whereas the objective is to maximize the number of QALYs a person accumulates over a lifetime, the objective with DALYs is to minimize the number lost.

In practice, calculation of DALYs also involves applying age-weights to time lived at different ages, so that the years of life lived as a young or middle-aged adult are given a higher weight than years lived in childhood or old age. These weightings were

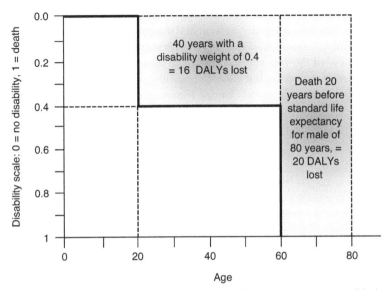

Fig. 5.7 DALY profile for a male injured in a road traffic accident at age 20, with death at age 60.

initially provided by a group of public health experts (Murray 1994). Thus DALYs lost after the age of 60 in Figure 5.7 would be given less weight than those lost between the ages of 20 and 60.

DALYs have been adopted by the WHO and the World Bank to quantify the global burden of disease, and the WHO has also used them to estimate the cost-effectiveness of a range of interventions, particularly in low- and middle-income country settings (Tan-Torres *et al.* 2003). However, although conceptually similar to QALYs in some respects, DALYs differ substantially in their use of age-weights, the health state classification system used, the way in which weights have been derived for health states, and the age-weighting principle and weights, and consequently their use in measuring patient-level outcomes and in detailed cost-effectiveness analyses has been limited.

5.8.2 **Capabilities**

As noted above and in Chapter 2, the QALY approach has affinities, if not direct theoretical links, with a particular strand of welfare economics that stresses the concept of utility. However, since the 1980s an alternative approach has been developed, particularly associated with the work of Amartya Sen (Sen 1985) and Martha Nussbaum (Nussbaum 2000), which lays much more emphasis on individuals having functional capabilities or 'substantive freedoms' to function in particular ways if they wish to, rather than focusing on their level of utility or access to resources. Typical capabilities might include being able to live a normal lifespan, having good health, being able to move around freely without threat or assault, being able to participate in political choices, and having property rights on an equal basis with others.

Although highly influential, there are many practical questions concerning how capabilities might be measured. A version of the approach was described and used in the 1990 United Nations Development Programme's Human Development Report, which introduced the concept of a human development index based not just on national income per person but also on capability measures such as life expectancy and educational enrolment rates (United Nations Development Programme 1990).

Table 5.7 Capability attributes and values of the ICECAP instrument

Attribute	Value
Attachment	
I can have all of the love and friendship that I want	0.2535
I can have a lot of the love and friendship that I want	0.2325
I can have a little of the love and friendship that I want	0.134
I cannot have any of the love and friendship that I want	−0.0128
Security	
I can think about the future without any concern	0.1788
I can think about the future with only a little concern	0.1071
I can only think about the future with some concern	0.0661
I can only think about the future with a lot of concern	0.0321
Role	
I am able to do all of the things that make me feel valued	0.1923
I am able to do many of the things that make me feel valued	0.1793
I am able to do a few of the things that make me feel valued	0.1296
I am unable to do any of the things that make me feel valued	0.0151
Enjoyment	
I can have all of the enjoyment and pleasure that I want	0.166
I can have a lot of the enjoyment and pleasure that I want	0.1643
I can have a little of the enjoyment and pleasure that I want	0.1185
I cannot have any of the enjoyment and pleasure that I want	0.0168
Control	
I am able to be completely independent	0.2094
I am able to be independent in many things	0.1848
I am able to be independent in a few things	0.1076
I am unable to be at all independent	−0.0512

Reproduced from Coast *et al.* (2008) with permission from Elsevier.

This was primarily intended as an aggregate measure of national development rather than an individual measure, but since then efforts have been made to derive person-specific capability measures. For example, Anand *et al.* (2009) have explored whether capabilities measures can be extracted from existing population surveys and have also proposed new survey instruments to measure capabilities.

Coast *et al.* (2008) have begun the development of an index of capability (ICECAP) for use with older people that is intended as an economic evaluation measure that could, for example, be used to evaluate public health interventions. The ICECAP measure incorporates five dimensions: attachment, security, role, enjoyment, and control. Initial valuation work using stated preference discrete choice experiments produced a set of valuations for the possible states or levels of capability that can be described by the instrument, rescaled so that the absence of capability sums to zero and full capability sums to 1. These are shown in Table 5.7.

Clearly, this type of approach has the potential to record broad changes in a person's life, brought about, for example, by a new social care programme or sheltered housing development, that would be less easily captured or possibly missed altogether by an instrument such as the EQ-5D. However, it also seems likely that an instrument such as the ICE-CAP might not detect health-specific changes such as better pain management. It is also worth noting that the issues involved in selecting attributes or domains, describing levels within them, and attaching valuations to them are no less complex with a capabilities index than with instruments such as the EQ-5D, SF-6D, or HUI. Indeed, it is clear that many respondents may have struggled with the ICE-CAP valuation procedure, with possibly as few as 26% of them conforming unequivocally in their stated preferences to the assumptions of conventional random utility theory (Flynn *et al.* 2008).

5.9 **Summary**

In this chapter we have considered non-preference-based and preference-based instruments to measure health status, and reviewed the main methods of obtaining valuations for health states. We have also considered some methods for mapping between instruments. We looked in more detail at the main preference-based generic instruments in widespread use—EQ-5D, HUI, and SF-6D—and at some proposed alternatives.

The next two chapters turn to the other side of the cost-effectiveness equation, and consider how information on resource use should be measured and valued to obtain estimates of cost.

References

Aaronson, N.K., Ahmedzai, S., Bergman, B., *et al.* (1993). The European Organization for Research and Treatment of Cancer Qlq-C30: a quality-of-life instrument for use in international clinical trials in oncology. *Journal of the National Cancer Institute*, **85**, 365–76.

Anand, P., Hunter, G., Carter, I., Dowding, K., and van Hees, M. (2009). The development of capability indicators. *Journal of Human Development and Capabilities*, **10**, 125–52.

Baron, J., Asch, D.A., Fagerlin, A., *et al.* (2003). Effect of assessment method on the discrepancy between judgments of health disorders people have and do not have: a web study. *Medical Decision Making*, **23**, 422–34.

Barry, M.J., Fowler, F.J., O'Leary, M.P., *et al.* (1992). The American Urological Association Symptom Index for benign prostatic hyperplasia. *Journal of Urology*, **148**, 1549–57.

Barton, G.R., Bankart, J., Davis, A.C., and Summerfield, Q.A. (2004). Comparing utility scores before and after hearing-aid provision : results according to the EQ-5D, HUI3 and SF-6D. *Applied Health Economics and Health Policy*, **3**, 103–5.

Boyd, N.F., Sutherland, H.J., Heasman, K.Z., Tritchler, D.L., and Cummings, B.J. (1990). Whose utilities for decision-analysis. *Medical Decision Making*, **10**, 58–67.

Brauer, C.A., Rosen, A.B., Greenberg, D., and Neumann, P.J. (2006). Trends in the measurement of health utilities in published cost-utility analyses. *Value in Health*, **9**, 213–18.

Brazier, J. and McCabe, C. (2007). 'Is there a case for using visual analogue scale valuations in CUA' by Parkin and Devlin: a response: 'Yes there is a case, but what does it add to ordinal data?' *Health Economics*, **16**, 645–7.

Brazier, J.E. and Roberts, J. (2004). The estimation of a preference-based measure of health from the SF-12. *Medical Care*, **42**, 851–9.

Brazier, J., Usherwood, T., Harper, R., and Thomas, K. (1998). Deriving a preference-based single index from the UK SF-36 Health Survey. *Journal of Clinical Epidemiology*, **51**, 1115–1128.

Brazier, J., Deverill, M., Green, C., Harper, R., and Booth, A. (1999). A review of the use of health status measures in economic evaluation. *Health Technology Assessment*, **3**(9).

Brazier, J., Roberts, J., and Deverill, M. (2002). The estimation of a preference-based measure of health from the SF-36. *Journal of Health Economics*, **21**, 271–92.

Brazier, J., Roberts, J., Tsuchiya, A., and Busschbach, J. (2004). A comparison of the EQ-5D and SF-6D across seven patient groups. *Health Economics*, **13**, 873–84.

Brazier, J., Ratcliffe, J., Tsuchiya, A., and Salomon, J. (2007). *Measuring and Valuing Health Benefits for Economic Evaluation*. Oxford University Press, New York.

Campbell, H., Rivero-Arias, O., Johnston, K., Gray, A., Fairbank, J., and Frost, H. (2006). Responsiveness of objective, disease-specific, and generic outcome measures in patients with chronic low back pain: an assessment for improving, stable, and deteriorating patients. *Spine*, **31**, 815–22.

Cassileth, B.R., Lusk, E.J., Strouse, T.B., *et al.* (1984). Psychosocial status in chronic illness: a comparative-analysis of 6 diagnostic groups. *New England Journal of Medicine*, **311**, 506–11.

Coast, J., Flynn, T.N., Natarajan, L., *et al.* (2008). Valuing the ICECAP capability index for older people. *Social Science and Medicine*, **67**, 874–82.

Daly, E., Gray, A., Barlow, D., McPherson, K., Roche, M., and Vessey, M. (1993). Measuring the impact of menopausal symptoms on quality of life. *British Medical Journal*, **307**, 836–40.

DCCT Research Group (1988). Reliability and validity of a diabetes quality-of-life measure for the Diabetes Control and Complications Trial (DCCT). *Diabetes Care*, **11**, 725–32.

Dolan, P. and Roberts, J. (2002). Modelling valuations for EQ-5D health states: an alternative model using differences in valuations. *Medical Care*, **40**, 442–6.

Dolan, P., Gudex, C., Kind, P., and Williams, A. (1995). *A Social Tariff for EuroQol: Results from a UK General Population Survey*, Discussion Paper 138, Centre of Health Economics, University of York.

Drummond, M. (2001). Introducing economic and quality of life measurements into clinical studies. *Annals of Medicine*, **33**, 344–9.

Drummond, M.F., Sculpher, M.J., Torrance, G.W., O'Brien, B.J., and Stoddart, G.L. (2005). *Methods for the Economic Evaluation of Health Care Programmes* (3rd edn). Oxford University Press.

EuroQol Group (1990). EuroQol—a new facility for the measurement of health-related quality of life. *Health Policy*, **16**, 199–208.

Feeny, D., Furlong, W., Torrance, G.W., *et al.* (2002). Multiattribute and single-attribute utility functions for the health utilities Index Mark 3 system. *Medical Care*, **40**, 113–28.

Flynn, T.N., Louviere, J.J., Marley, A.A.J., Coast, J., and Peters, T.J. (2008). Rescaling quality of life values from discrete choice experiments for use as QALYs: a cautionary tale. *Population Health Metrics*, **6**, 6.

Franks, P., Lubetkin, E.I., Gold, M.R., and Tancredi, D.J. (2003). Mapping the SF-12 to preference-based instruments: convergent validity in a low-income, minority population. *Medical Care*, **41**, 1277–83.

Franks, P., Lubetkin, E.I., Gold, M.R., Tancredi, D.J., and Jia, H. (2004). Mapping the SF-12 to the EuroQol EQ-5D Index in a national US sample. *Medical Decision Making*, **24**, 247–54.

Fryback, D.G., Lawrence, W.F., Martin, P.A., Klein, R., and Klein, B.E. (1997). Predicting quality of well-being scores from the SF-36: results from the Beaver Dam Health Outcomes Study. *Medical Decision Making*, **17**, 1–9.

Gold, M.R., Siegel, J.E., Russell, L.B., and Weinstein, M.C. (1996). *Cost-effectiveness in Health and Medicine*. Oxford University Press, New York.

Gray, A.M., Rivero-Arias, O., and Clarke, P.M. (2006). Estimating the association between SF-12 responses and EQ-5D utility values by response mapping. *Medical Decision Making*, **26**, 18–29.

Hadorn, D.C. (1991). The role of public values in setting health-care priorities. *Social Science and Medicine*, **32**, 773–81.

Hallan, S., Asberg, A., Indredavik, B., and Wideroe, T.E. (1999). Quality of life after cerebrovascular stroke: a systematic study of patients' preferences for different functional outcomes. *Journal of Internal Medicine*, **246**, 309–16.

Hawthorne, G., Richardson, J., and Osborne, R. (1999). The Assessment of Quality of Life (AQoL) instrument: a psychometric measure of health-related quality of life. *Quality of Life Research*, **8**, 209–24.

Health Survey (1998). *Health Survey for England 1996*. Stationery Office, London.

Herdman, M., Gudex, C., Lloyd, A., *et al.* (2009). *Development and Preliminary Testing of an Official Five-level Version of EQ-5D*. EQ-5D Group, Rotterdam.

Horsman, J., Furlong, W., Feeny, D., and Torrance, G. (2003). The Health Utilities Index (HUI): concepts, measurement properties and applications. *Health and Quality of Life Outcomes*, **1**, 54.

Johannesson, M. (1996). *Theory and Methods of Economic Evaluation of Health Care*. Kluwer Academic, Boston, MA.

Kaplan, R.M. and Anderson, J.P. (1988). A general health policy model: update and applications. *Health Services Research*, **23**, 203–35.

Kendrick, T., Simons, L., Mynors-Wallis, L., *et al.* (2006). Cost-effectiveness of referral for generic care or problem-solving treatment from community mental health nurses, compared with usual general practitioner care for common mental disorders: randomised controlled trial. *Bitish Journal of Psychiatry*, **189**, 50–9.

Long, J.S. (1997). *Regression Models for Categorical and Limited Dependent Variables*. Sage, London.

Lundberg, L., Johannesson, M., Isacson, D.G., and Borgquist, L. (1999). The relationship between health-state utilities and the SF-12 in a general population. *Medical Decision Making*, **19**, 128–40.

McDonough, C.M., Grove, M.R., Tosteson, T.D., Lurie, J.D., Hilibrand, A.S., and Tosteson, A.N.A. (2005). Comparison of EQ-5D, HUI, and SF-36-derived societal health state values among Spine Patient Outcomes Research Trial (SPORT) participants. *Quality of Life Research*, **14**, 1321–32.

Murray, C.J. (1994). Quantifying the burden of disease: the technical basis for disability-adjusted life years. *Bulletin of the World Health Organization*, **72**, 429–45.

Murray, C.J. (1996). Rethinking DALYs. In: Murray, J.A. and Lopez, A.d. (eds), *The Global Burden of Disease: A Comprehensive Assessment of Mortality and Disability from Diseases, Injuries, and Risk Factors in 1990 and Projected to 2020*. Harvard University Press, Cambridge, MA.

Murray, C.J., Lopez, A.D., and Jamison, D.T. (1994). The global burden of disease in 1990: summary results, sensitivity analysis and future directions. *Bulletin of the World Health Organization*, **72**, 495–509.

NICE (2008). *Guide to the Methods of Technology Appraisal*. National Institute for Health and Clinical Excellence, London.

Nord, E., Pinto, J.L., Richardson, J., Menzel, P., and Ubel, P. (1999). Incorporating societal concerns for fairness in numerical valuations of health programmes. *Health Economics*, **8**, 25–39.

Nussbaum, M.C. (2000). *Women and Human Development: The Capabilities Approach*. Cambridge University Press.

O'Brien, B.J., Spath, M., Blackhouse, G., Severens, J.L., Dorian, P., and Brazier, J. (2003). A view from the bridge: agreement between the SF-6D utility algorithm and the Health Utilities Index. *Health Economics*, **12**, 975–81.

Parkin, D. and Devlin, N. (2006). Is there a case for using visual analogue scale valuations in cost-utility analysis? *Health Economics*, **15**, 653–64.

Parkin, D. and Devlin, N. (2007). 'Is there a case for using visual analogue scale valuations in CUA? Yes there is a case, but what does it add to ordinal data'? A rejoinder. *Health Economics*, **16**, 649–51.

Pyne, J.M., Fortney, J.C., Tripathi, S., Feeny, D., Ubel, P., and Brazier, J. (2009). How bad Is depression? Preference score estimates from depressed patients and the general population. *Health Services Research*, **44**, 1406–23.

Rawls, J. (1971). *A Theory of Justice*. Belknap Press, Cambridge, MA.

Rivero-Arias, O., Campbell, H., Gray, A., Fairbank, J., Frost, H., and Wilson-MacDonald, J. (2005). Surgical stabilisation of the spine compared with a programme of intensive rehabilitation for the management of patients with chronic low back pain: cost utility analysis based on a randomised controlled trial. *British Medical Journal*, **330**, 1239.

Rivero-Arias, O., Gray, A., Frost, H., Lamb, S.E., and Stewart-Brown, S. (2006). Cost-utility analysis of physiotherapy treatment compared with physiotherapy advice in low back pain. *Spine*, **31**, 1381–7.

Rivero-Arias, O., Ouellet, M., Gray, A., Wolstenholme, J., Rothwell, P.M., and Luengo-Fernandez, R. (2010). Mapping the modified Rankin scale (mRS) measurement into the generic EuroQol (EQ-5D) health outcome. *Medical Decision Making*, **30**, 341–54.

Sen, A. (1985). *Commodities and Capabilities*. Oxford University Press, Oxford.

Shaw, J.W., Johnson, J.A., and Coons, S.J. (2005). US valuation of the EQ-5D health states: development and testing of the D1 valuation model. *Medical Care*, **43**, 203–20.

Shmueli, A. (1999). Subjective health status and health values in the general population. *Medical Decision Making*, **19**, (2) 122–127

Simon, J., Gray, A., Clarke, P., Wade, A., Neil, A., and Farmer, A. (2008). Cost-effectiveness of self-monitoring of blood glucose in the management of patients with non-insulin treated type 2 diabetes: economic evaluation of data from the randomised controlled DiGEM trial. *British Medical Journal*, **336**, 1177–80.

Sintonen, H. (2001). The 15D instrument of health-related quality of life: properties and applications. *Annals of Medicine*, **33**, 328–36.

Tan-Torres, E., Baltussen, R., and Adams, T. (2003), *Making Choices in Health: WHO Guide to Cost-Effectiveness Analysis*. World Health Organization, Geneva.

Tarlov, A.R., Ware, J.E., Greenfield, S., Nelson, E.C., Perrin, E., and Zubkoff, M. (1989). The Medical Outcomes Study: an application of methods for monitoring the results of medical care. *Journal of the American Medical Association*, **262**, 925–30.

Tengs, T.O. and Lin, T.H. (2003). A meta-analysis of quality-of-life estimates for stroke. *Pharmacoeconomics*, **21**, 191–200.

Torrance, G.W. (1976). Toward a utility theory foundation for health status index models. *Health Services Research*, **11**, 439–69.

Torrance, G.W. (1986). Measurement of health state utilities for economic appraisal: a review. *Journal of Health Economics*, **5**, 1–30.

Torrance, G.W., Thomas, W.H., and Sackett, D.L. (1972). A utility maximization model for evaluation of health care programs. *Health Services Research*, **7**, 118.

Torrance, G.W., Boyle, M.H., and Horwood, S.P. (1982). Application of multi-attribute utility-theory to measure social preferences for health states. *Operations Research*, **30**, 1043–69.

Torrance, G.W., Feeny, D.H., Furlong, W.J., Barr, R.D., Zhang, Y., and Wang, Q. (1996). Multiattribute utility function for a comprehensive health status classification system. Health Utilities Index Mark 2. *Medical Care*, **34**, 702–22.

United Nations Development Programme (1990). *Human Development Report 1990: Concept and Measurement of Human Development*. Oxford University Press.

von Neumann, J. and Morgenstern, O. (1944). *Theory of Games and Economic Behavior*. Princeton University Press, Princeton, NJ.

Walters, S.J. and Brazier, J.E. (2005). Comparison of the minimally important difference for two health state utility measures: EQ-5D and SF-6D. *Quality of Life Research*, **14**, 1523–32.

Ware, J.E. and Sherbourne, C.D. (1992). The MOS 36-Item Short-Form Health Survey (SF-36). 1. Conceptual framework and item selection. *Medical Care*, **30**, 473–83.

Ware, J.E., Kosinski, M., Bayliss, M.S., McHorney, C.A., Rogers, W.H., and Raczek, A. (1995). Comparison of methods for the scoring and statistical analysis of SF-36 health profile and summary measures: summary of results from the Medical Outcomes Study. *Medical Care*, **33**, AS264–79.

Ware, J.E., Kosinski, M., and Keller, S.D. (1996). A 12-item short-form health survey: construction of scales and preliminary tests of reliability and validity. *Medical Care*, **34**, 220–33.

Weinstein, M.C. and Stason, W.B. (1976). *Hypertension: A Policy Perspective*. Harvard University Press, Cambridge, MA.

World Bank (1993). *World Development Report, 1993: Investing in Health,* Oxford University Press for the World Bank, New York.

World Health Organization (1948). *Constitution of the World Health Organization.* World Health Organization, Geneva.

Zeckhauser, R. and Shepard, D. (1976). Where now for saving lives? *Law and Contemporary Problems,* **40**, 5–45.

Exercise

Quality-adjusted survival analysis

If you go to the website www.herc.ox.ac.uk/books/applied you will find an Excel file *Outcomes2.xlsx* which contains five worksheets. The first sheet, **Life Table**, and the second sheet, **Survival Times**, were used in the Exercises for Chapters 3 and 4. The third sheet, **EQ-5D survey data,** contains responses of Control Group and Treatment Group patients to an EQ-5D survey undertaken at entry to the study and then at five-yearly intervals.

(i) Use the EQ-5D algorithm on the worksheet entitled **EQ5D** to obtain tariff values for these patients.

(ii) Then use these tariff values to estimate the quality-adjusted survival time (QAS) for the Control and Treatment group patients on the **QAS** worksheet using the population based approach.

Step-by-step guide

The worksheet **EQ-5D survey data** contains the responses of these patients to an EQ-5D survey undertaken at entry to the study and then at five-yearly intervals. Use the EQ-5D algorithm on the fourth worksheet (**EQ5D**) to obtain tariff values for these patients. Use these tariff values to estimate the QAS for the Control Group and Treatment Group using the population based approach.

First, the utility values must be obtained for each patient. Go to the worksheet **EQ5D**. This worksheet contains the formula for calculating the EQ-5D tariff values. Calculate the utility values for the Control Group patients.

♦ Copy the data from the first survey in the worksheet **EQ-5D survey data** to this worksheet. You do not need to copy the patient numbers, which are just there as a check. You can copy the data by copying and pasting, or by linking the cells.

♦ Copy the formula for EQ-5D tariffs from cell G5 to G15, and then copy this formula down the column **Utility values**. NB: There may be some negative values since the tariff can be negative, indicating health states worse than death.

♦ Do the same for all five surveys.

♦ Once this has been completed, go to worksheet **QAS**. This worksheet contains a table of the utility values for each patient for each survey.

♦ The utility values calculated on **EQ5D** now need to be transferred to this worksheet. Again, you can copy and paste, making sure that you paste the values rather than the formula, or link the two sheets. To do this go to cell C7 which needs to contain the utility value for the first Control Group patient at the baseline survey.

To link it with the value previously calculated place the following formula in the cell: =EQ5D!G15.

♦ Copy this formula down the column.

♦ Repeat this for the rest of the time periods.

♦ Repeat all the steps above for the Treatment Group patients.

♦ Now calculate the average utility value in each time period. For example, for the Control Group patients the average utility at the baseline survey can be obtained using the formula: =AVERAGE(C7:C106).

♦ Copy these average values (mean utility weights) to the section **Calculating QALYs**.

♦ Link the survival probabilities with those calculated using the product limit method on the **Survival times** worksheet. Tip: the survival probability required for 5 years, for example, will be the value in column A of the sheet that is closest to but does not exceed 5.

♦ Apply the quality-adjusted survival formula:

$$QAS = \sum_{i=1}^{k}((Q_i + Q_{i+1})/2)((S_i + S_{i+1})/2)(t_{i+1} - t_i)$$

where Q_i are the mean quality weights and S_i are the survival probabilities. Intuitively, this is the quality of life averaged over two periods times the average survival probability times the length of the time period of interest.

♦ Calculate the total quality adjusted survival.

The discount rate should now be applied to these results. Insert the discount rate of 3.5% in cell C128. Then insert the discount formula in cells C130 to N130, referring to cell C128 for the rate. For example: =C124/(1+$C$128)^C118.

Finally, in cells C132 and K132, sum the results in the discounted cells to obtain total discounted quality adjusted survival in each group.

A completed version of this exercise is available from the website www.herc.ox.ac.uk/books/applied in the Excel file *Outcomes2 solutions.xlsx*

Chapter 6

Defining, measuring, and valuing costs

When estimating the relative cost-effectiveness of health-care interventions, reliable estimates of incremental costs are clearly important. Despite this importance, most methodological research on economic evaluation, especially throughout the 1980s and 1990s, focused on the outcome or effectiveness component of economic evaluation. However, by the late 1990s it was recognized that costing methods required both attention and improvement, especially with the increased use of economic evaluation alongside clinical trials and of cost-effectiveness results by policy-makers (NICE 2008). This has led to several advances in costing methodology, especially concerning data analysis (Glick *et al.* 2007).

In this chapter, we outline cost measurement and discuss how to define, measure, and value costs. Alternative costing perspectives (health service and societal) are described, and issues concerning the incorporation of productivity costs and informal costs are explored. A worked example illustrates how choice of perspective can result in different conclusions concerning the cost-effectiveness of health-care interventions. Next, we outline different ways of collecting data on resource use and unit costs, and show how to construct a cost dataset. Adjustments to costs that may be required, such as converting costs into common base years and currencies, are described, and the chapter concludes by describing the rationale behind event-based cost analysis, again with a worked example.

6.1 Costing in economic evaluation

In economic evaluation, costs are calculated by quantifying the different types of resources used in producing a particular good or service, and then multiplying these amounts by their respective unit costs. Resources can be measured on a patient-specific or a non-patient-specific basis. The former is an example of a **stochastic** analysis, in that the resources used by each patient are subject to variability and will be influenced by a range of known and unknown variables and cannot be predicted exactly. The latter is often dealt with **deterministically**, for example by assuming in a model that every patient having a myocardial infarction will on average spend 4 days in hospital, although in practice the variation might be substantial.

6.2 Identifying, measuring, and valuing costs

Performing a cost analysis typically involves three stages: first, identifying resources, then measuring these resources using appropriate physical units, and finally valuing them (Gold *et al.* 1996; Drummond *et al.* 2005). For instance, in a clinical trial comparing two different surgical interventions the three stages would be as follows:

- **Identify**: estimate the different categories of resource likely to be required (e.g. theatre staff, consumables and equipment, recovery time, surgical complications, re-admissions).

- **Measure**: estimate how much of each resource category is required (e.g. type of staff performing the surgery and time involved, post-surgery length of stay, re-admission rates).

- **Value**: apply unit costs to each resource category (e.g. salary scales from the relevant hospital or national wage rates for staff inputs, cost per inpatient day for the post-surgery hospital stay).

6.2.1 Identification

The process of identifying resource items can be seen as a study of the production function of the health-care programme (Brouwer *et al.* 2001). Identifying which items to include in a cost analysis requires consideration of the perspective of the study, the types of resource use likely to be relevant to the comparison (Drummond *et al.* 2005), and the target audience or user of the study (Gold *et al.* 1996). The main perspectives are the payer (often the health service) and the societal perspectives (discussed in more detail later in this chapter). The identification stage requires knowledge about the resources needed to perform the intervention and knowledge of the disease process itself, especially during and after treatment. It may also be important to identify whether the way in which care is delivered varies between different centres or settings: for example, some hospitals may routinely perform a procedure on a day-case basis, while others may require an overnight stay.

The approach to identifying resources used will also depend on the general approach to costing being adopted. The two main approaches are gross-costing and micro-costing (Brouwer *et al.* 2001; Gold *et al.* 1996), also referred to by some as top-down costing and bottom-up costing, respectively (Wordsworth *et al.* 2005). Broadly, with gross-costing the resources are viewed in bundles, such as a day in hospital following a surgical procedure. Alternatively, micro-costing requires the identification of all underlying activities, such as the consumables and staff time which form this hospital day. In practice the choice is often based on the ease of data collection, and many economic evaluations use a combination of the two approaches (Adam *et al.* 2003a). However, in some situations one approach could be preferred. For example, if there is a potential for a substitution effect from an intervention which is labour intensive (such as hospital haemodialysis for endstage renal disease) to a relatively cheaper and more consumable intensive intervention (continuous ambulatory peritoneal dialysis for treating the same disease), gross-costing might fail to detect important differences (Wordsworth *et al.* 2005). This suggests that it is important to have some a priori view on the kinds of resource-use differences that are likely to arise between two interventions being compared.

6.2.2 Measurement

The measurement of resource quantities often depends on the specific context of the evaluation. For instance, if the evaluation is being conducted alongside a clinical trial, data on resource quantities, such as types and amounts of drugs administered, may be routinely collected on case report forms for the trial. Alternatively, if the evaluation is a stand-alone economic evaluation, resource quantities could be estimated from data systems, such as hospital records or patient case notes. For some items of resource use, such as health visitor contacts, the difficulty of accessing routinely recorded information may necessitate asking patients to provide estimates of their use of these resource items, for example by completing questionnaires, giving interviews, or keeping diaries. An example of a standard one-page questionnaire to collect this type of data is presented in Figure 6.1. This example was used in the UK Prospective Diabetes Study (UKPDS), which has been drawn on for many of the exercises and examples in this book.

When asking patients to complete resource/time questionnaires (or answer interview questions), a particularly important issue is deciding on the optimum recall period. Two types of recall error can be distinguished: simply forgetting an entire episode, or incorrectly recalling when it occurred. If a study requires information on a specific period of time, for example if there is reason to think that an intervention may influence the number of GP visits immediately following a hospital procedure, a shorter recall period of a few weeks could be reasonable. However, if a study is trying to get a picture of resource use over a much longer time, such as 12 months, using a short recall period to provide a snapshot of typical resource use may be insufficient and misleading, as results from the short period will have to be extrapolated over the longer period. In summary, there is a trade-off between recall bias and complete sampling information. Clarke *et al.* (2008) set out this trade-off in a clear analytical framework, showing that the longer the period of recall the greater is the likelihood of recall error, but the shorter the recall period the greater is the problem of missing information. The authors suggest that there is no general answer to the question of optimal recall periods, as this question largely depends on the main objective for the data collection, but argue that there is no compelling reason why the default situation in survey design should be a short recall period (Clarke *et al.* 2008). The example in Figure 6.1 used a period of 4 months, but more recent repeat exercises using this type of questionnaire have usually asked for information over a 12-month period.

6.2.3 **Valuation**

When assigning unit costs to resources, the price for a resource should theoretically be its opportunity cost. In practice it will commonly have to be assumed that the market price is a reasonable approximation of the opportunity cost, and market prices are likely to be available for many resource items, in the form of list prices or routine purchase prices for drugs or agreed salaries for staff inputs.

A further consideration when using prices for costing health-care interventions is that they may include an element of profit. If this profit is above a perceived fair rate of return on investment, these prices cannot be considered as reflecting societal opportunity costs (Gold *et al.* 1996). One solution, adopted particularly in the USA, is to adjust market prices for the estimated excess profit using cost-to-charge ratios which indicate how the price could be deflated to reflect real opportunity costs more accurately (Gold *et al.* 1996). In other situations a market price may not exist for the resource item being costed, but there could be a comparable item for which a price does exist. The price of this second item could then be used as a 'shadow price'

Appendix – UKPDS Patient cost questionnaire
HEALTH CARE ASSESSMENT

We would like to know how often you have seen other doctors or nurses (apart from those in this clinic) during the past (***) months.

Please answer every question, even if the answer is '0'.

Please fill in both boxes, for example: ....0 1 if seen once

If you have any questions about this form, please ask a member of staff.

During the past month, how many times have you:

1. Visited your GP ? ....

2. Been seen at home by your GP ? ....

3. Visited a nurse ? ....

4. Been seen at home by a nurse ?............................

5. Visited a health visitor ? ....

6. Been seen at home by a health visitor ? ....

7. Visited an optician or eye clinic ? ....

8. Been seen by a chiropodist / podiatrist ? ....

9. Visited a diabetes clinic ? ....

10. Visited any other hospital clinic ? ....

11. Been in hospital overnight, for treatment or respite care?.......

If you have been in hospital overnight at least once over the last ** months, please enter the total number of all nights in hospital here:..............

Do you have any other comments that you would like to make?

....

....

Fig. 6.1 Example of a brief patient-completed resource use questionnaire.

(Drummond *et al.* 2005; McIntosh *et al.* 2010). Shadow pricing has been used in some circumstances, for example to place a valuation on the time of friends or family providing unpaid care (Posnett and Jan 1996; van den Berg *et al.* 2004), but otherwise is rarely encountered in cost-effectiveness studies.

Another way of approximating the opportunity cost of health-care resources is to use health-care tariffs or charges. For example, in the British National Health Service (NHS), the payment by results system gives hospitals specific payments for undertaking items of activity, such as particular surgical procedures (Department of Health 2010); these payments may be averaged over quite different types of patient, hospital, or procedure, and may also be intended to incentivize or disincentivize particular types of activity or behaviour, and so their relation to underlying costs may be indirect. Therefore the general advice is to use a tariff only if there is a clear indication that it represents a reasonable approximation of the actual costs (Brouwer *et al.* 2001).

There are several methods of gathering unit costs, including widely available data sources and primary data collection. At a national level there are several published datasets of unit costs within high-income countries. For instance in the USA, diagnosis-related group (DRG) payments, used to classify hospital cases into groups expected to have similar hospital resource use and developed for Medicare as part of the prospective payment system, are often used in cost analyses. In England, the Department of Health produces a national Reference Costs dataset, which provides a basis for comparison within (and outside) the NHS, at the level of individual treatments. Reference Costs publications show details of unit cost, average length of stay, and activity levels for a wide range of services. These are national average costs for all Healthcare Resource Groups (HRGs)—standard groupings of clinically similar treatments which use common levels of health-care resource and are similar to DRGs. In addition, a Reference Cost Index (RCI) is available for each NHS Trust in England, showing the average cost of an organization's aggregate activity compared with the same activity delivered at the national average cost (Department of Health 2008). The annual publication *Unit Costs of Health and Social Care* provides a compendium of estimates of national unit costs for a wide range of both health and social care services, and is another widely used source of unit costs in the UK (Curtis 2009).

Reference costs are useful approximations, which may be more relevant for a country (or other jurisdiction) than costs calculated in a specific context, such as within one hospital. However, such unit costs often provide less detail than may be required for specific economic evaluations. For example, DRG- or HRG-based costs are primarily based on a hospital episode or admission, and so will detect differences between patient groups in rates of hospitalization, but will not be sensitive to differences in lengths of stay. Use of readily available unit costs also means, in effect, accepting that differences in costs between two surgical procedures, for example, are real and not simply due to accounting methods or the original sampling frame. Where the results are highly dependent on specific unit costs, primary data collection may have to be considered.

Primary data collection may also be considered if a trial is being performed on a multi-centre basis, where it might be important to capture differences in the costs of resource units in different centres. If this type of costing is not possible, non-centre-specific alternatives (Table 6.1) will have to be considered. In essence, non-centre-specific approaches attach one agreed (standardized) unit cost before applying this to all centres.

One rationale for using centre-specific costing, rather than average or single-centre costing, is that different centres will face different unit costs for their input resources. For example, health-care labour inputs generally cost more in London than elsewhere in the UK. Therefore basic production theory would suggest that some substitution might occur from more expensive inputs to less expensive inputs. Average-centre costing would fail to account for these substitution effects. This issue was examined by Raikou *et al.* (2000), who studied the implications of centre-specific versus average unit costs in a series of simulation exercises. A production function was simulated using two inputs, with their respective unit costs, for a number of centres. The simulation showed that if centres were not responsive to relative price changes in their two inputs, there would be no difference between using centre-specific or average unit costs. However, if centres behaved according to economic theory and substituted inputs according to their relative prices, the centre-specific and average unit cost approaches produced small but significant differences, even if the substitution effect was low (Raikou *et al.* 2000).

6.3 **Alternative costing perspectives**

The perspective of the analysis affects the costs (and outcomes) that are included in an economic evaluation. The main alternative perspectives are the payer (often the health service) and societal. The former includes only costs incurred by the health service, while the latter considers all costs regardless of who incurs them, for example costs to patients, to social services, to employers in the form of productivity losses, and to family and friends via informal care costs, as well as health service costs. Productivity costs and informal care costs in particular are considered by some as an important input into the production of health, with an individual's time being a limited resource with opportunity costs (Luce *et al.* 1996). Several official guidelines for evaluating health-care technologies support the incorporation of such time costs (Pritchard and Sculpher 2000). There is also a strong theoretical argument for adopting a societal

Table 6.1 Centre-specific versus non-centre-specific unit cost approaches

Approach	Data collection level
Centre-specific	Unit costs collected from all centres
Non-centre-specific	
Single-centre	Unit cost from one centre applied to all other centres
Averaged	Unit costs of selected centres averaged and applied to remaining centres
Published	Reference costs or costs from published papers are applied to all

perspective in economic evaluations. According to welfare economics, a policy change could have a series of effects on different individuals and groups, and adopting a purely health service perspective could lead to inefficient changes in health-care delivery (Sculpher 2001).

However, there is no consensus on whether productivity costs should be included in cost-effectiveness analyses. For instance the National Institute for Health and Clinical Excellence (NICE) in England and Wales recommends that the cost perspective adopted for the primary analysis should be that of the NHS and personal social services (PSS) only (NICE 2008). The rationale for this is that the role of NICE is to maximize value for money from the NHS budget, thus excluding productivity costs.

This lack of agreement on whether to include productivity costs has led to this area of costing being described as one of the thornier issues in economic evaluation (Drummond *et al.* 2005). However, in the event that a societal perspective is adopted, the next section focuses on the measurement and valuation of productivity costs and informal care time.

6.3.1 Measuring productivity costs

The range of patient-related costs included in economic evaluations can vary considerably. Some studies include only the costs incurred by patients in travelling to a hospital or clinic for treatment; others may include a wider range of costs including over-the-counter purchases of medications or equipment. However, in some studies a much broader approach is taken, in which attempts are made to capture both the costs associated with treatment and the consequences of illness in terms of absence from or cessation of work.

Several data collection questionnaires are available to measure these productivity costs, including the Work and Productivity and Activity Impairment Questionnaire (WPAI) (Reilly *et al.* 1993) and the Health and Labor Questionnaire (van Roijen *et al.* 1996). One review (Lofland *et al.* 2004) identified and evaluated 11 such questionnaires. It was found that eight had been tested for reliability and validity, of which five measured both absence from work and lower productivity whilst at work, while the remainder measured absenteeism alone. Six of the instruments were specific to one particular disease, such as migraine (Osterhaus *et al.* 1992), four covered several disease areas, ranging from four with the Health and Labour Questionnaire to 25 with the WPAI Questionnaire, and it was not possible to determine a disease area for the remaining questionnaire. Obviously, these questionnaires may not cover the disease area required for a specific evaluation. Therefore researchers often have to use their own unvalidated questionnaires, making it more difficult to compare results across different studies.

6.3.2 Valuing productivity costs

There are three main approaches to valuing productivity costs: the human capital approach, the friction cost method, and the Washington Panel approach.

Historically, the human capital approach (HCA) has been the most widely used method for assigning monetary values to productivity costs, especially in cost-benefit analysis (Rice and Cooper 1967; Drummond *et al.* 2005). The approach estimates productivity costs as the expected or potential earnings lost due to illness. Recent cost-effectiveness analyses have used the HCA to value changes in the amount of time individuals are able to allocate to paid work as a result of illness or treatment (Lorgelly *et al.* 2008; Witt *et al.* 2008). Essentially the gross wage becomes the unit of value for changes in paid working time resulting from the patient receiving treatment. In the case of an intervention that reduces the risk of mortality, the change in productivity costs is represented by the present value of the additional days in paid work over the individual's lifetime, with these days valued using the gross wage rate. Some health economists have strongly supported the HCA as they perceive it to have a substantial 'theoretical foundation' (Weisbrod 1961). However, common concerns are that the approach discriminates against those outside the formal labour force, such as students, stay-at-home parents, and the elderly (whose value would be lower than that of wage-earners).

There is also concern that the HCA may not hold from a societal viewpoint because of the possibility of replacement, i.e. most economies have some unemployment or underemployment, from which, after some time, another person will fill the vacancy arising when an individual becomes ill (Koopmanschap *et al.* 1995).

The friction cost approach (FCA) was largely developed as a response to this perceived limitation of the HCA, and was put forward by a group of Dutch health economists known as the Erasmus Group (Koopmanschap *et al.* 1995). The FCA aims to adjust the human capital estimates of productivity changes so that the cost is calculated only with reference to the friction periods, i.e. the time required to replace a sick worker and reach the productivity level that the worker achieved before the illness. The main criticism of the FCA is its implied rejection of key assumptions in traditional micro-economic theory (Liljas 1998), such as the existence of involuntary unemployment which effectively reduces the opportunity cost of labour to zero after the friction period. Further, it is unlikely that those who are unemployed will always replace sick workers, particularly in economies with low unemployment levels. In practice, the FCA has been mainly used in the context of cost-of-illness studies (Koopmanschap *et al.*1995), rather than in evaluating health-care interventions from a societal perspective, although several recent cost-effectiveness studies have used the approach (Nielsen *et al.* 2007; Goossens *et al.* 2008).

The Washington Panel, also known as the US Panel (Gold *et al.* 1996), distinguishes between patients' time invested in treatment (time costs) and other time (morbidity costs). They recommend the HCA for the valuation of time costs (plus the costs of substitute labour) and health-related quality-of-life measures for the valuation of morbidity costs. The quality-of-life component is related to the fact that the Panel argues that, unless patients are specifically asked to exclude the impact of illness on income, morbidity costs will already be captured in the quality-of-life levels reported by patients, and so to ask about income loss due to illness separately would result in double counting. However, Liljas (1998) argues that morbidity costs cannot be assumed to be included in an individual's reported utility weight for a health state.

There are advantages and disadvantages associated with the three main schools of thought on valuing productivity costs. Such methodological uncertainty is reflected in the findings of a review of 1039 cost-effectiveness studies on the Health Economic Evaluation Database (HEED), where only 10.4% of the studies had incorporated productivity losses (Pritchard and Sculpher 2000). More detailed information on productivity costs is given by Posnett and Jan (1996), Sculpher (2001), and Drummond (2005).

6.3.3 Informal care

Informal care is often provided by family members, friends, and volunteers. Devoting time and resources to collecting this information may not be worthwhile for interventions where informal care costs are likely to form a very small part of the total costs. However, in other studies non-health-service costs could represent a substantial part of the total costs. For instance, dementia is a disease where the burden of care is likely to fall upon other care agencies and family members rather than entirely on the health and social care services, in which case considering such costs would be important.

To date most economic evaluations have not considered informal care costs. In many cases such costs would probably be minimal but, according to Gold *et al.* (1996), where these costs do exist they should at least be pointed out to the decision-maker even if they are not included in the primary analysis. In practice, some studies identify and measure the amount of treatment or care time from patients, volunteers, family, etc., but do not place a value on this time. These time estimates are then reported alongside health service cost results. This at least provides information to decision-makers on whether particular programmes rely heavily on volunteer or family support. Thorough discussions of informal care costs are given by Sculpher (2001) and McIntosh *et al.* (2010). The key point to note here is that if studies use different perspectives to address the same health-care question, this could lead to an intervention appearing more or less cost-effective depending on the choice of perspective. This point is illustrated in Worked Example 6.1.

Worked Example 6.1. Importance of perspective adopted: pertussis vaccine in children

This example illustrates the importance of including productivity costs in an economic evaluation exploring alternative vaccines for pertussis. In this case, because it is in the context of children, the parent's productivity costs are estimated.

Pertussis, also known as whooping cough, is a highly contagious infection of the respiratory tract, mainly affecting children. Acellular pertussis vaccines were introduced in Canada based on evidence of improved safety and efficacy over whole-cell vaccines, the current standard of care. Older vaccines are relatively inexpensive but are known to cause adverse events. Newer acellular vaccines, although safer, cost approximately twice as much (Iskedjian *et al.* 2001).

To explore the costs and consequences associated with the alternative vaccines, a decision analytic model was constructed which considered the passage of a hypothetical cohort of 100,000 children from birth through to the age of 8 (Iskedjian *et al.* 2001). The health-care costs and savings for this hypothetical cohort were

> **Worked Example 6.1. Importance of perspective adopted: pertussis vaccine in children** (continued)
>
> estimated from both a health service and a societal perspective, and the results are shown in Table 6.2 (rounded to the nearest million Canadian dollars). Over 8 years, for the cohort of 100,000 the new vaccine was estimated to prevent 10,500 cases of pertussis, avoiding 504 hospital admissions. When costs are attached to these figures, taking a narrow health-care perspective (Ontario Ministry), the cost savings are ambiguous with no overall difference between the two vaccines.
>
> However, productivity costs in the form of lost workdays by parents were also estimated in the study. These results showed that the new vaccine avoided an estimated 73,500 days of work absence (producing a net saving of almost CN\$9 million). This clearly illustrates the importance of the perspective adopted in certain situations, as adopting the health service perspective rather than the societal perspective in this case could have led to a different conclusion being drawn on the overall cost-effectiveness of the alternative vaccines.

Table 6.2 Economic impact of a new acellular vaccine in the Ontario pertussis immunization programme

Cost category	Cost (million CN\$)[*]		
	New vaccine	Old vaccine	Net cost of new vs. old vaccine
Vaccine and administration	8	5	3
Disease management costs	4	7	−3
Total costs: health-care perspective	12	12	−
Lost productivity costs	4	13	−9
Other indirect costs	−	1	−1
Total costs: societal perspective	16	26	−10

[*]Costs rounded to nearest million Canadian dollars.
Reproduced from Iskedjian et al. (2001) with permission.

6.4 Constructing a cost dataset

Once resource data and data on unit costs have been collected, the next step is to combine this information. Suppose hypothetically that we were interested in the cost of treating some form of cancer and that one of our categories was surgery costs. We would have collected data on resource use for surgery, such as the surgery itself and the number of days spent in hospital. If we take the number of days spent in hospital, we would also have collected the unit cost for a day in hospital. The resource use and

Table 6.3 Example cost dataset for cancer treatment

Patient ID	Cancer stage	Surgery (£)	Radio-therapy (£)	Chemo-therapy (£)	Hormone therapy (£)	Complications (£)	Inpatient palliative care (£)	Follow-up (£)	Total cost (£)
1	1	2147	2868	262	0	1195	0	402	6876
2	1	0	7465	0	0	7238	137	332	15173
3	1	0	7767	0	0	0	0	141	7908
4	1	0	2868	4482	0	3076	5965	40	16433
5	1	1952	0	0	186	0	0	1085	3224
6	2	0	2793	0	0	0	1784	91	4669
7	2	0	6418	0	42	0	873	199	7532
8	2	0	6418	0	0	0	0	356	6774
9	2	2343	0	1476	0	1206	0	1112	6138
10	2	0	6386	809	144	0	3706	229	11276
Sum for each category		6443	42,987	7031	373	12,717	12,466	3989	86,006
Average for each category		644.33	4298.70	703.14	37.30	1271.66	1246.62	398.86	8600.60

unit cost data could then be entered onto a spreadsheet such as Excel or a statistical software package such as STATA. If a patient spent 7 days in hospital related to their cancer surgery and each day in hospital cost £300, the cost for days in hospital would be 7 × £300 = £2100. This cost would then be added to the cost of the surgical procedure and other costs such as pre-surgical tests. The resultant cost would be the total cost of surgery for a particular patient.

Other categories of cost such as chemotherapy would be organized in the same manner for this and all other patients in this hypothetical example. Once information on resource use and unit costs have been combined for all resource categories and all patients, the resultant dataset will look like the one shown in Table 6.3 which shows a hypothetical dataset of 10 cancer patients. The first column shows each patient's unique identifying number and the second column shows the stage of cancer (1 or 2); subsequent columns show information on the costs of different treatment resources such as surgery, chemotherapy, radiotherapy, and inpatient palliative care. The rows provide information on the costs incurred by each individual patient, and the average cost per patient for each variable can be determined. As this dataset has complete data for all patients, with no missing data, the sum of the average cost per variable is the same as the average of the total cost per patient: £8600.60 (£86,006.01/10). However, if information was missing, for example on the radiotherapy costs of some patients, this would not be the case (this is discussed in Chapter 7).

6.5 Adjustments to cost data

Once data on resource use and unit costs have been collected, it is possible to undertake any other adjustments that may be required. For example, if data have been collected over a long period of time, costs may have been incurred at different times; they may also have been incurred in different countries and currencies. For differential timings, the two key adjustments that need to be considered relate to time preference and inflation. Time preference refers to the different valuation individuals tend to place on goods or services that are consumed now or at some point in the future. Inflation refers to the general upward movement of the nominal price of goods and services over time.

6.5.1 Discounting

Most economists agree that costs and benefits occurring at different times should not be given the same weighting. This is because of a preference to incur costs later in the future, rather than immediately (Cairns 2001). It is also because resources not spent now can be invested at a real rate of return, and therefore there is an opportunity cost of incurring them now. For example, if £100 was available to spend or invest now and the real rate of return was 5%, it could be invested and in 5 years would equal £128. By the same logic, if £100 was required in 5 years, only £77 would need to be invested now.

To account for time preference and opportunity cost, a discount rate is normally applied, using the formula

$$C_p = \frac{Cf_1}{(1+r)} + \frac{Cf_2}{(1+r)^2} + \frac{Cf_3}{(1+r)^3} \cdots\cdots + \frac{Cf_n}{(1+r)^n}$$

where C_p is the present value of costs, Cf_n is the future cost at year n, and r is the rate of discount (for ready-made discounting tables, see Drummond *et al.* (2005)). Currently, the UK Treasury recommends a discount rate of 3.5% for both costs and benefits for the first 30 years of an analysis and 3% thereafter, but other government departments and agencies and other countries use different rates, although many use 3% (Glick *et al.* 2007).

In the UK the different factors comprising the discount rate have been 'unbundled' in the current edition of the *Green Book* (HM Treasury 2004). The social time preference rate (STPR) is defined as the value society attaches to present as opposed to future consumption. This has two components:

• the rate at which individuals discount future consumption compared with present consumption on the assumption of no change in levels of income
• the effect of increased income over time.

As income increases over time we value a specific incremental rise less. Therefore we need to allow for the fact that gross domestic product (GDP) and overall wealth are expected to increase in the future.

The rate at which individuals discount future consumption includes uncertainty about the future (the expected returns may not materialize, or an individual may not survive to enjoy them) and pure time preference. This risk-adjusted time preference rate is estimated as 1.5% annually. The effect of increased income over time is estimated as 2% annually, so the UK government guidance is that the discount rate is now set at 3.5% per annum (HM Treasury 2004).

6.5.2 Inflation

Sometimes costs for a particular intervention could be incurred at different times, and trials running over many years may collect costs at different time periods. Therefore it is important to ensure that costs are all placed on a common base year, and if necessary adjusted to this year to eliminate the effects of inflation. This adjustment can be done using measures of domestic inflation such as consumer price indices or GDP deflators. The consumer price index (CPI) reflects the change in cost to the consumer of purchasing a fixed basket of goods and services. The GDP price deflator is a price index that measures the change in the price level of GDP relative to real output, i.e. it measures the average annual rate of price change in the economy as a whole.

Variants of these indices are producer- or industry-specific indexes, and an example is the Hospital and Community Health Services (HCHS) pay and price index in England. This is a weighted average of two separate inflation indices: the pay cost index (PCI) and the health service cost index (HSCI). The PCI measures pay inflation and is a weighted average of increases in unit staff costs for each of the staff groups within the HCHS sector. Pay cost inflation tends to be higher than pay settlement

Table 6.4 UK Hospital and Community Health Services pay and prices index

Year	Pay (%)	Prices (%)	Pay and prices (%)	Index (1996–1997 = 100)
1997–1998	2.5	0.4	1.7	101.7
1998–1999	4.9	2.5	4.0	105.8
1999–2000	6.9	1.2	4.5	110.5
2000–2001	7.2	−0.3	4.2	115.2
2001–2002	8.3	0.1	5.1	121.0
2002–2003	5.0	0.9	3.5	125.3
2003–2004	7.3	1.5	5.2	131.8
2004–2005	4.5	1.0	3.3	136.1
2005–2006	4.7	1.9	3.7	141.2
2006–2007	4.1	3.0	3.7	146.4
2007–2008	3.5	1.8	2.9	150.7

Source: UK Department of Health 2009.

inflation because of an element of pay drift within each staff group. Estimates of pay inflation are based on information supplied by the UK Department of Health based on pay awards to NHS staff and earnings surveys. The other component of the HCHS, the HSCI, is calculated monthly and measures changes in the price of each of 41 sub-indices of goods and services purchased by the NHS. The PCI and the HSCI are weighted together according to the proportion of expenditure on each. This provides an HCHS combined pay and prices inflation figure. Table 6.4 shows inflation figures for the years 1997 to 2008 from the HCHS index. The baseline year for the index can be varied, but is shown here as 1996–1997 = 100. To use these data, for example to convert a cost of £1500 in 1998–1999 prices to 2007–2008 prices, we would simply calculate £1500 × (150.7/105.8) = £1500 × 1.424 = £2137.

When analysing clinical trials that have run over many years, in practice it is common to undertake the cost analysis towards the end of the trial, and to apply unit costs prevailing at the end of the trial to resource use incurred at any point during the trial. This avoids the need to collect different unit costs for different years of the study and hence the need to adjust for inflation, but it also ignores the possibility that relative prices of different resources have changed over time.

6.5.3 Converting costs into a common currency

If an economic evaluation is being performed on a multinational basis or has to make use of unit costs from another country, it will be necessary to convert costs into a common currency base. To date, two main approaches have been used to convert cost data across countries: exchange rates and purchasing power parities (PPPs).

Exchange rates are the prices (rates) at which currencies are bought and sold on the international market. In the long run they will tend to equalize prices of internationally traded goods, but they may also be influenced by many other factors including macro-economic expectations and political uncertainty, and do not necessarily reflect the prices of non-tradables such as health care. As a result they are not necessarily a good way of translating the cost of a health intervention in one country into the comparable cost in another country. For example, between 2000 and 2010 the exchange rate between the UK (£) and the euro (€) varied between £1 = €0.59 and £1 = €0.98, but there is no reason to think that the actual cost of performing a hip replacement operation in Germany compared with the UK fluctuated by anything like this.

In contrast PPPs are an explicit attempt to circumvent such fluctuations in exchange rates by calculating how much it costs in different countries to purchase a standardized set of goods and services, such as the rental of a serviced two-bedroom apartment in a city centre. If the answer is £500 per week in London and €750 in Frankfurt, this suggests that €1.5 has the same purchasing power as £1, i.e. for every £1, one would need €1.5 to obtain a more or less identical good or service in Frankfurt compared with London. The PPP approach has been used extensively by the World Bank to make national income comparisons between countries across all components of GDP in international dollars (Heston *et al.* 2009). International dollars have the same purchasing power as the US dollar has in the USA and therefore provide a means of translating and comparing costs from one country to another using a common reference point. Various organizations such as the Organization for Economic Cooperation and Development (OECD) and the World Bank produce PPPs (OECD 2009; World Bank 2009), and these use the US dollar as the reference base, i.e. compared in national currency units per US dollar. Eurostat also produce PPPs using the euro as the reference base, with rates for all countries in the European Union and major economies such as the USA and Japan (Eurostat 2009).

Table 6.5 shows the PPP rates for selected countries for the year 2007, where US$1 is set as the reference figure. To use these rates, for instance to convert US$500 to British sterling, multiply the US$500 by the PPP rate for the UK: $500 \times 0.656 = £328$. The table also shows the average exchange rate for the same countries for 2007. It is evident that the exchange rate and the PPP rate differ significantly in some cases, such as the UK, Sweden, and Poland.

The World Health Organization's WHO-CHOICE project has developed an international dataset of health-care costs and input prices (Adam *et al.* 2003b; Johns *et al.* 2003) presented in international dollars.

A variant of the PPP approach is the Big Mac Index, introduced in *The Economist* in September 1986 as a light-hearted illustration of purchasing power variations and subsequently published by that journal annually. In the Big Mac Index, the basket of goods in question consists of just one item: a Big Mac hamburger, sold by the McDonald's fast food restaurants. The burger was chosen because it is available to a common specification in many countries around the world, but with local McDonald's franchisees having significant responsibility, at least in theory, for negotiating input prices. For these reasons, the index enables a comparison to be made between the currencies of many countries (Economist 2009). For example, using figures from

Table 6.5 Selected OECD purchasing power parity and exchange rates (2007)

Country	Exchange rate*	PPP rate†
USA (base)	1.00	1.00
UK	0.499	0.656
Sweden	6.76	9.10
Japan	118	120
Portugal	0.731	0.679
Spain	0.731	0.745
New Zealand	1.36	1.54
Australia	1.20	1.42
Poland	2.77	1.89

*Rates for Portugal and Spain are the same because they are in euros.
†Figures are shown in domestic currency units per $US
Sources: www.oanda.com (historical exchange rates); OECD Statistics Directorate (www.oecd.org).

July 2008, the price of a Big Mac averaged $3.57 in the USA and £2.29 in the UK, and so the implied purchasing power parity was $3.57/£2.29 = $1.56 to £1. This compares with an actual exchange rate of $2.00 to £1 at the time, suggesting that the exchange rate was overvaluing sterling against the dollar by approximately 22%. The Big Mac index has occasionally been used in multinational cost-effectiveness studies where OECD PPP rates are not available for all countries (Briggs *et al.* 2010).

Although the PPP approach has also been advocated as an improvement on exchange rate conversions for making health-care-specific comparisons (Kanavos 1999), there are several concerns with this approach. One important concern is that the relative weights within the basket of goods used to construct the PPP index are unlikely to be the same as the weights for specific health-care interventions (even with specific health-care PPPs). In response to this, some health economists have developed intervention-specific PPPs for use within particular multicentre studies that they are undertaking (Wordsworth and Ludbrook 2005). However, despite concerns over the contents of the PPP baskets, PPPs are likely to be less unreliable than exchange rates in comparing cost-effectiveness results across locations.

As a final note on costing adjustments, because inflation rates are likely to differ across countries, it is better to work in local currencies first (i.e. adjust for inflation using a country's own rate) and then convert to US dollars, international dollars, or another currency at a later stage (Fox-Rushby and Cairns 2005).

6.6 **Event-based cost analysis**

So far we have assumed that a cost analysis proceeds by first recording all relevant resource use, then attaching unit costs, and then calculating a total cost per patient in order to compare mean costs (e.g. between two groups in a trial). However, in some cases it may be desirable to isolate and quantify the effects on costs of a particular event such as a major complication, either because the events are relatively rare and their effect might otherwise be lost against a background of 'noise' generated by other costs, or because it is desired to extract estimates of the costs of particular events in order to use these estimates as parameter values in subsequent modelling. Similar issues arose in Chapter 4 in the context of quality of life, and the concept of 'event-based' quality-of-life estimation was introduced. For similar reasons, the same approach can be adopted to the analysis of cost data, and has been referred to as 'event-based cost analysis'. This type of cost analysis is illustrated in Worked Example 6.2.

Worked Example 6.2. Event-based cost analysis of magnesium sulphate for pre-eclampsia

A useful example of event-based costing is the economic analysis which accompanied the Magpie Trial (for trial methods see Altman *et al.* 2002). This 33-country multinational trial examined the effectiveness and cost-effectiveness of using magnesium sulphate ($MgSO_4$) for pre-eclampsia to prevent eclampsia. Pre-eclampsia is a multisystem disorder of pregnancy, generally associated with high blood pressure and protein in the urine, which affects 2–8% of pregnancies. Eclampsia is the occurrence of convulsions superimposed on pre-eclampsia and, although rare, has a high mortality rate. Magnesium sulphate is the main anticonvulsant used for treating eclampsia. The Magpie Trial included 9996 women with pre-eclampsia, across low-, middle-, and high-income countries. The study examined whether the treatment should be given to all women with pre-eclampsia as a prophylactic for reducing the number of women with eclampsia. The women were randomized into a magnesium sulphate treatment group or a control group (Altman *et al.* 2002).

The main outcome measure for the economic component of the trial (Simon *et al.* 2006) was the number of cases of eclampsia prevented. Hospital resource use data were available for the trial period, and country-specific unit costs were collected (US dollars, year 2001). Unit costs were combined with hospital resource use to calculate the cost per pregnancy, including both mothers and babies. Total cost was the sum of 'treatment cost' for magnesium sulphate and its administration, plus 'other costs'. These 'other costs' covered all other aspects of hospital care in the trial such as actually treating pre-eclampsia, eclampsia or treatment side-effects. Cost-effectiveness was estimated for three categories of countries grouped by gross national income (GNI) into high-, middle- and low-GNI countries.

Because of the high chance that the 'other costs' recorded would include many items that were not directly related to the trial intervention, and the relatively low frequency of eclampsia, it was highly probable that simply comparing 'other costs' in different arms of the trial would fail to reveal any statistically significant differences. Any signal would be hidden in the background noise. However, simply separating out hospital admissions directly related to eclampsia would have risked ignoring other reasons for hospitalization that may have

Worked Example 6.2. Event-based cost analysis of magnesium sulphate for pre-eclampsia *(continued)*

been indirectly related to eclampsia. To deal with this, the authors conducted an event-based cost analysis in which the influence of eclampsia on 'other costs' was estimated using multivariate regression analysis, with the occurrence of eclampsia as an explanatory variable.

The results showed that with the observed unadjusted cost data there was no statistically significant difference in 'other costs' or total costs between the intervention and the control arm in any of the GNI groups. However, when a regression approach was used to estimate other costs, true differences were much easier to identify. Table 6.6 presents the results for high-GNI countries (middle- and low-GNI countries showed similar results).

The table shows that when using observed costs, the 'other cost' and 'total cost' results showed large standard deviations within groups and wide confidence intervals around the estimated differences, suggesting a high level of non-trial-related variance in these data. In contrast, the results of the regression approach show much smaller standard deviations within groups and much tighter confidence intervals around the between-group differences. The applied regression model showed that the average hospital cost of a case of eclampsia was $6569 in the high-GNI countries. Using these estimates to adjust the observed 'other costs', the results showed a significant difference in 'other costs' of –$20 in the high-GNI countries (Simon *et al.* 2006).

Table 6.6 Magpie study: health service cost estimates per woman in high gross national income countries*

	MgSO$_4$ ($n = 597$) (mean (SD))	Control ($n = 598$)	Difference (mean, CI)
MgSO$_4$ treatment costs[†]	86 (39)	0	86
Drug	20 (12)	0	20
Administration	66 (29)	0	66
Other costs[†]			
Observed	12,678 (20,704)	12,926 (21,269)	–248 (–2630,2135)
Regression adjusted	12,818 (601)	12,839 (601)	–20 (–60,0)
Total costs[†]			
Observed	12,764 (20,709)	12,926 (21,269)	–162 (–2545, 2221)
Regression adjusted	12,904 (601)	12,839 (601)	65 (26,86)

SD, standard deviation; CI, confidence interval.
*Australia, Canada, Denmark, Israel, Italy, Singapore, The Netherlands, United Arab Emirates, UK, and USA.
[†]Costs are expressed in U.S dollar for year 2001.
Reproduced from Simon *et al.* (2006) with permission.

Further examples of studies using event-based cost analysis can be found in two diabetes studies (Clarke *et al.* 2003; O'Brien *et al.* 2003). Variants of the approach include separating the cost impact of an event into immediate and long-term effects, or separately estimating the effect of an event on different costs, for example the hospital cost impact and the primary care cost impact of a stroke (Clarke *et al.* 2003).

6.7 **Presenting cost results**

Once resource use information has been assembled, unit costs added, and total costs calculated, it is helpful to adopt clear reporting procedures. In particular, all sources of unit cost information should be clearly reported and documented, along with measures of mean resource use and variance for the main items of interest, and mean costs by main category with subtotals and totals. If the study is a randomized trial, between-group differences should also be clearly reported along with confidence intervals (as described in Chapter 7). Unit cost information is commonly presented in a separate table or even as an appendix or web table, while the number of tables required to report resource use and cost data will depend on the complexity of the study and the reporting constraints of the journal.

Table 6.7 reproduces a table from a study examining the costs and outcomes associated with using ultrasonography to diagnose and manage neonatal hip instability (Gray *et al.* 2005). The study was conducted in the UK but reported in an American journal, and so the costs are reported in US dollars. Detailed information on unit costs was given in an appendix, and the table concentrates on health-care resource use and costs in each group. Data are presented on the mean volume of each resource use category used in the ultrasonography group and in the clinical assessment only group, with accompanying standard deviations. The between-group difference is reported with 95% confidence. Similar information is reported for costs, along with an unadjusted total cost across all categories, and in this case a total cost adjusted for any differences in baseline prognostic factors.

It is evident that the only significant difference between the two groups was in the number and cost of ultrasonographs; there is a suggestion that this intervention led to fewer subsequent hospitalizations, fewer days of other treatment, and fewer splints, but these results were not statistically significant. Total costs were lower, but not significantly so, in the ultrasonography group, whether unadjusted or adjusted for baseline differences. The clear recommendation is that it is good practice to report clearly disaggregated information on resource use and costs.

6.8 **Summary**

The costing component of economic evaluation has seen considerable methodological development since the 1990s. In this chapter we have reviewed the basic elements of assembling cost information, including the identification, measurement, and valuation of resources used. We have also examined the different perspectives which can be adopted when deciding what costs to include, and we have considered methods for adjusting cost information for price differences over time and between countries.

Table 6.7 Example of reporting resource use and cost results from a trial-based economic evaluation

Item	Ultrasonography (n=254) (mean (SD))		Non-ultrasonography (n=267) (mean (SD))		Difference (mean (95% CI))	
	Number	Cost	Number	Cost	Number	Cost
Ultrasonographs	2.7 (2.8)	86 (91)	1.4 (2.9)	43 (94)	1.3 (0.8, 1.8)	43 (26, 58)
Radiographs	2.3 (1.9)	85 (70)	2.3 (1.8)	87 (66)	-0.1 (-0.4, 0.3)	-2 (-14, 10)
Outpatient visits	6.0 (3.9)	630 (416)	6.0 (4.3)	615 (448)	0 (-0.7, 0.7)	15 (-54, 91)
Home visits	0.1 (0.9)	19 (133)	0.2 (1.2)	34 (168)	-0.1 (-0.3, 0.1)	-15 (-25, 8)
Hospital admissions	0.3 (1.0)	–	0.3 (1.0)	–	0 (-0.2, 0.1)	–
Days in hospital	0.7 (3.2)	331 (1605)	1.1 (4.6)	535 (2291)	-0.4 (-1.1, 0.3)	-204 (-542, 136)
Splints	0.4 (0.6)	31 (42)	0.5 (0.6)	37 (42)	-0.1 (-0.2, 0.0)	-6 (-14, 2)
Other treatments	0.2 (0.8)	–	0.2 (0.7)	–	0.0 (-0.1, 0.1)	–
Days/other treatment	12.4 (45.0)	40 (144)	15.7 (64.9)	50 (130)	-3.2 (-12.8, 6.3)	-10 (-42, 21)
Primary care contacts	2.4 (6.9)	75 (211)	2.7 (7.0)	86 (213)	-0.3 (-1.5, 1.9)	-11 (-48, 26)
Total		1298 (2168)		1488 (2912)		-190 (-630, 250)
Total adjusted for baseline prognostic factors*						-171 (-602, 261)

*Ethnic group; maternal age; unilateral/bilateral level of clinical suspicion; family history of congenital dislocation of hip; parity of mother.

Reproduced from Gray et al. (2005) with permission.

Finally, we have introduced the event-based cost analysis approach as a way of identifying and isolating the effects of events of interest on costs.

In the next chapter we turn to the analysis of cost data, particularly concerning skewed data, missing data, and variation at the centre or hospital level as well as between patients.

References

Adam, T., Koopmanschap, M.A., and Evans, D.B. (2003a). Cost-effectiveness analysis. Can we reduce variability in costing methods? *International Journal of Technology Assessment in Health Care*, **19**, 407–20.

Adam, T., Evans, D.B., and Murray, C.J. (2003b). Econometric estimation of country-specific hospital costs. *Cost Effectiveness and Resource Allocation*, **1**, 3.

Altman, D., Carroli, G., Duley, L., *et al.* (2002). Do women with pre-eclampsia, and their babies, benefit from magnesium sulphate? The Magpie Trial: a randomised placebo-controlled trial. *Lancet*, **359**, 1877–90.

Briggs, A., Glick, H., Lozano-Ortega, G., *et al.* (2010). Is treatment with ICS and LABA cost-effective for COPD? Multinational economic analysis of the TORCH study. *European Respiratory Journal*, **35**, 532–9.

Brouwer, W., Rutten, F., and Koopmanscap, M.A. (2001). Costing in economic evaluations. In: Drummond, M. and McGuire, A. (eds). *Economic Evaluation in Health Care: Merging Theory with Practice*. Oxford University Press.

Cairns, J. (2001). Discounting in economic evaluation. In: Drummond, M. and McGuire, A. (eds). *Economic Evaluation in Health Care: Merging Theory with Practice*. Oxford University Press.

Clarke, P., Gray, A., Legood, R., Briggs, A., and Holman, R. (2003). The impact of diabetes-related complications on healthcare costs: results from the United Kingdom Prospective Diabetes Study (UKPDS Study No. 65). *Diabetic Medicine*, **20**, 442–50.

Clarke, P.M., Fiebig, D.G., and Gerdtham, U.G. (2008). Optimal recall length in survey design. *Journal of Health Economics*, **27**, 1275–84.

Curtis, L. (2009). *Unit Costs of Health and Social Care 2009*. Personal Social Services Research Unit, University of Kent (available online at: www.pssru.ac.uk).

Department of Health. (2008). *Reference Cost Index*. Department of Health, London (available online at: www.dh.gov.uk/en/Publicationsandstatistics).

Department of Health (2009). Hospital and Community Health Services (HCHS) Pay and Prices Index. Department of Health, London.

Department of Health (2010). *Payment by Results*. Department of Health, London (available online at: http://www.dh.gov.uk/en/Managingyourorganisation/Financeandplanning/NHSFinancialReforms/DH_900).

Drummond, M.F., Sculpher, M.J., Torrance, G.W., O'Brien, B.J., and Stoddart, G.L. (2005). *Methods for the Economic Evaluation of Health Care Programmes* (3rd edn). Oxford University Press.

Economist (2009). The Big Mac index. London, The Economist (available online at: http://www.economist.com/markets/indicators/displaystory).

Eurostat (2009). *Purchasing Power Parities* (available online at: http://epp.eurostat.ec.europa.eu/portal/page/portal/hicp/data/database).

Fox-Rushby, J. and Cairns, J. (2005). *Understanding Public Health. Economic Evaluation.* Open University Press, Milton Keynes.

Glick, H., Doshi, J.A., Sonnad, S.S., and Polsky, D. (2007). *Economic Evaluation in Clinical Trials.* Oxford University Press.

Gold, M.R., Siegel, J.E., Russell, L.B., and Weinstein, M.C. (1996). *Cost-effectiveness in Health and Medicine.* Oxford University Press, New York.

Gray, A., Elbourne, D., Dezateux, C., King, A., Quinn, A., and Gardner, F. (2005). Economic evaluation of ultrasonography imaging in the diagnosis and management of developmental hip dysplasia. *Journal of Bone and Joint Surgery (American Volume)*, **87**, 2472–9.

Goossens, L.M., Standaert, B., Hartwig, N., Hövels, A.M., and Al, M.J. (2008). The cost-utility of rotavirus vaccination with Rotarix (RIX4414) in the Netherlands. *Vaccine*, **26**, 1118–27.

Heston, A., Summers, R., and Aten, B. (2009). *Penn World Tables Version 6.3.* Center for International Comparisons of Production, Income and Prices at the University of Pennsylvania, Philadelphia, PA.

HM Treasury (2004). *Green Book: Appraisal and Evaluation in Central Government.* Stationery Office, London (available online at: http://greenbook.treasury.gov.uk/).

Iskedjian, M., Einarson, T.R., O'Brien, B.J., *et al.* (2001). Economic evaluation of a new acellular vaccine for pertussis in Canada. *Pharmacoeconomics*, **19**, 551–63.

Johns, B., Baltussen, R., and Hutubessy, R. (2003). Programme costs in the economic evaluation of health interventions. *Cost Effectiveness and Resource Allocation*, **1**, 1.

Kanavos, P. and Mossialos, E. (1999). International comparisons of health care expenditures: what we know and what we do not know. *Journal of Health Services Research and Policy*, **4**, 122–6.

Koopmanschap, M.A., Rutten, F.F., van Ineveld, B.M., and van Roijen, L. (1995). The friction cost method for measuring indirect costs of disease. *Journal of Health Economics*, **14**, 171–89.

Liljas, B. (1998). How to calculate indirect costs in economic evaluations. *Pharmacoeconomics*, **13**, 1–7.

Lofland, J.H., Pizzi, L., and Frick, K.D. (2004). A review of health-related workplace productivity loss instruments. *Pharmacoeconomics*, **22**, 165–84.

Lorgelly, P.K., Joshi, D., Iturriza Gómara, M., Gray, J., and Mugford, M. (2008). Exploring the cost effectiveness of an immunization programme for rotavirus gastroenteritis in the United Kingdom. *Epidemiology and Infection*, **136**, 44–55.

Luce, B.R., Manning, W.G., Siegel, J.E., *et al.* (1996). Estimating costs in cost-effectiveness analysis. In: Gold, M.R., Siegel, J.E., Russell, L.B., and Weinstein, M.C. (eds), *Cost-Effectiveness in Health and Medicine.* Oxford University Press, New York.

McIntosh, E. (2010). Shadow pricing in health care. In: McIntosh, E., Louviere, J.J., Frew, E., and Clarke, P.M. (eds), *Applied Methods of Cost-Benefit Analysis in Health Care.* Oxford University Press.

NICE (2008). *A Guide to the Methods of Technology Appraisal.* National Institute for Health and Clinical Excellence, London.

Nielsen, M., Hes, F.J., Vasen, H.F., and van den Hout, W.B. (2007). Cost-utility analysis of genetic screening in families of patients with germline *MUTYH* mutations. *BMC Medical Genetics*, **8**, 42.

O'Brien, J.A., Patrick, A.R., and Caro, J. (2003). Estimates of direct medical costs for microvascular and macrovascular complications resulting from type 2 diabetes mellitus in the United States in 2000. *Clinical Therapeutics*, **25**, 1017–38.

OECD (2009). *Comparative Price Levels 2009*. OECD, Paris (available online at: http://www. oecd.org/dataoecd/48/18/18598721.pdf).

Osterhaus, J.T., Gutterman, D.L., and Plachetka, J.R. (1992). Healthcare resource and lost labour costs of migraine headache in the US. *Pharmacoeconomics*, **2**, 67–76.

Posnett, J. and Jan, S. (1996). Indirect cost in economic evaluation: the opportunity cost of unpaid inputs. *Health Economics*, **5**, 13–23.

Pritchard, C. and Sculpher, M. (2000). *Productivity Costs: Principles and Practice in Economic Evaluation*. Office of Health Economics, London.

Raikou, M., Briggs, A., Gray, A., and McGuire, A. (2000). Centre-specific or average unit costs in multi-centre studies? Some theory and simulation. *Health Economics*, **9**, 191–8.

Reilly, M.C., Zbrozek, A.S., and Dukes, E.M. (1993). The validity and reproducibility of a work productivity and activity impairment instrument. *Pharmacoeconomics*, **4**, 353–65.

Rice, D.P. and Cooper, B.S. (1967). The economic value of life. *American Journal of Public Health*, **57**, 1954–66.

Sculpher, M. (2001). The role and estimation of productivity costs in economic evaluation. In: Drummond, M. and McGuire, A. (eds). *Economic Evaluation in Health Care: Merging Theory with Practice*. Oxford University Press.

Simon, J., Gray, A., Duley, L., *et al.* (2006). Cost-effectiveness of prophylactic magnesium sulphate for 9996 women with pre-eclampsia from 33 countries: economic evaluation of the Magpie Trial. *British Journal of Obstetrics and Gynaecology*, **113**, 144–51.

van den Berg, B., Brouwer, W.B.F., and Koopmanschap, M.A. (2004). Economic evaluation of informal care: an overview of methods and application. *European Journal of Health Economics*, **5**, 36–45.

van Roijen, L., Essink-Bot, M., Koopmanschap, M., Bonsel, G., and Rutten, F. (1996). Labor and health status in economic evaluation of health care. The Health and Labor Questionnaire. *International Journal of Technology Assessment in Health Care*, **12**, 405–15.

Weisbrod, B. (1961). The valuation of human capital. *Journal of Political Economy*, **69**, 425–36.

Witt C.M., Reinhold, T., Jena, S., Brinkhaus, B., and Willich, S.N. (2008). Cost-effectiveness of acupuncture treatment in patients with headache. *Cephalalgia*, **28**, 334–45.

Wordsworth, S., Ludbrook, A., Caskey, F., and Macleod, A. (2005). Collecting unit cost data in multicentre studies: creating comparable methods. *European Journal of Health Economics*, **6**, 38–44.

Wordsworth, S. and Ludbrook, A. (2005). Comparing costing results in across country economic evaluations: the use of technology specific purchasing power parities. *Health Economics*, **14**, 93–9.

World Bank (2009). *Global Purchasing Power Parities and Real Expenditures 2005*. World Bank International Comparison Program, Washington, DC (available online at: http://siteresources.worldbank.org/ICPINT/Resources/icp-final.pdf).

Chapter 7

Analysing costs

In Chapter 6 we considered the rationale behind costing in economic evaluation and some basic steps in undertaking a costing study. In this chapter we explore issues surrounding the analysis of cost data once collected and entered into a spreadsheet such as Excel or statistical software packages such as STATA, SAS or SPSS. We begin by highlighting the importance of providing basic descriptive statistics on costs, with measures of central tendency (such as the mean) and measures of variability and precision to support the mean cost. Next, we examine the issue of skewness in cost data, and review different options that have been proposed to handle this problem such as transformations, generalized linear models, and the non-parametric bootstrap. We then explore the problem of missing cost data, along with potential ways to handle this common problem, including a worked example on the use of imputation. Worked examples are then presented to demonstrate two popular methods to deal with the issue of censored costs data: the Kaplan–Meier sample average (KMSA) estimator and the inverse probability weighting (IPW) estimator. We then discuss the use of multi-level modelling to deal with hierarchical data, and finish with two exercises, the first on bootstrapping and the second on KMSA.

7.1 Description and basic statistical analysis of cost data

The previous chapter described the steps involved in constructing a cost dataset, with each patient in a separate row and categories of costs specified in different columns. Because no data were missing this was a rectangular dataset. Prior to performing any formal analysis on cost datasets, such as calculating differences between treatment groups, basic descriptive information should be reported. These descriptive statistics include measures of central tendency, variability, and precision.

7.1.1 Measures of central tendency

Measures of central tendency include the arithmetic mean, the median, and the mode. The arithmetic mean (also known as sample mean or average) is the sum of the data values divided by the number of values contributing to that total:

$$\bar{x} = \frac{1}{n}\sum_{i=1}^{n} x_i$$

where $\bar{x}$ represents the arithmetic mean, x_i the individual data values, and n the sample size. The sample mean is considered an unbiased and efficient estimator for the population mean but it is sensitive to the presence of outliers.

The median is the value of the observation that divides the distribution of the data into two equal fractions. It is sometimes used to describe skewed or non-normal data because it is not sensitive to outliers. The mode is the value that occurs most frequently in the variable under evaluation. The application of the mode to cost data is very limited, partly because it is not necessarily unique as more than one value may be equally frequent. Overall, the crucial information for cost data is usually the arithmetic mean, i.e. the average cost. This is largely because the mean times the sample size, or the mean times the population of interest, will give the best estimate of the total cost of a programme or intervention, and policy-makers will almost invariably need information on the total cost of implementing a programme or intervention (Thompson and Barber 2000; Briggs and Gray 1998).

7.1.2 Measures of variability

Information on the variability or range of cost values permits the analyst to judge to what extent the average cost data are representative of the patients studied. There are several descriptive statistics that report variability, including percentiles, the range, the interquartile range, variance, and standard deviation.

Percentiles are values of a variable that define the percentage of observations below those values. For example, the 20th percentile is the value below which 20% of the observations are located. The 25th percentile is known as the first quartile, the 50th percentile is the median or second quartile, and the 75th percentile is known as the third quartile.

The range is a measure of distance from the lowest to the highest value of a variable. It is an easy measure to calculate, but the presence of outliers may result in the range giving a distorted picture of variability. To account for this, the interquartile range is often used, which is obtained by discarding the upper and lower 25% of the distribution of values. It is the difference between the 75th and 25th percentiles.

The sample variance (S^2) is the sum of the squared deviations from the mean divided by $n - 1$. Formally, the sample variance is defined as

$$S^2 = \frac{1}{n-1} \sum_{i=1}^{n} (x_i - \overline{x})^2$$

where $\overline{x}$ represents the arithmetic mean, x_i the individual data values, and n the sample size.

The sample standard deviation (S) is simply the square root of the sample variance, i.e. $\sqrt{S^2}$. Like the variance, it is a widely used measure of variation and is measured in the same units as the mean. For instance, in the analysis of cost data, the standard deviation will be expressed in monetary units and will typically be denoted by SD next to the mean.

7.1.3 Measures of precision

In the statistical analysis of cost data, we are primarily interested in inferences around the mean and mean differences between groups. Therefore evaluating the precision of the sample mean is extremely useful. Standard errors and confidence intervals both reflect the precision of the estimated mean.

The standard error (SE) of the mean is the standard deviation of the sampling distribution of the mean. It is obtained by dividing the sample standard deviation S by the square root of the sample size n, i.e. $SE = S/\sqrt{n}$.

The standard error and the sample standard deviation are often confused. However, the sample standard deviation is a measure of variability between individuals whereas the standard error is a measure of the uncertainty of the sample statistic, for instance the mean derived from individual measurements.

Confidence intervals (CIs) are a range of values that are likely to cover the true yet unknown population mean value, and are based on the notion of repetition of a study. For instance, if a study were to be repeated 100 times, the calculated 95% CI (which would differ for each of these samples) could be expected to include the true population mean on 95 occasions. CIs are formally defined as follows:

$$\bar{x} \pm t_{1-\alpha/2} \times SE(\bar{x})$$

where $\bar{x}$ is the mean, $t_{1-\alpha/2}$ is the appropriate value from the t-distribution with $n-1$ degrees of freedom associated with a confidence of $100(1-\alpha)\%$, α is the significance level and $SE(\bar{x})$ is the standard error of the mean. When a 95% CI is constructed around a mean difference between two groups, $t_{1-\alpha/2}$ is the appropriate value from the t-distribution with $n_1 - n_2 - 2$ degrees of freedom, where n_1 is the sample size in the first group and n_2 is the sample size in the second group.

7.2 The distribution of the data

The methods described in the previous section, such as parametric confidence interval estimation and measures of central tendency, rely for their validity on the underlying distribution of the data. As any introduction to medical statistics makes clear, standard parametric methods are typically based on the assumption of a normal distribution. However, as experience has accumulated on the analysis of data for economic evaluation of health interventions, it has become increasingly apparent that cost and outcome data may not be normally distributed. This in turn has led to a great deal of interest in parametric and non-parametric methods that might address this problem.

In this section we examine the distribution of data, considering the normal distribution and departures from it such as skewness. Potential solutions for dealing with the problem of skewed cost data are then put forward.

7.2.1 Normal and skewed distributions

To understand the underlying distribution of a variable, we can display the data graphically, with histograms being particularly useful. A histogram is a graphical display of tabulated frequencies plotted using bars. Each bar represents the frequencies or proportions of cases that are included in a particular bin (an interval). The histogram in Figure 7.1 plots a typical variable that might form an important part of a cost analysis: time in theatre for patients undergoing surgery. In this hypothetical example

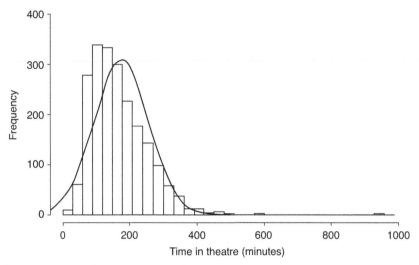

Fig. 7.1 Histogram for time in theatre for patients undergoing surgery.

there are 2097 patients, each having time in theatre. The horizontal axis shows information on theatre time (in minutes) and the vertical axis shows how frequently particular times occur. The figure shows the actual data for the patients (the bars) and superimposed on this is a line indicating the shape of the normal distribution. The normal distribution is a pattern for the distribution of data which has a bell-shaped curve. For a large population of independent random numbers the majority of the population often cluster near a central value, and the frequencies of the higher and lower values taper off smoothly on either side, creating the bell shape. The normal distribution is sometimes called the Gaussian distribution in honour of Carl Friedrich Gauss, a famous mathematician who used the distribution to analyse astronomical data. Important features of this distribution are that the curve is symmetric, the probability of deviations from the mean is comparable in each direction, and the data are less likely to produce unusually extreme values compared with other distributions.

In contrast, if we now look closely at the bars on Figure 7.1 we can see that, although most patients are clustered in the same bins, there is a long right-hand tail, with a small number of patients spending much longer than average in theatre. This indicates that the data do not follow the normal distribution particularly well. This distributional shape is described as right-skewed or positively skewed.

7.2.2 Skewed cost data

Skewness measures the asymmetry of a distribution. The expected value of skewness for a symmetric distribution (e.g. the normal distribution) is zero. A skewness value greater than 1 generally indicates a distribution that differs significantly from a normal distribution. Formally, this is defined as follows:

If m_r is the rth moment about the mean $\bar{x}$:

$$m_r = \frac{1}{n}\sum_{i=1}^{n}(x_i - \bar{x})^r$$

where n is the sample size and x_i are the individual data values; the coefficient of skewness is defined as $m_3 m_2^{-\frac{3}{2}}$.

Cost data often have distributions that are skewed to the right. The main reasons for this are as follows:

- The cost incurred by a participant in a study cannot be negative, thus placing a bound on the lower tail of the distribution.
- There could be many patients with zero costs.
- There may be a few study participants who require much more health care than the average individual, creating a long right tail.

Skewness needs to be explored before conducting any further analysis, because if skewness is large, it has the potential to affect the measures of precision presented earlier and any subsequent statistical analysis. Several methods have been proposed to help deal with skewed data, including the median, data transformations, the non-parametric bootstrap and non-parametric tests, generalized linear models, and reliance on the central limit theorem. These methods are considered below.

7.2.3 Median cost

The mean and median are identical in normally distributed data, but differ with skewed data. With right-skewness the median is smaller than the arithmetic mean, and vice versa for left-skewness. The median is sometimes considered an attractive statistic to present with skewed data, partly because it is less influenced by outliers than the mean. The median can be useful for purely descriptive purposes. However, it will not be helpful to health-care policy-makers, who require information on the total cost of implementing a health-care intervention which, as noted earlier, cannot be obtained by multiplying the median cost by the total number of patients.

7.2.4 Data transformations

An alternative way of dealing with skewness is to transform the data, for example by using a log transformation. Individual health-care resource use or cost data that are skewed on the normal scale may well be log-normally distributed, in which case parametric methods can be used on the transformed data without violating the assumption of normality (Briggs and Gray 1998). Unfortunately, although transformations provide potentially more efficient estimates of cost data (Manning and Mullahy 2001; O'Hagan and Stevens 2003), they have been called into question for use in cost-effectiveness analysis for several reasons. Firstly, the method could perform badly if inappropriate transformations are used (Briggs et al. 2005). Secondly, many transformations cannot be used if there are zero costs in the data, which is common with health-care resource use; the method of replacing zero by a small number is no longer recommended. Thirdly, if we are interested in making estimates and inferences about differences in the arithmetic means of untransformed costs, it is necessary to back-transform the point estimates of central tendency and variation (Duan 1983; Ai and Norton 2000). However, once back-transformed, inferences about the log of costs translate into inferences about differences in the geometric rather than arithmetic mean. The geometric mean is similar to the arithmetic mean, except that instead of adding the set of numbers and then dividing the sum by the count of numbers in the set (n), the numbers are multiplied and then the nth root of the resulting product is taken, which, with variable cost data, will be a downward-biased estimate of the arithmetic mean (Chiang and Wainwright 2005). Although methods to deal with this, such as smearing, have been proposed (Duan 1983; Manning 1998), these in turn are dependent on the appropriate transformation having been made in the first place. These issues are described and illustrated in detail by Glick *et al.* (2007).

7.2.5 **Non-parametric methods**

Non-parametric tests which make no assumptions about the underlying distribution of the data are available. Examples include the Mann–Whitney (or Wilcoxon rank–sum) tests, the singular Kolmogorov–Smirnov test, and the Kruskall–Wallis test. The problem with using these tests is that although they can tell us that some measure of the cost distribution differs between the treatment groups, such as its shape or location, they do not necessarily tell us whether the arithmetic means differ between groups. As such, they are rarely used in cost analysis.

However, a non-parametric approach that has gained more widespread use is the bootstrap. In essence bootstrapping mimics a real-world sampling approach. In reality we typically have just one sample of data (our observed sample) and calculate our statistic of interest (such as the mean) from that observed sample. The bootstrap treats the observed sample as an empirical distribution, draws another sample from the observed sample, and calculates the parameter of interest, such as the mean, from the new sample. Crucially, when we take a sample from the observed distribution, each case is returned to the sample every time it is drawn out and so is available to be sampled again. Without this step, known as sampling with replacement, each sample would simply replicate the original sample each time.

The sampling process is then repeated many times to provide a series of resamples or bootstrap datasets, each of which is the equivalent of a repetition of the original data, and all of which have treatment groups of size n_i. Between 25 and 200 resamples are recommended to estimate bootstrap SEs and at least 1000 resamples to estimate bootstrap CIs (Efron and Tibshirani 1993). Figure 7.2 illustrates this re-sampling procedure using a hypothetical dataset with costs for 10 patients.

These bootstrap samples are different from each other because they have been drawn with replacement, and this means that a bootstrap sample may include the costs for some patients more than once, while excluding the costs for others. For example, in Figure 7.2 there are 10 hypothetical patients (column 1), with their corresponding original sample costs (column 2). The mean from this original sample is £20. A bootstrap resample is created by randomly selecting with replacement 10 values

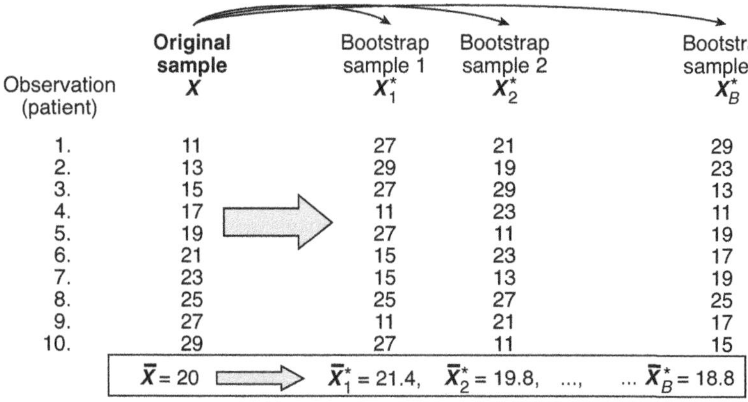

Observation (patient)	Original sample X	Bootstrap sample 1 X_1^*	Bootstrap sample 2 X_2^*	Bootstrap sample B X_B^*
1.	11	27	21	29
2.	13	29	19	23
3.	15	27	29	13
4.	17	11	23	11
5.	19	27	11	19
6.	21	15	23	17
7.	23	15	13	19
8.	25	25	27	25
9.	27	11	21	17
10.	29	27	11	15

$\bar{X} = 20 \implies \bar{X}_1^* = 21.4, \quad \bar{X}_2^* = 19.8, \quad ..., \quad ... \bar{X}_B^* = 18.8$

Fig. 7.2 A bootstrapping example.

from the original sample. In the first resample, patient 9 (who incurred a cost of £27) appears four times, while patient 2 (who incurred a cost of £13) does not appear at all. In the final sample, patient 9 (£27) does not appear. This process gives a vector of bootstrap estimates of the statistic of interest, which is an empirical estimate of the sampling distribution of the statistic of interest, such as the mean. As Figure 7.2 shows, this mean is varying around the original mean of £20, with bootstrap values of £21.4, £19.8, and £18.8.

Once the procedure has been repeated many times, the bootstrap estimates produce a sampling distribution of the mean which can be plotted using a histogram of the vector of bootstrapped statistics. This distribution can also be used to estimate mean costs, SEs, or CIs. Several approaches exist to estimate CIs using bootstrapping, but the simplest is the percentile approach. With this approach, the upper and lower CI are obtained using the $(\alpha/2) \times 100$ and $(1 - \alpha/2) \times 100$ percentiles of the empirical sampling distribution. For 95% CIs, values for the confidence limits are chosen which correspond to the 26th and 975th points in the rank-ordered vector. These points are chosen because this excludes 25 values ($25/1000 = 2.5\%$) at either end of the estimated distribution (Briggs *et al.* 1997). The exercise on bootstrapping at the end of this chapter demonstrates how to produce CIs using bootstrapping.

Although for a while bootstrapping became a recommended technique for dealing with skewed cost data, or at least for testing whether the normal distribution was a reasonable assumption (Barber and Thompson 2000), it has increasingly been recognized that the conditions the bootstrap requires to produce reliable parameter estimates are not fundamentally different from the conditions required by parametric methods (see O'Hagan and Stevens (2003) and Chapter 11). However, bootstrapping has been found to be particularly useful for dealing simultaneously with issues such as censoring, missing data, and skewness, and for producing SEs and CIs. Other uses have recently been proposed for bootstrapping including estimating net benefits and computing cost-effectiveness acceptability curves (Nixon *et al.* 2010). Some of these will be considered in more detail in Chapter 11. An exercise on bootstrapping is presented at the end of this chapter.

7.2.6 Generalized linear models

Another method of handling skewness which overcomes some of the disadvantages associated with transformations is to use a generalized linear model (GLM) to model the mean of the distribution directly rather than focusing on transformation methods (Glick *et al.* 2007). GLMs are essentially a generalization of the linear model which, in its most straightforward form, specifies the (linear) relationship between a dependent (or response) variable Y and a set of predictor variables X. For example, from a dataset with measures of height, weight, and gender, we could estimate an individual's weight as a function of their height and gender, using linear regression to estimate the respective regression coefficients.

A major difference between a simple linear model and a GLM is that with the latter the distribution of the dependent or response variable can be (explicitly) non-normal. GLMs also permit flexible modelling of covariates and enable inferences to be made directly about the mean cost (Manning and Mullahy 2001; Barber and Thompson 2004). The dependent variable values are predicted from a linear combination of predictor variables, which are 'connected' to the dependent variable via a link function. Various link functions (McCullagh and Nelder 1989) can be chosen, such as normal, log, gamma, inverse normal, and Poisson distributions, depending on the assumed distribution of the values of the y variable. A gamma distribution is often used for cost data. The link function directly characterizes how the mean $E(y/x)$ on the untransformed scale is related to the predictors $X\beta$. For instance, if a GLM model is used with a log link, this is modelling the log of the arithmetic mean, i.e. $\ln[E(y/x)]=X\beta$. This is different from log ordinary least squares, where rather than modelling the log of arithmetic mean cost, the arithmetic mean of log cost is modelled: $E[\ln(y)/x] = X\beta$ (Glick *et al.* 2007). An illustration of how the log of the mean does not equal the mean of the log and can produce different results can be found in Glick *et al.* (2007). For detailed discussions of the use of GLMs with cost data see Manning and Mullahy (2001), Barber and Thompson (2004), and Glick *et al.* (2007).

7.2.7 The central limit theorem

In a recent review of various methods of analysing skewed cost data, Mihaylova *et al.* (2010) identified several alternatives to bootstrapping, including models based on the normal distribution, models based on normality following a transformation of the data, semi-parametric and non-parametric methods, and single-distribution generalized linear models (Blough *et al.* 1999).

One of their recommendations was that simple methods should be preferred where sample sizes are sufficiently large for the central limit theorem to exert itself. The central limit theorem states that, given a distribution with a mean μ and variance σ^2, the sampling distribution of the mean approaches a normal distribution with mean μ and variance σ^2/N as the sample size N increases, irrespective of the shape of the original distribution.

Therefore the challenge for analysts is to judge whether the sample size is adequate to justify an assumption of normality. A number of contributions have thrown light on this, including O'Hagan and Stevens (2003) and Nixon et al. (2010). Nixon and colleagues found that, even when data were highly skewed, methods reliant on the central limit theorem and bootstrapping both accurately estimated the true standard errors when sample sizes were moderate to large (defined as $N > 50$), and also provided 'good' estimates for small datasets with low skewness. However, when sample sizes were relatively small and the data highly skewed, methods reliant on the central limit theorem led to slightly more accurate standard errors compared with bootstrapping.

7.3 **Missing data**

We now turn to another problem that is likely to confront the analysts of a cost dataset: missing data. The problem of missing data arises when data on some variables and/or patients are not available. The problem is not new and has received considerable attention from statisticians for many years, not least concerning health outcome data in clinical trials, where missing data could invalidate the study results (Altman and Bland 2007). Data from a trial or other study design collected for use in economic evaluations are also likely to suffer from this problem, primarily because the economic analysis has to draw on all aspects of the study, including the main clinical outcomes, other patient-reported outcomes, and resource information on treatments and complications, some of which may have had to be collected by questionnaire. Hence, even if a study is very carefully designed, data on resource use and costs for all patients in a trial are unlikely to be complete.

Another example of missing data arises when, for example, hospital resource use data are complete for the first two follow-up visits, but subsequently missing for the remaining follow-ups. These data are referred to as censored rather than simply missing, because some process related to the passage of time means that past a certain time point there is no information on a patient's outcomes and/or their resource consumption.

Although the problem of missing data probably arises in most economic evaluations using patient-level data, it is not common for authors to detail the extent of the problem and how it was handled (Briggs et al. 2003). As standard statistical techniques have been designed to deal with rectangular datasets (where data are complete), they may not be directly applicable. Hence it is important for researchers to detail the completeness of the dataset and how the missing values were dealt with when reporting costing results.

7.3.1 **Why are data missing?**

Why might cost data be missing/censored? Rubin (1976) highlights three missing data mechanisms.

- ◆ **Missing completely at random (MCAR)** Here missing data are random cells from the rectangular dataset and bear no relation to the value of any of the variables. This implies that the costs for study participants who have incomplete follow-up are the same as the costs for those with complete data except for random variation.

For example, temporary staffing difficulties during the conduct of the trial may have resulted in some patients not being sent follow-up questionnaires on certain days of the week; the pattern of missingness resulting from this is likely to be random. In the context of censored cost data, an example would be censoring occurring in a study which has rolling admission and a fixed stopping date. In this case patients with shorter follow-up were simply recruited at a slightly later date and are unlikely to be different in other ways; their duration of follow-up is likely to be unrelated to anything that may have happened to them.

♦ **Missing at random (MAR)** This occurs when missing data are correlated in an observable way with the mechanism that generates the cost, i.e. after adjusting the data for observable differences between complete and missing cases, the cost for those with missing data is the same, except for random variation, as for those with complete data. For example, men could be more difficult to locate than women during follow-up in a trial. However, if gender is controlled for, those with missing data may have the same cost as those with complete data (Glick *et al.* 2007).

♦ **Not missing at random (NMAR)** This may also be called non-ignorably missing or censored data (Rubin 1976). This describes the case where missing values depend on unobserved variables, in that the values of the missing observations are conditional on the mechanism that created the missing values. This implies that the costs of participants with missing data differ in unpredictable ways from the costs of those without missing data. For example, NMAR could occur where study participants who have serious adverse events discontinue treatment within a study and do not have subsequent resource use documented despite the likelihood that it is higher than average. This type of missingness cannot be ignored without running the risk of obtaining a biased result. Consequently, this type of missingness/censoring is considered the most serious.

In practice the difference between these mechanisms is quite subtle, particularly with MCAR and MAR. For example, if a questionnaire were administered to patients asking them about their use of health-care resources following treatment, it is possible that not all the questionnaires would be returned. MCAR would be the reason why questionnaires were not completed if completely unrelated to any variables being examined. However, it is often hard to rule out some connection. For example, retired patients may find more time to complete the questionnaire than those still in full-time employment. As the elderly tend to make greater use of health-care resources, one would have to condition on the age of patients and their retirement status when dealing with study non-response to ensure that missing data are then MAR.

7.3.2 Missing data patterns

The pattern of missing cost information within an actual dataset can be classified in the following four ways:

♦ **univariate missingness**—a single variable in a dataset is causing a problem through missing values, while the remaining variables contain complete information

♦ **unit non-response**—no data are recorded for any of the variables for some patients

- **monotone missing**—caused, for example, by drop-out in panel or longitudinal studies, resulting in variables observed up to a certain time point or wave but not beyond that

- **multivariate missing**—also called item non-response or general missingness, where some but not all of the variables are missing for some of the subjects.

In analyses of cost information, monotone and multivariate are the most common types of missingness which health economists have to deal with. Briggs *et al.* (2003) observed that, faced with missing data, health economists have tended to use very simple ad hoc approaches, especially complete-case analysis and available-case analysis. This is also true for censored costs. These approaches are briefly described in the next section, and several methods of addressing missing data by imputing values for the missing observations are considered before moving on to considering specifically how to deal with costs that are censored.

7.3.3 Complete-case analysis

Complete-case analysis (CCA) or listwise deletion of cases is the default technique in many statistical packages, and involves discarding cases where any variables are missing. Advantages of the approach are that it is simple to perform and the same dataset (although reduced) is used for all analyses. The main disadvantage with this approach is that it excludes potentially informative data, and that it could be biased if the complete cases differ systematically from the original sample. If small amounts of data are missing, CCA could be acceptable, but it is difficult to determine at what point the level of missing data becomes a problem. For general missingness patterns in multivariate datasets, relatively small amounts of missing data points can result in the listwise deletion of a large number of cases using CCA, potentially resulting in the elimination of most cases and the loss of a large proportion of data.

7.3.4 Available-case analysis

Available-case analysis (ACA) estimates the mean for the complete cases for each variable and then sums the means. As with CCA, it is simple to perform. However, the major disadvantage of this approach is that different samples are used across the analysis; hence the sample base varies from one variable to another. This leads to problems of comparability across variables, in particular regarding the covariance structure between variables in the dataset (the covariance determines the extent to which two variables are related or how they vary together). Since the purpose of cost analysis is to calculate total cost per patient across the resource use variables, ACA can lead to difficulty in performing statistical analysis of per patient cost differences.

7.3.5 Imputation

An alternative method of addressing missing data is to estimate missing values using some form of imputation. Imputation can take several forms. At its simplest, an unconditional mean value is calculated with observed data for each variable, and the mean is then imputed in place of every missing observation for that variable.

Table 7.1 shows a hypothetical dataset for 10 patients undergoing cancer treatment, who are at two different stages of cancer (denoted by 1 or 2 in the cancer stage column). Some data on their subsequent treatment and follow-up care were missing.

If in the first instance, unconditional mean imputation was used to address the missing observations in this dataset, the mean cost for each resource use category would be inserted in place of the missing values: for example, £963 for surgery costs for patient 7. By definition this would not affect the mean value in each category, but it would affect the standard deviation: for example, the standard deviation around the mean cost for surgery falls from £1147 to £1081, simply because missing values are imputed using the mean across a particular variable.

The main advantage of mean imputation is its simplicity and transparency. However, it also has some major limitations. First, imputing the mean value for missing values will cause the estimated variance or standard deviation for that variable to be underestimated, as we have seen. Secondly, estimates of covariance and correlation (a single number that describes the degree of relationship between two variables) between variables, or regression analyses, are also affected, as the imputed values will dilute the observed correlation structure of the data.

One response to the above concerns is to make the imputation conditional. For example, the imputation of missing data on cancer treatment costs could be conditional

Table 7.1 Worked example for mean imputation, unconditional replacement

Patient ID	Cancer stage	Surgery	Radio-therapy	Chemo-therapy	Hormone	Complications	Follow-up
1	1	2147	–	262	0	1195	402
2	1	0	7465	0	–	7238	–
3	1	0	7767	0	0	0	141
4	1	2227	2868	4482	0	3076	–
5	1	1952	0	0	186	0	1085
6	2	0	2793	0	0	1098	91
7	2	–	–	0	–	0	–
8	2	0	6418	0	0	–	–
9	2	2343	–	1476	0	–	–
10	2	0	6386	809	144	1223	229
Mean		963	4814	703	41	1729	390
SD		1147	2939	1416	77	2452	406
Mean with unconditional mean replacement		963	4814	703	41	1729	390
SD		1081	2400	1416	68	2162	271

on cancer stage, as shown in Table 7.2. The shaded cells show values that have been replaced.

. The conditional mean could be calculated either by simple regression methods or by calculating mean values in the relevant subsets of patients. In this instance, the imputation was performed using the following steps:

1 split the dataset into subgroups, here two different stages of cancer

2 calculate the mean for each variable within each subgroup

3 insert the conditional means back into the missing data cells and recalculate variance.

As Table 7.2 shows, the standard deviations for stages 1 and 2 combined have increased compared with unconditional mean imputation, but remain lower than in the original sample.

The conditional mean approach addresses some of the problems identified above, but calculation of conditional means based on what are effectively subsamples may give rise to spurious differences based on small numbers. Therefore a further step in mean or conditional mean imputation would be to incorporate uncertainty, for example by calculating the mean value of the variable of interest and the observed variance around it, and then drawing values from that distribution as in a probabilistic sensitivity

Table 7.2 Worked example for mean imputation, conditional replacement

Patient ID	Cancer stage	Surgery	Radio-therapy	Chemo-therapy	Hormone	Complications	Follow-up
1	1	2147	4525	262	0	1195	402
2	1	0	7465	0	47	7238	543
3	1	0	7767	0	0	0	141
4	1	2227	2868	4482	0	3076	543
5	1	1952	0	0	186	0	1085
6	2	0	2793	0	0	1098	91
7	2	586	5199	0	36	0	160
8	2	0	6418	0	0	774	160
9	2	2343	5199	1476	0	774	160
10	2	0	6386	809	144	1223	229
Mean, stage 1		1265	4525	949	47	2302	543
SD		1159	3255	1978	81	3033	345
Mean, stage 2		586	5199	457	36	774	160
SD		1015	1473	669	62	476	49
Mean, stages 1+2		925	4862	703	41	1538	351
SD		1088	2408	1416	68	2199	307

analysis (see Chapter 10 for more details). For instance, the follow-up costs of patients 7, 8, and 9 in Table 7.2 have all been given the same value of £160. Instead, it would be possible to draw values randomly from a distribution based on a mean of £160 and a standard deviation of £49, thus engendering variation in the imputed figures while leaving the mean value unaffected. However, this approach still neglects the likely existence of covariance between variables. A further alternative to deal with missing data which incorporates uncertainty is to perform multiple imputation.

7.3.6 Multiple imputation

The idea behind multiple imputation is to incorporate covariance and uncertainty around the imputed values in an incomplete dataset. Instead of filling in a single value for each missing value, Rubin's (1987) multiple imputation replaces each missing value with a set of plausible values, thus creating multiple datasets. The number of replications needed to obtain reliable estimations is relatively small; between three and ten datasets should be enough (Schafer 1999). In general, multiple imputation techniques require that missing observations are missing at random.

Performance of multiple imputation requires three steps: imputation, analysis, and combination. At the imputation stage the missing entries of the incomplete datasets are imputed (filled in), not once, but *m* times. These imputed values are drawn from a distribution (which can be different for each missing entry). The imputation step could be done using regression methods, where a regression model is fitted for each variable with missing values, with the previous variables as covariates. Based on the resulting model, a new regression model is then estimated and used to impute the missing values for each variable. This process is repeated several times, producing a new dataset with each new imputation.

Working with imputed datasets requires conducting the analysis separately in each dataset and combining the result from each dataset using Rubin's rules (Rubin 1987). These rules ensure that the uncertainty around the parameter of interest is correctly represented. Multiple imputation is typically performed using statistical software packages such as STATA or SAS and cannot easily be undertaken in spreadsheets such as Excel. For further information on multiple imputation see Schafer (1999), and consult STATA and SAS manuals. For applied examples of studies using multiple imputation see Ratcliffe *et al.* (2006), Richardson *et al.* (2008) and Grieve *et al.* (2009).

7.4 Censored cost data

As mentioned earlier, censoring can be viewed as a particular type of missing data. Ignoring the issue of censoring could result in downward-biased mean estimates of costs or outcomes, and so it is important to address this issue. Therefore in the next section we focus on how to estimate costs in the presence of censoring, and include worked examples for two popular methods, the Kaplan–Meier sample average (KMSA) estimator and the inverse probability weighting (IPW) estimator.

7.4.1 **Why are data censored?**

Censoring arises when follow-up information on some study subjects is not available for the full duration of interest. This may occur for a number of reasons:

◆ There may be **attrition** of patients within a study, because they move to another area or withdraw from the study, resulting in incomplete follow-up information

◆ The final date of follow-up occurs before all patients reach the endpoint of interest, which could be death or some intermediate outcome

As economists are typically interested in lifetime analysis, this means that what happens after the censor date is of interest but unknown.

These are both examples of right-censoring, where time is progressing from left to right and events after a certain point are unknown. Left-censoring may also occur, for example when someone is known to have survived for less than a specified period, but their exact point of death is unknown. However, economic analysis and survival analysis are more typically concerned with right-censoring.

7.4.2 **Dealing with censored costs**

There is no clear guidance on the amount of censored data that would make censor adjustment of costs absolutely necessary. The ISPOR RCT-CEA taskforce states that 'ignoring small amounts of missing data is acceptable if a reasonable case can be made that doing so is unlikely to bias treatment group comparisons' (Ramsey *et al.* 2005), but does not specify what 'small' might be.

In the past, analysts frequently ignored the effects of censoring on cost estimation, or deployed simple methods such as complete-case or available-case analysis. However, complete-case analysis is likely to result in dropping large amounts of information, and available-case analysis, in effect assuming that no further costs were incurred by the patient after he/she was censored, produces biased results, as those costs incurred after censoring are not accounted for. As a result of these limitations, more appropriate techniques such as non-parametric interval methods have been proposed (Briggs *et al.* 2003).

7.4.3 **Non-parametric interval methods**

The KMSA estimator (also known as the product limit estimator), proposed by Lin *et al.* (1997), and the IPW estimator, proposed by Bang and Tsiatis (2000), have become popular methods for dealing with censored cost data. Both are non-parametric interval methods and assume that at any follow-up time the probability of censoring is independent of the future outcomes of individuals (they assume non-informative censoring).

7.4.4 **Kaplan–Meier sample average estimator**

In this method, the study period is partitioned into smaller periods; for example a 5-year study period is broken down into five distinct 1-year periods. For each time period, the mean costs of those patients still alive and not censored at the beginning of each period are estimated. These mean estimates are then weighted by the KMSA estimator, i.e. the probability of survival in a given time period, conditional on having survived the previous time period. The weighted estimates are then summed over all periods to obtain an estimate of the mean censored adjusted costs.

It is important to note at this point that KMSA is not appropriate for dealing with censoring due to attrition, unless the attrition is MCAR which is almost never the case. KM, and hence by extension KMSA, has the fundamental assumption that censoring is independent of the event of interest.

Table 7.3 presents a cost dataset for a hypothetical study where 20 patients started a study which lasted for 10 years (denoted as time periods t_1–t_{10}). The cost information for each patient in each time period is shown, together with the total cost. The penultimate column shows whether the patient was then censored or died (denoted by c or d), with the final column showing survival time. The mean costs for each time period are shown on the bottom row together with the total cost. The average total cost per patient of £13,798.70 (produced by summing the total cost per patient column and dividing by the number of patients in the dataset ((20,493 + 8549 ... + 13,951 + 21,487)/20) is not adjusted for censoring at this point.

Box 7.1 outlines the steps required to undertake the KMSA estimator, many of which are the same as the KM information provided in Chapter 4.

Table 7.4 then takes the information from Table 7.3 and adjusts for censoring using the steps required to undertake the KMSA estimator as described above. As Table 7.4 shows, the total cost once adjusted for censoring is £15,219.81, compared with the uncensored cost of £13,798.70.

7.4.5 Inverse probability weighting estimator

As with KMSA, with IPW the study period is partitioned into smaller time intervals. The total cost incurred for all patients alive at the beginning of each period is calculated. The estimated total costs of patients with complete costs in each time period are then weighted by the KMSA estimator using reverse censoring (i.e. the probability of not being censored at the beginning of each time period). These weighted total costs are then summed over all time periods and divided by the total number of patients (i.e. all the patients included in the study) to obtain an estimate of the mean censor-adjusted cost.

In contrast with KMSA, IPW is able to handle attrition, since the weights can be covariate adjusted. An example of a study that used IPW to handle censoring that was due to attrition is given by Briggs et al. (2010). The steps required to undertake the IPW are outlined in Box 7.2.

Table 7.5 now takes the information from Table 7.3 and adjusts for censoring using the IPW approach as described above.

Comparisons of the IPW and KMSA estimators have shown that they both perform well over different levels of censoring (O'Hagan and Stevens 2004; Raikou and McGuire 2004), and both are considered reasonable approaches for dealing with censoring.

Further methods allow for adjustments for covariates whilst adjusting for censoring (Carides et al. 2000; Lin 2000) and have been used in cost-effectiveness studies (Willan et al. 2005; Pullenayegum and Willan 2007). Extensions to better adjust for

Table 7.3 Hypothetical dataset illustrating censoring

Patient	t_1	t_2	t_3	t_4	t_5	t_6	t_7	t_8	t_9	t_{10}	Total cost	d/c*	Survival time (yr)
1	4830	3461	91	627	2978	1788	513	2269	1330	2606	20493	c	10
2	2636	525	3154	374	1481	379	.	.	.	.	8549	c	6
3	4398										4398	d	1
4	2840	2740	3477	440	12	962	1407	2286	942	669	15775	c	10
5	4398	3966	.	.	.						8364	c	2
6	3512	3122	4288	172	1376	2462	1575	2930	565	2173	22175	c	10
7	2103	4024	1091	1990	2600	1111	193	.	.	.	13112	c	7
8	3088	2414	4881	2671	2290	1071	1474	1882	2740	.	22511	c	9
9	2639	1024	2676	459	2373	165	2484	1776	624	30	14250	c	10
10	2429	1049	3193								6671	d	3
11	3578	3540	1564	2520	1745	2710	791	2255	2979	370	22052	c	10
12	4253	4119	1695	1301	2508	.	.	.	.	.	13876	c	5
13	3153	751	4290	1880	983	541	2707	569	1616	410	16900	c	10
14	2436	777	1488	211	1314	1099	376	98	1301	1120	10220	c	10

(continued)

Table 7.3 (continued) Hypothetical dataset illustrating censoring

Patient	t_1	t_2	t_3	t_4	t_5	t_6	t_7	t_8	t_9	t_{10}	Total cost	d/c*	Survival time (yr)
15	3898	2359	431	2450	.	.	.	.	.	.	9138	c	4
16	3207	4476									7683	d	2
17	2182	4714									6896	d	2
18	2159	3477	4033	1211	1202	2715	1799	877			17473	d	8
19	3855	2984	234	731	2288	2046	1813	.	.	.	13951	c	7
20	2960	2630	3297	2936	102	1903	2677	1683	841	2458	21487	c	10
Mean	3227.70	2744.84	2492.69	1331.53	1660.86	1457.85	1484.08	1662.50	1437.56	1229.50	13798.70		

*d/c, died or censored.

Box 7.1 Steps required to undertake the KMSA estimator

1. Time period—partition the whole time period into smaller intervals
2. Number at risk in each time period—number of people who are alive and at risk of death at the beginning of each period (i.e. number at risk in the previous period minus number of deaths and censored cases in that period)
3. Number of deaths and censored patients
4. Hazard rate $(H(t))$—observed deaths divided by the number at risk at the beginning of the period
5. The probability of survival in time interval $(P(t))$: $P(t) = 1 - H(t)$
6. Overall probability of survival to time t $(S(t))$: $S(t) = P(t)_1 \times P(t)_2 \times P(t)_3 \times \dots P(t)$

Then incorporate the costing information:

7. Mean cost data for each time period
8. Mean cost for period times survival probability
9. Finally calculate the total costs (sum the per period product)

Table 7.4 Calculating the KMSA estimator

Time period (yr)	No of individuals at risk	Deaths	Censored	$H(t)^*$	$P(t)^†$	$S(t)^‡$	Mean cost (£)	KMSA cost (£)
0	20	0	0	0	1	1		
1	20	1	0	0.05	0.95	0.95	3227.70	3066.32
2	19	2	1	0.1053	0.8947	0.85	2744.84	2333.12
3	16	1	0	0.0625	0.9375	0.7969	2492.69	1986.36
4	15	0	1	0	1	0.7969	1331.53	1061.07
5	14	0	1	0	1	0.7969	1660.86	1323.50
6	13	0	1	0	1	0.7969	1457.85	1161.72
7	12	0	2	0	1	0.7969	1484.08	1182.63
8	10	1	0	0.1	0.9	0.7172	1662.50	1192.32
9	9	0	1	0	1	0.7172	1437.56	1031.00
10	8	0	8	0	1	0.7172	1229.50	881.78
							Censor-adjusted mean cost	15,219.81

$^*H(t)$, observed deaths/number at risk (e.g. 1/16=0.0625).
$^†P(t) = H(t)_1$, probability of survival in a certain time interval t (e.g. 1 –0.0625 = 0.9375).
$^‡S(t) = P(t)_1 \times P(t)_2 \times P(t)_3 \times \dots$, overall probability of survival to time t.

Box 7.2 Steps required to undertake the IPW

1. Time period—partition the whole time period into smaller intervals
2. Number at risk—number of people who are alive and at risk of death at the beginning of each period (i.e. number at risk in the previous period minus number of deaths and censored cases in that period)
3. Number of deaths and censored patients
4. Hazard rate ($H(t)$), observed censored cases divided by number at risk at the beginning of the period
5. The probability of not being censored in the time interval ($P(t)$): $P(t) = 1 - H(t)$
6. Overall probability of not being censored to the beginning of time t ($S(t)$)

Then incorporate the costing information,

7. Total cost data for each time period
8. Total cost for period divided by survival probability
9. Total cost—sum the per period product and divide by the patient sample at the beginning of the study.

Table 7.5 Calculating the inverse probability weighting (IPW)

Time period (yr)	No of individuals at risk	Deaths	Censored	$H(t)^*$	$P(t)^†$	$S(t)^‡$	Total cost (£)	IPW§ (£)
0	20	0	0	0.000	1.000	1.000		
1	20	1	0	0.000	1.000	1.000	64,554	64,554
2	19	2	1	0.053	0.947	1.000	52,722	52,722
3	16	1	0	0.000	1.000	0.947	39,883	42,115
4	15	0	1	0.067	0.933	0.947	19,973	21,091
5	14	0	1	0.071	0.929	0.883	23,252	26,317
6	13	0	1	0.077	0.923	0.821	18,952	23,089
7	12	0	2	0.167	0.833	0.758	17,809	23,507
8	10	1	0	0.000	1.000	0.631	16,625	26,343
9	9	0	1	0.111	0.889	0.631	12,938	20,501
10	8	0	8	1.000	0.000	0.561	9,836	17,532
							Sum of periods	317,770
							Censor adjusted mean cost	15,888

*$H(t)$, censored cases/number at risk (e.g. 1/19=0.053).
†$P(t) = 1 - H(t)$, probability of not being censored in a certain time interval t (e.g. 1 -0.053 = 0.947).
‡$S(t) = P(t-1) \times S(t-1)$, overall probability of not being censored at the beginning of each time period (e.g. $S(t)$ at time 5 = 0.933 × 0.947)
§IPW = total cost per period/$S(t)$.

survival time (Liu *et al.* 2007) and two-part models for costs (Tian and Huang 2007) have also been proposed. Multiple imputation methods have also been improved for use with censored cost data (Lavori *et al.* 1995; Oostenbrink *et al.* 2003), and regression based methods have also been proposed (Oostenbrink and Al 2005). However, to date the basic KMSA and IPW estimators are the most common methods used to handle censored cost data.

7.5 **Analysing hierarchical data**

Cost-effectiveness analysis is increasingly undertaken alongside studies (observational or randomized controlled trials) performed across multiple sites (either within a country or across different countries). The resultant data may be hierarchical (i.e. clustered), where data have several levels which can be arranged in a tree-like structure. A simple hierarchical structure might be patients nested within hospitals. This structure has two levels: patients are level 1, grouped within hospitals at level 2. Clinical trials that randomize by location rather than by patient are termed cluster-randomized trials. In these studies, even with randomization, the treatment site (e.g. the hospital) may have an impact on trial outcomes irrespective of the patients' treatment (Rice and Jones 1997). This may be due to several reasons such as differences in clinical practice by individual clinicians, patient case-mix, or the unit costs of delivering health care at each site (Manca *et al.* 2005).

In studies which have involved several sites, cost (and effect) data have often been analysed using ordinary least squares (OLS) regression. However, OLS requires that random errors are independently distributed. This assumption clearly fails in this context, as observations within clusters will be correlated (Manca *et al.* 2005). This is because patients' resource use (and costs) within a particular site may be more similar than resource use and costs between different sites.

Multilevel models, in contrast with OLS regression, are able to incorporate the hierarchical structure of the data, as the inclusion of site as a level in a multilevel analysis can ensure that the clustering effects within sites will be adequately controlled for (Rice and Jones 1997; Carey 2000; Grieve *et al.* 2005). The technique has been used for some time in areas such as education and health services research (Goldstein 1995; Leyland and Goldstein 2001). There are many areas in health economics where the use of multilevel modelling could be useful, for instance exploring medical practice variation. However, in cost-effectiveness analysis the technique has tended to be used in the context of multicentre and multi-country evaluations. A useful applied example of using a multilevel model is provided by Johnston *et al.* (2003) in the context of a UK-based cluster randomized trial assessing three methods of promoting secondary prevention of coronary heart disease. The approach has also been used in the context of analysing the cost (and effect) data from multinational trials and compared with other main approaches: fixed-effect models and tests of homogeneity (Willke *et al.* 1998; Cook *et al.* 2003; Glick *et al.* 2007). For examples and discussions of the advantages of multilevel models, especially in multi-country cost-effectiveness analyses, see Grieve *et al.* (2005, 2007), Manca *et al.* (2005), Nixon and Thompson (2005), Pinto *et al.* (2005), and Willan *et al.* (2005).

7.6 **Summary**

In this chapter we have described some of the key approaches to consider when analysing cost data. This area of cost-effectiveness analysis has been moving rapidly in recent years, and the chapter has tried to reflect this. We have highlighted the importance of providing basic descriptive information on costs, notably the mean supported by measures of variability and precision. We then looked at the problems of skewed data, and then missing data generally and censored costs specifically. Finally, we introduced the potential use of multilevel models to analyse data that are hierarchical in nature.

In the next chapter we turn to the use of modelling in cost-effectiveness analysis. Before moving on to modelling, you may wish to work through the exercise on the bootstrap approach, followed by an exercise on the KMSA estimator.

References

Ai, C. and Norton, E.C.J. (2000). Standard errors for the retransformation problem with heteroscedasticity. *Health Economics*, **19**, 697–718.

Altman, D.G. and Bland, J.M. (2007). Statistics notes: missing data. *British Medical Journal*, **334**, 424.

Bang, H. and Tsiatis, A.A. (2000). Estimating medical costs with censored data. *Biometrika*, **87**, 329–43.

Barber, J.A. and Thompson, S.G. (2000). Analysis of cost data in randomized trials: an application of the non-parametric bootstrap. *Statistics in Medicine*, **19**, 3219–36.

Barber, J.A. and Thompson, S.G. (2004). Multiple regression of cost data, use of generalised linear models. *Journal of Health Services Research and Policy*, **9**, 197–204.

Blough, D.K., Madden, C.W., and Hornbrook, M.C. (1999). Modeling risk using generalized linear models. *Journal of Health Economics*, **18**, 153–71.

Briggs, A. and Gray, A. (1998). The distribution of health care costs and their statistical analysis for economic evaluation. *Journal of Health Services Research and Policy*, **3**, 233–45.

Briggs, A.H., Wonderling, D.E., Mooney, C.Z. (1997). Pulling cost-effectiveness analysis up by its bootstraps, a non-parametric approach to confidence interval estimation. *Health Economics*, **6**, 327–40.

Briggs, A., Clark, T., Wolstenholme, J., and Clarke, P. (2003). Missing ... presumed at random, cost-analysis of incomplete data. *Health Economics*, **12**, 377–92.

Briggs, A., Glick, H., Lozano-Ortega, G., *et al.* (2010). Is treatment with ICS and LABA cost-effective for COPD? Multinational economic analysis of the TORCH study. *European Respiratory Journal*, **35**, 532-9.

Carey, K. (2000). A multi-level modelling approach to analysis of patient costs under managed care. *Health Economics*, **9**, 435–46.

Carides, G.W., Heyse, J.F., and Iglewicz, B. (2000). A regression-based method for estimating mean treatment cost in the presence of right-censoring. *Biostatistics*, **1**, 299–313.

Chiang, A.C. and Wainwright, K. (2005). *Fundamental Methods of Mathematical Economics* (4th edn). McGraw-Hill, London.

Cook, J.R., Drummond, M., Glick, H., and Heyse, J.F. (2003). Assessing the appropriateness of combining economic data from multinational clinical trials. *Statistics in Medicine*, **22**, 1955–76.

Duan, N. (1983). Smearing estimate, a nonparametric retransformation method. *Journal of the American Statistical Association*, **78**, 605–10.

Efron, B. and Tibshirani, R.J. (1993). *An Introduction to the Bootstrap*. Chapman & Hall, New York.

Glick, H.A., Doshi, J.A., Sonnad, S.S., and Polsky, D. (2007). *Economic Evaluation in Clinical Trials*. Oxford University Press.

Goldstein, H. (1995). *Multilevel Statistical Models*. Edward Arnold, London.

Grieve, R., Nixon, R., Thompson, S.G., and Normand, C. (2005). Using multilevel models for assessing the variability of multinational resource use and cost data. *Health Economics*, **14**, 185–96.

Grieve, R., Nixon, R., Thompson, S.G., and Cairns, J. (2007). Multilevel models for estimating incremental net benefits in multinational studies. *Health Economics*, **16**, 815–26.

Grieve, R., Cairns, J., and Thompson, S.G. (2009). Improving costing methods in multicentre economic evaluation, the use of multiple imputation for unit costs. *Health Economics*, **19**, 939–954.

Johnston, K., Gray, A., Moher, M., Yudkin, P., Wright, L., and Mant, D. (2003). Reporting the cost-effectiveness of interventions with nonsignificant effect differences: example from a trial of secondary prevention of coronary heart disease. *International Journal of Technology Assessment in Health Care*, **19**, 476–89.

Lavori, P.W., Dawson, R., and Shera, D. (1995). A multiple imputation strategy for clinical trials with truncation of patient data. *Statistics in Medicine*, **14**, 1913–25.

Leyland, A.H. and Goldstein, H. (eds) (2001). *Multi-level Modelling of Health Statistics*. John Wiley, Chichester.

Lin, D.Y. (2000). Linear regression analysis of censored medical costs. *Biostatistics*, **1**, 35–47.

Lin, D.Y., Feuer, E.J., Etzioni, R., and Wax, Y. (1997). Estimating medical costs from incomplete follow-up data. *Biometrics*, **53**, 419–34.

McCullagh, P. and Nelder, J.A. (1989). *Generalised Linear Models* (2nd edn). Chapman & Hall, London.

Manca, A., Rice, N., Sculpher, M.J., and Briggs, A.H. (2005). Assessing generalisability by location in trial-based cost-effectiveness analysis, the use of multilevel models. *Health Economics*, **14**, 471–85. Erratum in: *Health Economics*, **14**, 486.

Manning, W.G. (1998). The logged dependent variable, heteroscedasticity, and the retransformation problem. *Journal of Health Economics*, **17**, 283–95.

Manning, W.G. and Mullahy, J. (2001). Estimating log models: to transform or not to transform? *Journal of Health Economics*, **20**, 461–94.

Mihaylova, B., Briggs, A.H., O'Hagan, A., and Thompson, S. (2010). Review of statistical methods for analysing healthcare resources and costs. *Health Economics*, in press.

Nixon R.M. and Thompson, S.G. (2005). Methods for incorporating covariate adjustment, subgroup analysis and between-centre differences into cost-effectiveness evaluations. *Health Economics*, **14**, 1217–29.

Nixon, R.M., Wonderling, D., and Grieve, R.D. (2010). Non-parametric methods for cost-effectiveness analysis, the central limit theorem and the bootstrap compared. *Health Economics*, **19**, 316–33.

O'Hagan, A. and Stevens, J.W. (2003). Assessing and comparing costs. How robust are the bootstrap and methods based on asymptotic normality? *Health Economics*, **12**, 33–49.

O'Hagan, A. and Stevens, J.W. (2004). On estimators of medical costs with censored data. *Journal of Health Economics*, **23**, 615–25.

Oostenbrink, J.B., Al, M.J., and Rutten-van Mölken, M.P. (2003). Methods to analyse cost data of patients who withdraw in a clinical trial setting. *Pharmacoeconomics*, **21**, 1103–12.

Oostenbrink, J.B. and Al, M.J. (2005). The analysis of incomplete cost data due to dropout. *Health Economics*, **14**, 763–76.

Pinto, E.M., Willan, A.R., and O'Brien, B.J. (2005). Cost-effectiveness analysis for multinational clinical trials. *Statistics in Medicine*, **24**, 1965–82.

Pullenayegum, E.M. and Willan, A.R. (2007). Semi-parametric regression models for cost-effectiveness analysis: improving the efficiency of estimation from censored data. *Statistics in Medicine*, **26**, 3274–99.

Raikou, M. and McGuire, A. (2004). Estimating medical care costs under conditions of censoring. *Journal of Health Economics*, **23**, 443–70.

Ramsey, S., Willke, R., Briggs, A., *et al.* (2005). Good research practices for cost-effectiveness analysis alongside clinical trials: the ISPOR RCT-CEA Task Force report. *Value in Health*, **8**, 521–33.

Ratcliffe, J., Thomas, K.J., MacPherson, H., and Brazier, J. (2006). A randomised controlled trial of acupuncture care for persistent low back pain: cost effectiveness analysis. *British Medical Journal*, **333**, 626.

Rice, N. and Jones, A. (1997). Multilevel models and health economics. *Health Economics*, **6**, 561–75.

Richardson, G., Kennedy, A., Reeves, D., *et al.* (2008). Cost effectiveness of the Expert Patients Programme (EPP) for patients with chronic conditions. *Journal of Epidemiology and Community Health*, **62**, 361–7.

Rubin, D.B. (1976). Inference and missing data. *Biometrika*, **63**, 581–92.

Rubin, D.B. (1987). *Multiple Imputation for Nonresponse in Surveys*. John Wiley, New York.

Schafer, J.L. (1999). Multiple imputation: a primer. *Statistical Methods in Medical Research*, **8**, 3–15.

Thompson, S.G. and Barber, J.A. (2000). How should cost data in pragmatic randomised trials be analysed? *British Medical Journal*, **320**, 1197–1200.

Tian, L. and Huang, J. (2007). A two-part model for censored medical cost data. *Statistics in Medicine*, **26**, 4273–92.

Willan, A.R., Pinto, E.M., O'Brien, B.J., *et al.* (2005). Country specific cost comparisons from multinational clinical trials using empirical Bayesian shrinkage estimation, the Canadian ASSENT-3 economic analysis. *Health Economics*, **14**, 327–38.

Willke, R.J., Glick, H.A., Polsky, D., and Schulman, K. (1998). Estimating country-specific cost-effectiveness from multinational clinical trials. *Health Economics*, **7**, 481–93.

Understanding a cost dataset and the concept of bootstrapping

Introduction

An overview and instructions to complete the exercise are given. A step-by-step guide is also provided for readers who would prefer more detailed instructions.

Overview

On the Health Economics Research Centre website www.herc.ox.ac.uk/books/applied you will find the Excel file *Bootstrap Exercise.xlsm* that you will need for this exercise. Once you have downloaded this spreadsheet you will see that it includes a dataset with the long-term costs associated with 200 simulated patients, of whom 100 were assigned to treatment and the remainder were in the control group.

The aim of this exercise is to calculate the mean difference in cost between the groups and compute the 95% confidence interval associated with this difference.

The spreadsheet also includes a macro that will generate 1000 bootstrap replicates of the mean cost difference for this dataset, from which you can calculate 95% confidence intervals. To help you complete the exercise successfully, the cells that you need to complete are coloured light yellow.

Exercise instructions

- Using the **Raw Data** spreadsheet calculate descriptive statistics for each group to familiarize yourself with the dataset.
- Calculate the mean cost difference between groups and the 95% confidence interval associated with this difference (applying the central limit theorem).
- Set up a spreadsheet to create bootstrap replicates of the dataset using the built-in bootstrap macro.
- Compute 1000 bootstrap replicates of the mean cost difference between groups.
- Compute descriptive statistics and examine the distribution of the 1000 replicates using a histogram.
- Calculate 95% confidence intervals for the mean difference using the percentile method.

Step-by-step guide

After obtaining the file *Bootstrap Exercise.xlsm* from www.herc.ox.ac.uk/books/ applied, please check two important things on your computer to ensure that you are able to complete the exercise. First, check that macros are enabled, so that you can run the macro that will be used later in the exercise. Secondly, ensure that your **Data Analysis** package is installed to allow you to create a histogram. These two steps take a couple of minutes to complete on your computer and instructions are shown below.

Enabling macros to run

To enable macros in Excel 2007, click the **Microsoft Office** button (top left-hand corner of your screen), then click **Excel Options** (bottom right of the box). Then click **Trust Centre** and then **Trust Centre Settings**. Once in Trust Settings click on **Macro Settings** and then **Enable all macros**. Because enabling macros lowers your computer security, remember to change back to disable macros once you have completed the exercise. If your computer will not let you change your macro settings, it is possible that the computer administrator in your organization has prevented you from doing this and you will need to ask for this to be allowed.

Creating a histogram

You will need to ensure that the Data Analysis option is selected. Click the **Microsoft Office** button, and then click **Excel Options**. Click **Add-Ins**. In the **Manage** box, click **Excel Add-ins** and then click **Go**. In the **Add-Ins available** box, do one of the following. To load the Analysis ToolPak, select the **Analysis ToolPak** check box and then click **OK**. To include Visual Basic for Applications (VBA) functions for the Analysis ToolPak, select the **Analysis ToolPak-VBA** check box, and then click **OK**.

Once your macros are enabled and the Data Analysis package is added, the Excel file includes the following worksheets: **Raw Data**, **Summary Statistics**, **Bootstrapping**, **Histogram**, and **Confidence Interval**. These worksheets provide all the data that you will need to complete the exercise. All cells that need to be completed are coloured light yellow.

Step 1. Familiarizing yourself with the data
Excel commands required

=COUNT(...)	N
=AVERAGE(...)	Mean
=STDEV(...)	Standard deviation (SD)
=SKEW(...)	Skew
=SQRT(...)	Square root

Formulae

The standard error of the mean is equal to the standard deviation divided by the square root of the sample size

$$SE = \sqrt{\frac{SD^2}{n}} = \frac{SD}{\sqrt{n}}$$

Spend some time familiarizing yourself with the data in the **Raw Data** worksheet. The data represent a hypothetical clinical trial of a drug therapy with two arms, a treatment group, and a control group. The trial includes 200 patients in total, with 100 patients in each group. The total cost per patient discounted at an annual rate of 3.5% over 20 years is included in this exercise and corresponds to unadjusted censored estimates (where data are missing after a certain time period).

Move to the **Summary Statistics** worksheet and using the Excel commands above calculate the following:

◆ sample size (n)

◆ mean

◆ standard deviation (SD)

◆ standard error (SE)

◆ skewness of the cost variable in the control and treatment groups.

Step 2. Calculating mean differences and applying the central limit theorem

Excel commands required

=NORMINV(0.975,0,1)	t_α assuming a normal distribution. This formula should return a value of 1.96.
=TDIST(t-value,(n_1+n_2-2),2)	p value associated with the t-value entered, based on a two-tailed test and $n_1 + n_2 - 2$ degrees of freedom. Note that the Excel command TDIST does not work on negative values of t. Therefore you need to use absolute values for t, making use of the symmetrical property of the distribution.
=ABS(…)	Returns absolute value

Formulae

Variance sum law: the variance of the sum of or difference between two independent variables is equal to the sum of their variances. If we assume that the groups have equal sample sizes and equal variance, the variance sum law indicates that the standard error of the difference is given by

$$SE_{diff} = \sqrt{\frac{SD_1^2}{n_1} + \frac{SD_2^2}{n_2}} = \sqrt{SE_1^2 + SE_2^2}$$

The 95% confidence interval around the mean difference is defined as

$$mean\ difference \pm t_\alpha \times SE_{diff}$$

Alternatively, a parametric t-test (assuming equal variances) can be conducted by calculating a t-value and the associated p-value. The t-value is defined as follows:

$$t\ value = \frac{mean\ difference}{SE_{diff}}$$

- ◆ Calculate the mean difference in costs between the control and treatment group (simply the difference between the two means).
- ◆ Estimate the standard error (using standard error information from the control and treatment groups) and 95% confidence interval around the mean difference (using the information on mean and standard error around the mean difference).
- ◆ Use the t-test to calculate a p-value for the difference in mean cost between the groups.

Step 3. Setting up a spreadsheet to create bootstrap replicates of the cost dataset

Excel commands required

=INT(number)
The function 'INT' rounds a number down to the nearest integer. For example, INT(8.9) equals 8; INT(–8.9) equals –9.
=RAND()
Returns a uniformly distributed random number ≥0 and <1. A new random number is returned every time the worksheet is calculated. To generate a random number between 1 and 100 (inclusive), use RAND()*100+1
=**VLOOKUP**(lookup_value,table_array,col_index_num,range_lookup)
The function VLOOKUP has the arguments lookup_value, table_array, col_index_num and range_lookup where:
Lookup_value is the value to be found in the first column of the array. Lookup_value can be a value, a reference, or a text string.
Table_array is the table of information in which data is looked up. You can enter a reference to a range of cells or a range name, such as 'control' or 'treatment' if you have named ranges in your spreadsheet.
Col_index_num is the column number in table_array from which the matching value must be returned. A col_index_num of 1 returns the value in the first column in table_array; a col_index_num of 2 returns the value in the second column in table_array, and so on.
Range_lookup is a logical value (TRUE or FALSE) that specifies whether you want VLOOKUP to find an exact match (FALSE) or an approximate (closest) match (TRUE).

Step 4. Now go to the worksheet **Bootstrapping**

(a) In columns A and E, we will create a random number generator. In cell A7 insert the formula, =INT(RAND()*(100)+1). Copy the formula in cell A7 down until you have 100 random numbers (i.e. until cell A106). Do the same with cell E7 (i.e. until E106). However, this time the random number needs to be included in the interval (101–200). Therefore insert the formula =INT(RAND()*(100)+101) in cell E7.

(b) In columns B and F create the lookup table. In cell B7, open the dialogue box for the command VLOOKUP included in the Lookup and Reference category.
MS Excel 2007: click on the Formulas button at the top of your screen and then pick the Lookup and Reference category. Next find the VLOOKUP command which is usually at the bottom of the list.

(c) In the dialogue box insert the following information:

- ◆ Lookup_value: A7
- ◆ Table_array: 'Raw Data'!$B$5:$C$104
- ◆ Col_index_num: 2
- ◆ Range_lookup: FALSE

The formula should look as follows: =VLOOKUP(A7,'Raw Data'!$B$5:$C$104,2, FALSE)

Drag to copy from cell B7 to B106.

In cell F7 open the dialog box for the VLOOKUP command and insert the following information:

- ◆ Lookup_value: E7
- ◆ Table_array: 'Raw Data'!$E$5:$F$104
- ◆ Col_index_num: 2
- ◆ Range_lookup: FALSE

The formula should look as follows: =VLOOKUP(E7,'Raw Data'!$E$5:$F$104,2, FALSE)

Drag to copy from cell F7 to F106.

(d) In cell B109 calculate the mean value of the total cost per patient in the control group using =AVERAGE(B7:B106). In cell D109 calculate the mean cost per patient for the treatment group. These are the means of this bootstrap replicate. Press F9 to change the random numbers and observe how new samples are drawn from the raw data each time. See how the bootstrap means change with each press of F9.

Step 5. Running the bootstrap simulation

Excel macro

To save you time, the macro to run the simulation has been programmed for you. However, the details of the code included in the macro are provided below for your information.

To look at the macro in MS Excel 2007:

- Go to **View, Macros,** and select **View Macros.**
- Click on the macro **Bootstrap** and click on the **step into** button.

_____**Visual Basic Code**_____

```
Sub Bootstrap()
'Bootstrap Macro
'Macro recorded 14/04/2009 and based on the work by Andrew Briggs and Joanna
    Swaffield
Sheets("Bootstrapping").Select
Index = 0
Range("B109:D109").Select
Selection.Copy
Do While Index < 1000
Range("K7").Select
ActiveCell.Offset(Index, 0).Range("A1").Select
Selection.PasteSpecial Paste: =xlValues, Operation: =xlNone, SkipBlanks: = _
    False, Transpose: =False
Index = Index + 1
Loop
Range("A2").Select
End Sub
```

Click on the **Run Bootstrap Macro** button. After a few seconds (or minutes depending on the processor and RAM memory of your computer), columns K7:K1006 and M7:M1006 should have been filled with 1000 bootstrap means for the control and treatment groups, respectively.

In cell O7, calculate the mean difference in costs between the groups for the first bootstrap replicate with the formula =M7–K7. Copy cell O7 down until O1006.

Step 6. Evaluating the results from the bootstrap analysis
Excel commands required

=MEDIAN(…)	Median
=PERCENTILE(…, 0.025)	2.5th percentile
=PERCENTILE(…, 0.975)	97.5th percentile
=MIN(…)	Minimum value
=MAX(…)	Maximum value

(a) Still in the worksheet **Bootstrapping**, fill the cells R7:R13 with the appropriate summary statistics for the 1000 bootstrap replicates of mean cost differences.

(b) Create a histogram of the 1000 replicates so that you can study its distribution. To do this, you first need to construct the frequency table that will be plotted in the histogram (in MS Excel 2007, it can be found through **Data, Data Analysis, Histogram**). NB: if you are unable to see the **Data Analysis** option at the top right hand corner of your screen, it could be that there was a problem when you added the **Data Analysis** option at the start of the exercise. If so, please go back to the first page of instructions for this exercise, read the section on creating a histogram, and try again.

- ♦ In the histogram dialogue box, you are required to enter three items of information.

  - • The **Input range**, which is the vector of bootstrapped mean cost differences. Select the button with the red arrow, then highlight the cells showing the mean cost difference for each of your 1000 bootstrap replicates, and press Enter to return to the histogram dialogue box.

  - • The **Bin range**, which represents the cut-off values for the categories at which Excel will evaluate the frequency of the data. For example, the top bin –£2000 will include all values ≤–£2000, while the bin below (–£1800) will include all values ≥–£2000 and ≤–£1800. Click the red arrow adjacent to **Bin range** and select cells Q17:Q57.

  - • The final information required is the **Output range**. Press the button next to **Output range**, then press the red arrow and select the single cell R16, and then press Enter to return to the dialogue box.

  Now press OK to start the histogram calculation. In a few seconds, Excel will generate a frequency table.

- ♦ Move to the **Histogram** worksheet to create a bar chart of the frequencies calculated in the previous step. The formatting of the histogram has been done for you. In MS Excel 2007 click the right-hand mouse button and choose **Select Data**. Press the red arrow next to **Data range** and select the frequency data that you have just calculated for the bootstrap means in the **Bootstrapping sheet** (column S). Press Enter to return to the dialogue box.

  Click on the **Edit** button in the box labelled **Horizontal (Category) Axis Labels**. In the dialogue box that opens, press the red arrow next to **Axis label range**; now select the values adjacent to the frequency data labelled **Bin** (column R) and press Enter to return to the dialogue box. Finally, press OK to enter the information and generate the chart.

Step 7. Calculating 95% confidence intervals using the percentile method

(a) Move to the **Confidence Interval** worksheet. Paste the 1000 bootstrap mean differences from the worksheet **Bootstrapping** into column A starting in cell A2. Copy the values using **paste special** rather than paste to avoid copying the formulae.

(b) Sort these means into ascending order. Do not expand the selected range. In Excel 2007 this is done by selecting the data (the bootstrapped means). Then on the **Data** tab, in the **Sort and Filter** group, do one of the following:

- to sort from low numbers to high numbers, click **Sort Smallest to Largest**.

- to sort from high numbers to low numbers, click **Sort Largest to Smallest**.

The 95% confidence intervals are the 26th and 975th values (i.e. excludes the top and bottom 25 values). These should equal the values that you calculated in cells R10:R11 on the **Bootstrapping** worksheet.

A completed version of this exercise is available from the website www.herc.ox.ac.uk/books/applied in the Excel file ***Bootstrap Exercise Solution.xlsm***.

Analysis of censored cost data using the KMSA estimator

Introduction

An overview and instructions to complete the exercise are given. A step-by-step guide is also provided for readers who would prefer more detailed instructions.

Overview

On the Health Economics Research Centre website www.herc.ox.ac.uk/books/applied you will find the Excel file *KMSA.xlsm* that you will need for this exercise. Once you have downloaded this spreadsheet you will see that it includes data which were simulated from the UKPDS outcome model, in which long-term costs were modelled during 20 years for a sample of 200 patients of whom 100 were assigned to treatment and the remainder were in the current practice (control group). The aim of this exercise is to adjust the cost dataset for censoring using the KMSA.

The file comprises six spreadsheets: **Raw data control group**, **Raw data treatment group**, **KM survival control**, **KM survival treatment**, **KMSA**, and **Statistics**. The **Raw data control group sheet** gives you the raw data for the 100 patients receiving current practice, whereas the **Raw data treatment group sheet** gives you the raw data for the 100 patients receiving the new intervention. Each dataset has cost data over 20 time periods (Year 1 to Year 20).

In the control group there are 33 deaths (for each death, the column 'Year death' shows the year in which the patient died) and 67 censored observations (for each patient censored, the column 'Year censored' shows the year in which the patient was censored). In the treatment group there are 26 deaths and 74 censored observations (again, the year in which the patient died/censored are given in columns 'Year death' and 'Year censored', respectively).

For the control group, the sample mean of observed costs is £8,708. For the treatment group, the sample mean of observed costs is £12,002. However, both these sample means will be an underestimate of the true average cost per patient, as the costs incurred after censoring have not been accounted for.

To help you complete the exercise successfully, the cells that you need to complete are coloured light yellow.

Exercise instructions

In the **KM survival** worksheets, use the Kaplan–Meier method to estimate the following, for both patient groups:

1 The number of deaths and censored cases for each time period. NB: In order to save time these have already been filled in for you using the Excel command =COUNTIF(…).

2 The number at risk (NB: at time period 0 the number at risk is 100).

3 The hazard rate $H(t)$: $H(t)$ = observed death/number at risk.

4 The probability of survival $P(t)$ in a certain time interval t: $P(t) = 1 - $ (observed death/number at risk).

5 The overall probability of survival to time t $(S(t))$: $S(t) = P(t)_1 \times P(t)_2 \times P(t)_3\ldots$.

The time period 0 has been completed for you in both patient groups.

In sheet **KMSA**, fill in the following, for both patient groups:

1 Calculate the number at risk for each time period (you have already worked these out and can get them from sheet **KM survival**).

2 Calculate the probability of survival $(P(t))$ in each time interval t: $P(t) = 1 - $ (observed death/number at risk).

3 Calculate the overall probability of survival to time t $(S(t))$: $S(t) = P(t)_1 \times P(t)_2 \times P(t)_3\ldots$.

4 Enter the mean cost for each time period from the **Raw data** sheet.

5 Calculate the KMSA = sum of the survival-adjusted mean costs.

Step-by-step guide

Use file **KMSA exercise.xlsm** obtainable from www.herc.ox.ac.uk/books/applied. This file comprises six worksheets: **Raw data control group, Raw data treatment group, KM survival control, KM survival treatment, KMSA, Statistics.**

The **Raw data control group** sheet gives you the raw data for the 100 patients receiving current practice, whereas the **Raw data treatment group** sheet gives you the raw data for the 100 patients receiving the new intervention. Each dataset has cost data over 20 time periods (Year 1 to Year 20).

In the control group there are 33 deaths (for each death, column 'Year death' shows the year in which the patient died) and 67 censored observations (for each patient censored, column 'Year censored' shows the year in which the patient was censored). In the treatment group there are 26 deaths and 74 censored observations (again, the year in which the patient died/censored are given in columns 'Year death' and 'Year censored', respectively).

For the control group, the sample mean of observed costs is £8708. For the treatment group, the sample mean of observed costs is £12,002. However, both these sample means will be an underestimate of the true average cost per patient, as the costs incurred after censoring have not been accounted for.

Move to the **KM survival control** worksheet, where you will find two tables containing the following information.

1 The table on the right of the worksheet, **Kaplan–Meier Product Limit Table**, reports the KM product limit method used in the Health Outcomes exercise to estimate the survival function in the control group. All patients were ranked in terms of their time to death or censoring. The number of deaths and/or censored cases occurring at that precise time period are provided together with the number of patients still at risk at the end of each time period. The KM estimator of survival to time t is provided in the last column.

2 The table on the left has information on:

- The number of deaths and censored cases for each of the annual time periods used to estimate the costs. NB: In order to save time these have already been filled in for you using the Excel command =COUNTIF(...).

- The number at risk at the end of the time period (NB: at time period 0 the number at risk is 100).

- The Kaplan–Meier estimate of the survival function to time t ($S(t)$) for each of the time periods used in the cost analysis.

Most of the Kaplan–Meier estimates have been already completed for you. What you need to do is the following.

1 Obtain the missing estimates from the **Kaplan-Meier Product Limit Table**. For this, identify the KM estimate (i.e. column KM $S(t)$) corresponding to the period immediately before the period of interest. For example, for time period 6 the corresponding KM estimate to be obtained from the **Kaplan-Meier Product Limit Table** refers to time 5.72 years.

2 Move to the **KM survival treatment** worksheet and calculate the missing KM estimates using the same approach as above.

3 Move to the worksheet **KMSA** and fill in the following for both patient groups:

- Enter the KM survival estimator from the **KM survival control** and **KM survival treatment** sheets.

- Enter the mean cost for each time period from the **Raw data** sheet. Copy the mean costs for years 1 to 20, and then use paste special (values and transpose) to convert the row of formulae into a column of values.

- Calculate the KMSA which is equal to the sum of the survival-adjusted mean costs.

4 Discounting

(a) Using the formula for discounting $1/(1 + r)^n$ where r is the rate of interest (3.5%) and n is the number of years into the future, estimate the average censor-adjusted discounted cost for each treatment group. (Tip: For the first cell in the control group (H5), use the formula =G5/(1+$K$1)^(A5 − 1) and copy this down for the rest). The −1 is added because we are assuming that Year 1 rather than Year 0 is the present.

(b) Finally, move to the worksheet **Statistics**. Using the undiscounted estimates, fill in the following for both patient groups:

- enter the mean observed costs for each group under the **Mean unadjusted costs** column

- enter the mean adjusted costs for each group under the **Mean adjusted costs** column

- estimate the mean difference in costs for both groups and discuss the findings.

A completed version of this exercise is available from the website www.herc.ox.ac.uk/books/applied in the Excel file *KMSA Exercise Solutions.xlsm*.

Chapter 8

Decision analytic modelling: decision trees

The aim of this chapter is to provide an overview of decision analysis and modelling in the economic evaluation of health care. It explores the rationale for modelling and briefly introduces the types of models available for use in economic evaluation. The focus of the chapter is on decision tree models. The use of decision trees in economic evaluation is discussed using a worked example, with a guide to the steps that a researcher has to undertake in order to construct, analyse, and evaluate such a decision tree.

8.1 Economic evaluation in health care and decision analysis

Decision analysis is an approach used to construct and structure decisions. It includes a multitude of methods and tools for identifying, clearly representing, and formally assessing the important aspects of a decision situation. Decision analysts provide quantitative support for decision-makers in a wide range of disciplines such as marketing, law, and engineering (Raiffa 1968). Decision analysis has been widely applied in health-care decision-making, and decision analytic modelling is increasingly being used in the economic evaluation of health-care interventions (Sox *et al.* 1998; Hunink *et al.* 2001). Decision analysis encompasses the representation of alternative options available to the decision-maker, quantification of the uncertainty in the decision problem, and evaluation of alternatives in terms of the objectives or outcomes of interest.

A decision analysis model for the purpose of economic evaluation in health care is a systematic quantitative approach to decision-making under uncertainty where at least two decision options and their respective consequences are compared and evaluated in terms of their expected costs and expected outcomes. The aim is to provide decision-makers with a guide to health-care resource-allocation questions. Examples include: Should we increase the age range for the national breast screening programme? What is the most cost-effective drug to be given for a particular disease? Should the NHS fund a new intervention for Parkinson's disease?

The application of decision modelling in the economic evaluation of health care arises from the barriers and limitations that other frameworks have for conducting such an evaluation. Randomized clinical trials (RCTs) are increasingly used as a framework for the purpose of conducting an economic evaluation. Their advantages include that they provide an opportunity to prospectively collect and analyse patient-specific resource use and outcome data, and provide an unbiased assessment of the effects of an intervention on these outcomes. However, clinical trials may have limitations as the main basis of a well-designed economic evaluation, for some of the following reasons:

1 **RCTs might not compare all the relevant alternatives** As described in Chapter 2, economic evaluation is a comparative methodology for assessing the value of one course of action compared with another action (or range of options). A randomized trial may provide evidence on two or three options, but is unlikely to be able to provide evidence on all the relevant options available.

2 **Information from RCTs and other studies may have to be combined** As discussed above, a single trial is unlikely to provide all the information required, and it might be necessary to combine evidence from a range of sources. It is important that all available evidence is scrutinized and assessed for its applicability to the evaluation being undertaken. In the case of economic evaluation this means evidence on resource utilization, unit costs, effectiveness, and, where available, health-related quality of life. The range of sources from which this information could be drawn may include trials but also cohort studies, surveys, or patient records, and decision models can provide an organizing framework within which these different types of data can be synthesized.

3 **RCTs might not encompass the appropriate time horizon** The appropriate time period for the purpose of an economic evaluation should be long enough to capture in full the differences in resource use, costs, and benefits between the alternative options being evaluated. Often, as is the case for interventions for chronic diseases, this requires a time horizon that captures the patient's lifetime. Trials rarely provide evidence over the lifetime of all patients (except in cases of interventions for terminal illness). Therefore it is necessary to extrapolate beyond the trial evidence, and decision models can provide a vehicle to extrapolate evidence from trials to a longer and more appropriate time horizon.

4 **RCTs might not provide information on final endpoints** Related to the problem of limited time horizons, trials often provide evidence on intermediate clinical endpoints such as numbers of events or changes in risk factors. For example, a trial may collect, or even have as its pre-defined endpoint, information on HbA1c levels in patients with type 2 diabetes. It is unlikely that they will collect comprehensive information for all patients on final outcomes such as mortality, or that they will collect detailed health-related quality of life data that could be combined with survival data to provide quality-adjusted life-years (QALYs). As a result there will often be a need to link these intermediate endpoints to the long-term outcomes of interest to health economists, and this usually involves combining evidence from a number of sources. In the example given above, clinical trials may provide information on changes in HbA1c levels in patients with type 2 diabetes subsequent to an intervention, and the analyst would then have to extrapolate this information into life expectancy and quality-adjusted life expectancy using a survival model incorporating data from a range of sources including other trials and cohort studies.

5 **RCTs might not provide evidence specific to a particular setting or group of patients** Trials tend to provide evidence specific to a particular setting or group of patients, and this may not represent patients commonly seen in clinical practice or reflect the requirements for the particular decision problem being posed. If there is a need to generalize to other settings or patient subgroups, additional modelling of the trial baseline risks and resource usage informed by other sources may be required to make the results generalizable.

8.2 Uses of decision modelling

Given these limitations or barriers to using data from a single RCT, an alternative or supplementary approach is to use a decision analytic model as the framework for undertaking an economic evaluation. Modelling aims to overcome the limitations of conducting an economic evaluation alongside a randomized trial and can be used instead of, or as a complement to, the patient-specific trial-based approach. Even with a trial-based approach, some modelling may still be required, for example to explore external validity or generalizability of results or to extrapolate results over a longer time horizon.

Models and trials can best be seen as complements rather than substitutes in research design: trials and other studies provide data and estimates of particular parameters, while decision models provide an analytical framework within which the evidence can be synthesised to address the decision problem (Sculpher *et al.* 2006).

The use of decision modelling for the purpose of economic evaluation can:

- structure the economic question
- provide pre-trial modelling and generate study hypotheses (Chilcott *et al.* 2003)
- extrapolate beyond observed data
- link intermediate and final endpoints
- generalize results to other settings or patient groups
- synthesize evidence (Sutton and Abrams 2001; Ades *et al.* 2006) and permit head-to-head comparisons where RCTs do not exist by using indirect and mixed-treatment comparisons (Ades 2003; Lu and Ades 2004; Griffin *et al.* 2006)
- indicate the need for and value of further research (Claxton *et al.* 2001, 2004; Ginnelly *et al.* 2005).

8.3 Stages in the development of a decision analytic model

The development of any decision analytic model requires a number of analogous stages independent of model type. These have been outlined in a number of guidelines to decision analytic modelling for economic evaluation in health care (Sonnenberg *et al.* 1994; Halpern *et al.* 1998; Akehurst *et al.* 2000; Sculpher *et al.* 2000; Weinstein *et al.* 2001; Soto 2002; Weinstein *et al.* 2003; Philips *et al.* 2004, 2006). Each of the steps involved is considered in this section.

8.3.1 Defining the question

Before developing any decision model, the problem that needs to be addressed should be clearly defined. It is important to define the range and details of the alternative options available for evaluation, the recipient population, and the location and setting of the interventions being evaluated. It must also be remembered that, while the model should reflect reality as closely as possible, in essence all models represent a simplification of the real world. Therefore the way in which the question is defined must be realistic, but must also acknowledge and reflect data availability. Finally, the way the question is set out must reflect a set of methodological decisions on the appropriate perspective (e.g. patient or societal), time horizon, measures of costs and benefits, and more broadly the scope or boundaries of the model.

8.3.2 Decide on the type of decision model most appropriate for use in the economic evaluation

The next step in the process of developing a decision model is to decide on the appropriate type of decision model to use. Researchers have provided guidance on selecting the appropriate model type for the purpose of modelling in the economic evaluation of health care (Barton *et al.* 2004; Brennan *et al.* 2006; Cooper *et al.* 2007). Barton and colleagues have developed a flowchart recommending the best model to use depending on the answers to four questions; an adapted version is set out in Figure 8.1. They propose that the key consideration faced by modellers is whether the individuals in the model can be thought of as independent of each other (i.e. can be treated in a homogenous way within the model). Where interaction between individuals is not thought to be of importance, the choice is between decision trees, Markov models, and individual sampling models. These represent the main approaches to modelling that have been used in the economic evaluation of health care.

In general, if the timeframe is short and recurring events are not important, the decision tree is usually appropriate. Where recurrent events are required to be modelled, the Markov model is the model of choice. In cases where Markov models require a lot of health states in an attempt to overcome the Markovian assumption (see Chapter 9), the analyst might consider using an individual sampling model which samples individuals with specific attributes and follows their progress over time.

The assumption of independence between individuals may break down in certain circumstances, for example in infectious diseases where the risk of the individual contracting the disease will depend in part on the number of individuals with the disease, or where there are limitations on the rate at which treatments can be given and therefore choosing to treat one patient impacts on what can be given to another (e.g. liver transplant, where there is a shortage of organs). In these circumstances it becomes essential to capture interaction between individuals, and other model structures such as discrete event simulation (DES) or system dynamic modelling (SD) have been proposed (Karnon and Brown 1998; Barton *et al.* 2004; Caro 2005; Brennan *et al.* 2006) and indeed utilized (Edmunds *et al.* 1999; Brisson and Edmunds 2003; Karnon 2003). DES works at the individual level and allows full representation of each individual's history, whereas SD models operate at the aggregate level and only allow a limited

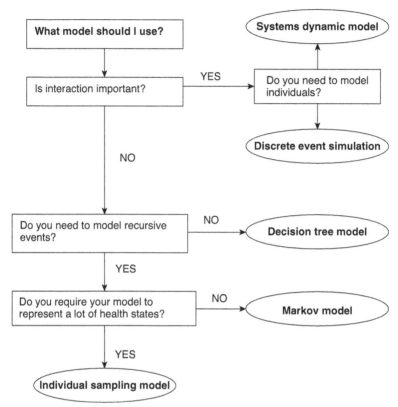

Fig. 8.1 How to decide on the appropriate model. Adapted from Barton *et al.* 2004 with permission.

representation of individuals' histories. Brennan *et al.* (2006) have extended the taxonomy provided by Barton *et al.* (2004) by emphasizing which features and assumptions of the decision problem (e.g. timing, randomness, patient heterogeneity) are most important.

In this chapter and in Chapters 9 and 10 we will concentrate on the two types of decision analytic model most frequently used by health economists when undertaking economic evaluations: the decision tree and the Markov model.

8.3.3 Identifying the evidence and populating the model

Although there are a number of guidelines for researchers undertaking decision models for the purpose of conducting an economic evaluation (Sonnenberg *et al.* 1994; Halpern *et al.* 1998; Akehurst *et al.* 2000; Sculpher *et al.* 2000; Weinstein *et al.* 2001; Soto 2002; Weinstein *et al.* 2003; Philips *et al.* 2004, 2006), very little has been written on how researchers should go about identifying and deciding what evidence to use when populating their model (but see Nuijten 1998; Petitti 2000; Philips *et al.* 2004, 2006; Golder *et al.* 2005).

There are well-known methods for identifying and assessing the quality of effectiveness data (NHS Centre for Reviews and Dissemination 2001; Cochrane Collaboration 2008). However, there is no guidance on how a similar strategy should be conducted for other model parameter inputs, such as resource use, unit costs, probabilities, quality of life, and utilities, except for the suggestion of being based on 'high-quality' evidence (Halpern *et al.* 1998; Soto 2002). Philips *et al.* (2004), in a review of good practice guidelines for decision analytic models, have proposed that methods for identifying data should be transparent and that it should be clear that the data identified are appropriate, given the objectives of the model. Where choices have been made between data inputs they should be justified appropriately and the quality described. They also emphasize that it should be clear that particular attention has been paid to identifying data for key parameters (i.e. those that are believed to impact most on the results of the model). They argue that data identification should be undertaken in a systematic yet not necessarily comprehensive manner. In fact, Golder and colleagues state that:

> Decision models for technology assessments are often undertaken within a relatively short period of time on a limited budget and have more numerous and varied data requirements than systematic reviews. The search techniques used in systematic reviews, therefore, may be impractical for the development of strategies to identify information to populate all the parameter estimates in a decision-analytic model.
>
> Golder *et al.* 2005, p.306

Philips *et al.* (2004) also discuss how data should be incorporated into the model, arguing that the process of data incorporation should be transparent, and should be described and referenced in sufficient detail.

8.3.4 Synthesizing evidence

When using decision models, the data are likely to come from a number of sources, such as RCTs, epidemiological or observational studies, databases, medical records, previously published literature (systematic reviews, meta-analyses) and expert opinion. The source and type of data should be defined, and in cases where expert opinion has been used the methods and sources should be described and justified (Philips *et al.* 2004). Leal *et al.* (2007) have provided an applied example of how expert opinion can be elicited for the purpose of economic models. Given the fact that a specific model input parameter might be based on a number of sources of evidence, there has been increasing support for a move towards more formal evidence synthesis. This has been well formulated for use with measures of effectiveness (Sutton *et al.* 2000), but less so for other cost-effectiveness parameter inputs (Cooper *et al.* 2005). In fact the use of multi-parameter evidence synthesis techniques (a generalization of meta-analysis in which multiple parameters are estimated jointly (Ades and Sutton 2006) for the purpose of health economic decision modelling remains an under-researched area.

Cooper and colleagues have taken this idea forward and proposed a method used by previous analysts (Matchar *et al.* 1997; Parmigiani *et al.* 1997; Fryback *et al.* 2001a,b) for simultaneously addressing all the individual components of undertaking a decision model in one Bayesian model, which they have called 'comprehensive decision analytical modelling' (Cooper *et al.* 2004). These models purport to reflect all available evidence along with a complete picture of the parameter uncertainty while maintaining the correlation coefficients between the parameters within the model. Ades *et al.* (2006) describe the technique as 'effectively integrating statistical evidence synthesis and parameter estimation with probabilistic decision analysis in a single unified framework'. Examples of cost-effectiveness analyses developed as comprehensive decision models are now appearing in the published literature (Fryback *et al.* 2001a; Iglesias and Claxton 2006; Bravo *et al.* 2007).

8.3.5 Analysing the model

The analysis of the model is dependent on the type of model chosen to undertake the cost-effectiveness analysis. Later in this chapter and in Chapter 9 there will be an in-depth discussion of how decision tree and Markov models are analysed in order to provide evidence on cost-effectiveness.

8.3.6 Model evaluation

Evaluation of the model is an important step in the development of a decision model and should be centred around the assumptions and model structure, the input parameters and any distributions used to reflect uncertainty, and the output and conclusions. There are several published articles on model evaluation; however, all vary in the breadth and terminology used to explain the processes involved (Eddy 1985; Halpern *et al.* 1998; McCabe and Dixon 2000; Sculpher *et al.* 2000; Weinstein *et al.* 2003; Ades and Sutton 2006; Philips *et al.* 2006). Here we define three key processes that summarize model evaluation: face or descriptive validity, internal validity/consistency, and external validity/consistency, which incorporate between-model (cross-model) validation and predictive validity. Calibration should be considered as part of the evaluation process, namely internal validity.

Face or descriptive validity

The 'descriptive validity' or 'face validity' of a decision model entails checking whether its assumptions, structure, and results are reliable, sensible, and can be explained intuitively (McCabe and Dixon 2000; Weinstein *et al.* 2003).

Internal validation and calibration

Internal validity/consistency relates to the logic of the model and whether the model inputs relate to its outputs. Testing for this relies on 'debugging' the model using sensitivity analysis by incorporating extreme or null values of parameter inputs to assess whether the results are moving in the expected direction. It may also involve getting another researcher to replicate the model using the same data to ensure comparability of results, or using a different software platform to replicate the model.

Internal validity/consistency also relates to how accurate the model is when compared with the evidence used for its development (Weinstein *et al.* 2003; Philips *et al.* 2006). Currently, there are a limited number of published examples where an internal model validation process has been described (Clarke *et al.* 2004; Mihaylova *et al.* 2006; Mueller *et al.* 2006; Kim *et al.* 2007). Eddy (1985) provided some of the first advice in this area, arguing that reproducing the results of a trial on which the model is based provides some corroboration of the model. Kim *et al.* (2007) undertook an internal validation of their decision model developed for the multicentre aneurysm screening study (MASS). They compared key outputs from the model after 4 years in terms of overall numbers and timing of events (ruptures, operations, and deaths), and costs and benefits, with the observed MASS trial data after 4 years follow-up. Similarly, Mihaylova *et al.* (2006) used an internal validation process to compare their outputs in terms of annual rates of death from vascular disease, major vascular events, and all vascular events from their Markov state transition model with trial data from the Heart Protection Study.

Model calibration is emerging as a method of aiding researchers in model development. It forms a central part of the internal validation and is particularly useful in the assessment of disease processes such as the natural history of disease, where key parameters in this process are unobservable. In essence calibration is the practice of determining the values of unobservable parameters by forcing the model output to replicate observed data. In a review of calibration methods used in cancer models, Stout *et al.* (2009) identified five components of model calibration: calibration targets (the observed data that the model attempts to replicate during calibration), goodness-of-fit (GOF) metric (quantitative measure of the ability of the model to replicate the target data given a particular set of parameter values), search algorithms (methods for selecting alternative parameter values), acceptance criteria (specification of the acceptable levels of fit based on the GOF metric), and stopping rules (the rationale for ending the search procedure and calibration process). They propose that their 'Calibration Reporting Checklist' be adopted as standard practice for modellers (Stout *et al.* 2009, p.539, Figure 2).

Some suggest that the data used for calibration of external consistency should be independent of the data used to populate the model. Kim *et al.* (2007) and van Houwelingen (2000) have compared external data with the expected data from the model to assess the consistency. However, others have argued that calibration can lead to an ad hoc search for parameter values until the model appears to fit the data, a practice that makes it impossible to characterize the uncertainty in the model parameters or outputs correctly (van Houwelingen and Thorogood 1995; Kennedy and O'Hagan 2001; Ades and Cliffe 2002). This is an important consideration for health economic models. They suggest that all the data, including the validating/calibrating data, should be incorporated when building a model as opposed to using 'validating' data as external sources only for comparison with the model outputs. The Bayesian Monte Carlo Markov Chain (MCMC) framework and other developed model criticism tools can then be applied to determine whether the evidence is statistically consistent (Ades and Cliffe 2002; Ades and Sutton 2006). This will help to inform the explicit clinical judgement decision of whether or not to include specific data sources in the model. Ades and Cliffe (2002) illustrate the use of model criticism tools using an HIV prenatal screening model. Furthermore, Welton and Ades (2005) provide a worked example of how Bayesian MCMC methods could be used to synthesize and calibrate data on the parameters of a Markov model to a particular study of interest. They represent a way of achieving the calibration within a probabilistic decision-modelling framework, correctly propagating the uncertainties in both the parameters and the study to which the model is to be calibrated and incorporating any correlations between parameters that are induced by the data structure.

External validation: between-model validation and predictive validity

External validation of a model concerns the extent to which the model results can be generalized beyond the evidence used for its development into the population of interest and other populations. This type of validation is more difficult to perform, as the data against which the model will be compared are not available during its development. External validation entails predictive validity and between-model validation. Predictive validity refers to the ability of the model to make accurate predictions of future events. However, a more useful model characteristic would be its ability to incorporate new evidence as it becomes available (Weinstein *et al.* 2003). Between-model validation can be assessed when models have been developed independently from one another, permitting tests of between-model corroboration (convergent validity), i.e. a process by which a model is validated by comparing the results with those from other independent models that have addressed the same question. This type of validation is integral to collaborative modelling projects such as the Cancer Intervention and Surveillance Modelling Network (CISNET) group (CISNET 2010). In the prostate cancer CISNET group three models have been developed by separate teams using diverse methods, and these models have then been calibrated to the incidence of prostate cancer by age, stage, and calendar year using SEER data. This has facilitated a direct comparison of the methods and results of each model (Draisma *et al.* 2009).

The Mount Hood Challenge has been one example of a successful approach to assessing both predictive validity and cross-model validation. Named after Mount Hood in Oregon where the first meeting was held, the challenge consisted of gathering eight diabetes modelling groups and asking them to compare model outputs systematically by predicting clinical trial outcomes on the basis of risk factor changes and then comparing the predictions against each other and against 'real' data from the clinical trial (Mount Hood 2007). In other exercises, modellers were asked to simulate lifetime outcomes for a hypothetical patient with specified characteristics. This systematic approach to validating models has enabled the identification of key differences among models in their performance, as well as possible causes for differences and directions for future improvement.

8.3.7 **Handling uncertainty**

Uncertainty exists in all economic evaluations and has to be appropriately accounted for. Briggs (2000) provides a useful discussion of how to deal with uncertainty when undertaking a cost-effectiveness analysis. For the purpose of decision modelling the focus has been on methodological, structural, and parameter uncertainty (Akehurst *et al.* 2000). The methods for handling the different types of uncertainty and the implications when undertaking a decision analytic model are discussed in detail in Chapter 10.

8.4 **Properties of good decision models and critical appraisal**

Evidence from research conducted by Cooper *et al.* (2005) suggests that reporting of the structure, data inputs, and outputs of health care decision models has been poor in the past, and that a more structured, transparent, and reproducible format for analysing and reporting should be developed. Perhaps the development of good practice guidelines for health-care decision models will have a positive impact on this (NICE 2008). In developing a synthesized best practice guideline for decision analytic modelling in health technology assessment, Philips *et al.* (2004, 2006) used major themes that emerged from 15 previously published guidelines as a basis for their best practice guideline. They provide a framework by which models can be quality assessed under the general themes of structure, data, and consistency. Table 8.1 outlines the basics of the checklist developed by Philips and colleagues.

These checklists and guidelines are also likely to be adapted as more decision models are constructed for the economic evaluation of health and health care interventions. For example, Karnon *et al.* (2007) have recently demonstrated that at least three specific issues not routinely included in modelling guidelines can have a significant impact on cost-effectiveness results: the inclusion of incident cases over the course of a specified time-horizon, the use of a non-lifetime time horizon, and the handling of age-specific patient subgroups.

8.5 **Decision tree models**

As already discussed, various types of decision analytic models can be used to undertake an economic evaluation of a health-care intervention. In this section we explore in more detail one of the most common: the decision tree. A decision tree, which is a representation of a decision analysis, is a branching structure in which each branch represents an event that may take place in the future. Identifying alternatives and specifying the sequence and linkage of events are essential steps in constructing such a model, but are also in themselves of great value in clarifying complex decisions.

The steps involved in developing, analysing, and evaluating a decision tree as part of an economic evaluation are set out below using a simple illustrative example: a hypothetical policy question concerning whether to introduce a breast cancer screening programme.

8.5.1 **Tree structure**

In the illustrative example the researcher has been commissioned to ascertain whether it would be cost-effective to screen for breast cancer. Therefore the first point in the decision tree represents this decision question with a decision node (representing the first point of choice), usually drawn as a square (Figure 8.2). The decision in this example is whether screening for breast cancer every two years compared to not screening at all represents a cost-effective alternative. It is possible for a decision node to have more than two alternatives emanating from it, for example a third alternative of screening every 5 years could have been added to this decision problem. Decision trees are by

Table 8.1 A checklist for the quality assessment of decision analytic modelling in health technology assessment

Themes	Quality dimension	Quality assessment questions
Structure	Statement of decision problem/objective	◆ Is there a clear statement of the decision problem? ◆ Is the objective of the evaluation and the model specified, and is it consistent with the decision problem? ◆ Is the primary decision-maker specified?
	Statement of the scope/perspective	◆ Is the model perspective stated? ◆ Are the model inputs consistent with the stated perspective? ◆ Has the scope of the model been stated and justified? ◆ Are the model outcomes consistent with the scope, perspective, and objectives of the model?
	Rationale for structure	◆ Is the model structure consistent with the theory of the health condition being evaluated? ◆ Are the data sources used to develop the model structure specified? ◆ Are the causal relationships within the model structure justified?
	Strategies and comparators	◆ Is there a clear definition of the options under evaluation? ◆ Have all the feasible options been evaluated? ◆ If feasible options have been excluded this requires justification
	Model type	◆ Is the model type specified? ◆ Given the problem is the chosen model type appropriate?
	Time horizon	◆ Is the time horizon of the model sufficient to reflect all important differences between the options? ◆ Are the time horizon of the model, the duration of treatment and the duration of treatment effect described and justified?
	Disease states/ pathways	◆ Do the disease states or pathways reflect the underlying biological process of the disease in question and the impact of the interventions?
	Cycle length	◆ Is the cycle length defined and justified?
Data	Data identification	◆ Are the data identification methods transparent and appropriate? ◆ Where choices have been made between data sources, are they appropriately justified? ◆ Has particular attention been paid to identifying data for the important parameters of the model? ◆ Has the data quality been assessed appropriately? ◆ Where expert opinion has been used, are the methods described and justified?

(continued)

Table 8.1 (continued) A checklist for the quality assessment of decision analytic modelling in health technology assessment

Themes	Quality dimension	Quality assessment questions
	Data modelling	♦ Is the data modelling methodology based on justifiable statistical and epidemiological methods?
	Baseline data	♦ Is the choice of baseline data described and justified?
		♦ Are transition probabilities calculated appropriately?
		♦ Has a half-cycle correction been applied to costs and outcomes?
		♦ If there is no half-cycle correction, is this justified?
	Treatment effects	♦ If relative treatment effects are from trial data, have they been synthesized using appropriate techniques?
		♦ Have the methods and assumptions used to extrapolate short-term results to final outcomes been documented and justified and alternative assumptions explored using sensitivity analysis?
		♦ Have the assumptions regarding the continuing effect of treatment once treatment is complete been documented and justified, and alternative assumptions explored in sensitivity analysis?
	Costs	♦ Are the costs described and justified?
		♦ Has the source of cost data been documented?
		♦ Have the discount rates been documented and justified?
	Quality of life weights (utilities)	♦ Are the utilities documented and appropriate?
		♦ Has the source of utility data been documented?
		♦ Are the methods for deriving utility data described and justified?
	Data incorporation	♦ Have all data incorporated in the model been described and referenced?
		♦ Have the assumptions and choice of data been made explicit and justified?
		♦ Is the process of data incorporation transparent?
		♦ If distributions have been used for the parameters, are these described and justified?
	Assessment of uncertainty	♦ Have the four principal types of uncertainty (methodological, structural, parameter, and heterogeneity) been addressed?
		♦ If not, has their omission been justified?
	Methodological	♦ Have methodological uncertainties been addressed by running the model with alternative methodological assumptions?
	Structural	♦ Have structural uncertainties been assessed using sensitivity analysis?

(continued)

Table 8.1 (continued) A checklist for the quality assessment of decision analytic modelling in health technology assessment

Themes	Quality dimension	Quality assessment questions
	Heterogeneity	◆ Has heterogeneity been addressed by running the model for separate subgroups?
	Parameter	◆ Are the methods of assessing parameter uncertainty appropriate?
		◆ If parameters are represented by point estimates, are the ranges used in the sensitivity analysis documented and justified?
Consistency	Internal consistency	◆ Is there evidence that the mathematical logic of the model has been tested?
	External consistency	◆ Are counter-intuitive results explained and justified?
		◆ If the model results are compared with independent data, are the differences explained and justified?
		◆ Have the results been compared with results from other models and any similarities or differences justified?

Adapted from Philips *et al.* (2004) with permission.

convention constructed from left to right, starting with the decision node and ending with the outcomes on the right, and follow the logical structure of the decision problem, usually following the sequence of events over time.

Once the comparators have been chosen, any events that follow from this decision are 'chance' events and are characterized by probabilities. These events are represented by chance nodes (circular symbols) in the decision tree diagram. Each outcome from each chance node is denoted by a line (branch) attached to the chance node and labelled.

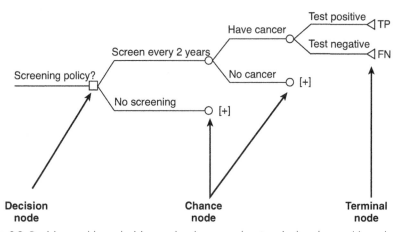

Fig. 8.2 Decision problem, decision node, chance nodes, terminal nodes, and branches.

The likelihood of the event is represented by the branch probability (see section 8.5.3). The events stemming from a chance node must be mutually exclusive, and the probabilities should sum exactly to 1. In this example, the introduction of a policy to screen for breast cancer every 2 years is followed in the tree by the possibility of either the uncertain event of the patient having breast cancer or the uncertain event of the patient not having cancer (it is possible to have more than two uncertain events emanating from a chance node as long as they are mutually exclusive and exhaustive).

Moving from left to right along the decision tree, the addition of chance nodes corresponds to the addition of subsequent uncertain events. In this example, if someone has cancer, there follows a subsequent chance node with branches relating to the screening test either returning a positive result or a negative result, with the final outcomes from these alternative decision tree pathways ending in terminal nodes (characterized by a triangle) and giving a true-positive screening result or a false-negative screening result conditioned on the pathway probabilities. Each terminal node has a value or payoff assigned to it (see section 8.5.4).

In Figure 8.2 there is a [+] sign at the end of some of the nodes; this simply means that there is more to come beyond this point in the tree diagram.

8.5.2 Order of events in the decision tree

The best way of ordering the decision tree should be considered. Although order makes no difference in terms of the expected value of the strategies (see section 8.5.5), it does have implications for how easy it is to perform the sensitivity analysis and deal with complex treatment and disease pathways.

In general, the order of the events in the decision tree usually follows the sequence of events over time according to the logical progression of the decision pathway. However, the structure of the tree may depend on the available probabilities. This can be illustrated by considering the nature of the screening outcomes in the example. Table 8.2 indicates four potential outcomes of any screening programme. A true-positive case occurs where the screening verdict is positive and cancer is present. A false-negative case occurs where the screening verdict is negative and cancer is present. The sensitivity of the test (the true-positive rate) is the probability of a test being positive given that the disease is present, $P[T+|D]$, and is obtained from $A/(A + C)$. A false-positive case occurs where the screening verdict is positive and cancer is not present. Finally, a true-negative case occurs where the screening verdict is negative and cancer is not present. The specificity of the test (the true-negative rate) is the probability of a test being negative given that the disease is not present, $P[T-|D-]$, and is obtained from $D/(B + D)$. The positive predictive value is the probability that the person has the disease given that he/she tests positive, $P[D+|T+]$, or $A/(A + B)$. The negative predictive value is the probability that the person is disease free given he/she tests negative, $P[D-|T-]$, and is obtained from $D/(C + D)$. Finally, the prevalence of the disease, $P[D+]$, is $(A + C)/(A + B + C + D)$.

Hence, the first way of ordering the tree in the illustrative example is as shown in Figure 8.3. Screening initially divides people into two groups, according to the result of the test (positive or negative). Subsequent tests would divide the population into

Table 8.2 Classification of screening outcomes

Screening verdict	True diagnosis		Total
	Cancer	No cancer	
Positive	True positive (A)	False positive (B)	A+B
Negative	False negative (C)	True negative (D)	C+D
Total	A+C	B+D	A+B+C+D
	Sensitivity = A/(A+C)	Specificity = D/(B+D)	

true- and false-positive cases. This order follows the sequence by which clinical decisions are taken. The disease status is to the right of the test result, and the subsequent branch probabilities required are then the probability of disease, conditional on the test results (e.g. $P(D+|T+)$).

An alternative order is to begin with the assumption that there is a proportion of people with and without disease and to divide the decision tree into two branches at this point (see Figure 8.4). This approach tends to be much simpler to populate, especially when the underlying disease and treatment pathways are complex, but the disadvantage is that it is slightly less intuitive for clinicians. In the initial branches, the probability represents the probability of a patient within the specific population having the disease, which is the incidence or prevalence of the disease in the population. Subsequent probabilities are the proportion of each test result conditional on the disease itself (i.e. the sensitivity and specificity). The following relationships are obtained for the four screening outcomes or payoffs:

true positive = sensitivity × prevalence
false negative = (1 − sensitivity) × prevalence
true negative = specificity × (1 − prevalence)
false positive = (1 − specificity) × (1 − prevalence).

8.5.3 Estimating probabilities

Once the structure of the model has been developed, the next step in the process is to start populating the model (see sections 8.3.3 and 8.3.4 for a more general discussion of identifying, incorporating, and synthesizing evidence for the model). Probabilities

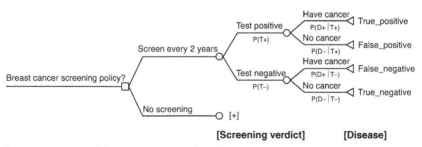

Fig. 8.3 Structure of the tree: process ordered.

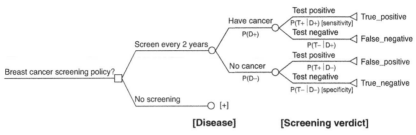

[Disease]   **[Screening verdict]**

Fig. 8.4 Structure of the tree: according to disease status.

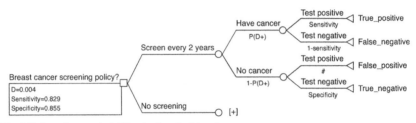

Fig. 8.5 Entering probabilities in the decision tree.

are usually derived from published studies. A systematic search of the literature should be performed and the validity of the results of published studies should be considered. When there is more than one source of information on a probability, information will need to be synthesized. The results of a meta-analysis undertaken by others can be used as the source of a probability estimate or data can be synthesised by the analyst. Alternative data sources include data from routinely collected databases, or if no estimates are found in the literature or from routine data sources, expert opinion may be sought. The best estimate for each probability is known as the 'base-case' estimate. Since there will be uncertainty about the best estimate, a range of reasonable estimates should be documented for later use in the sensitivity analysis.

By convention, probabilities (branch probabilities) are entered under the branches emanating from a chance node to represent the probability/likelihood of the uncertain event occurring (Figure 8.5). Since the events at a chance node must be mutually exclusive and exhaustive, the sum of the probabilities at each chance node must equal 1. If one of two outcomes has been specified, the remaining outcome is sometimes referred to as a residual or complementary probability and represented by the symbol #, although it can also be written as 1 minus the other, e. g. 1 – sensitivity in Figure 8.5:

$P(D+)$ = probability of having cancer = 0.004
$1 - P(D+)$ = probability of not having cancer = (1–0.004)
Sensitivity = probability of returning test positive result conditioned on having cancer = 0.829
Specificity = probability of returning test negative result conditioned on not having cancer = 0.855

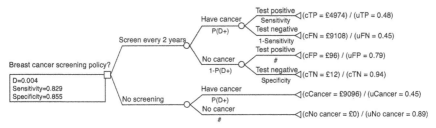

Fig. 8.6 Values attached to the payoffs: costs and outcomes.

1 – sensitivity = probability of returning test negative result conditioned on having cancer

= probability of returning test positive result conditioned on not having cancer.

8.5.4 **Payoffs**

Once all the probabilities have been identified and entered into the decision tree, the payoffs can be identified and entered. Payoffs include the costs related to the events in the decision tree and the final outcomes (life-years, utilities, quality-adjusted life-years), and are entered at the terminal node. Each terminal node requires one or more values to be assigned to it; in our worked example we are estimating cost-effectiveness, and so the values to be assigned are costs and utilities (Figure 8.6).

The costs associated with a true-positive result are sum of the cost of a screen, assessment, and treatment for early-stage breast cancer. The costs associated with a false-negative result are the sum of the cost of a screen, assessment, and treatment for late-stage breast cancer. The costs associated with a false-positive result are the sum of the costs of a screen and assessment. The costs associated with a true-negative result are the costs associated with a screen. In the no screening arm of the model, the costs of the cancer outcome are the sum of assessment and treatment for late-stage breast cancer. The costs of a no cancer outcome are assumed to be zero. The utilities, which come from a study by Gerard *et al.* (1999), give a value of 0.48 for a true positive, 0.45 for a false positive, 0.79 for a false negative, and 0.94 for a true negative. The utility of a cancer outcome is assumed to be the same as a false negative and the utility of a no cancer outcome is 0.89.

8.5.5 **Analysing the decision tree: expected values and cost-effectiveness**

Once the probabilities and payoffs have been entered, it is possible to perform the analysis. The decision tree is 'averaged out' and 'folded back' (or 'rolled back'). By folding back the tree, the expected values of each strategy are calculated. The folding-back process starts at the right-hand side of the tree and then averages back. The expected value is the sum of products of the estimates of the probability of events occurring and the consequence of the events, their outcomes, or their costs, i.e. the weighted average of the outcome or cost values. The value of the outcome of each branch is multiplied by its respective probability. At each chance node, the products for the entire branch are summed. Expected values are first calculated for each branch of the tree at chance nodes and then for each branch of a decision tree at decision nodes moving from right to left. This process is conducted separately for costs and effects. The concept of expected value corresponds to the mean value of an endpoint when using patient-specific data.

Using the example shown in Figure 8.7, the expected costs and expected outcomes are calculated separately by reading the decision tree from right to left and calculating the expected values at each chance node sequentially. The expected cost of having cancer in the option of screening every 2 years is £5680.91. This is calculated by multiplying the probability of the event occurring by the consequence of the event (e.g. cost and utility/life-years/QALYs) and summing these values at the chance node, for example

$$(0.829 \times £4974) + [(1 - 0.829) \times £9108] = £5680.91.$$

Similarly, the expected cost of not having cancer in the screening every 2 years option is calculated as

$$(0.855 \times £12) + [(1 - 0.855) \times £96] = £24.18.$$

To obtain the expected cost of screening every 2 years requires the decision tree to be calculated one more branch to the left, for example

$$(0.004 \times £5680.91) + [(1 - 0.004) \times £24.18] = £46.81.$$

The expected outcomes are calculated in the same way, resulting in an expected QALY of 0.92 for the screening every 2 years option. This process is replicated to obtain the expected costs and QALYs for the no screening option, and it can be seen from Figure 8.7 that the option to screen every 2 years has a higher expected cost and higher expected QALYs than the option of no screening. These expected values now enable the researcher to calculate an incremental cost effectiveness ratio (ICER) for screening every 2 years compared with no screening (Table 8.3). The incremental cost of implementing a biennial screening programme is £10.42 and the incremental effect is 0.0282 QALYs, resulting in an ICER of £369.13.

8.5.6 Model evaluation

Once the decision tree model has been constructed and analysed, it is important for the developer to assess its validity and check it for consistency. Issues surrounding validation and consistency of decision models have already been discussed earlier in this chapter (see section 8.3.6). It is suggested that the model developer use the checklist of quality assessment of decision analytic models compiled by Philips *et al.* (2004, 2006).

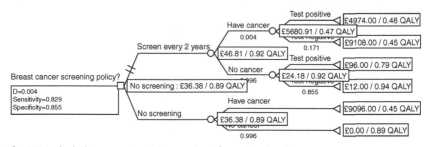

Fig. 8.7 Calculating expected values: output from TreeAge Pro.

Table 8.3 Calculating the incremental cost effectiveness ratio (ICER) for screening every 2 years compared with no screening using the expected values from the decision tree

Strategy	Mean cost	Incremental cost	Mean effect (QALY)	Incremental effect (QALY)	ICER
No screening	£36.38		0.8882		
Screen every 2 years	£46.81	£10.42	0.9165	0.0282	£369.13

8.5.7 Explore uncertainty

Even if the results show that one particular strategy is the best, given that there is undoubtedly uncertainty about the structure of the decision tree and the parameter values used within the model, there is a question as to how much confidence can be placed in this finding. Sensitivity analysis can be used to address the problems of structural and parameter uncertainty. The structure of the decision tree can be altered and re-analysed to assess the overall impact on the base-case results. To assess the impact of parameter uncertainty, researchers have traditionally reported a range of values for the parameter inputs to their decision tree models, and then used these ranges to assess the impact on the base-case results of altering a single parameter value (univariate or one-way sensitivity analysis) or a combination of parameters (multivariate or scenario sensitivity analysis). Although these forms of sensitivity analysis are still recommended, they have been largely superseded by the use of probabilistic sensitivity analysis (PSA), whereby each parameter is assigned a distribution and the cost-effectiveness results from simultaneously selecting a random value from the distributions around the parameter inputs using Monte Carlo simulation are recorded. The results of the PSA can provide 95% confidence limits for the expected outcome. This process is explained in greater detail in Chapter 10. Here we will use the decision tree example to explore the use of univariate sensitivity analysis.

In order to address the uncertainty in the base-case results, a one-way sensitivity analysis is conducted looking at the impact of alternative estimates of the test sensitivity and specificity. From the literature, the range of values around the base-case probability value for the sensitivity of the test is given as between 0.740 and 0.890, and the result of the sensitivity analysis shows that as the sensitivity of the test increases the ICER of biennial versus no screening falls, implying an improved cost-effectiveness (Figure 8.8a). Similarly, the range of values around the base-case estimate for specificity is given as between 0.839 and 0.901. Figure 8.8b shows that as the specificity of the test increases, the ICER falls from £455.06 to £187.26, again implying an improved cost-effectiveness.

8.6 Summary: advantages and limitations

Although decision trees are relatively simple to develop, and are transparent and easy to interrogate/communicate, there are some basic limitations which mean that in certain circumstances other decision analytic modelling techniques may be more appropriate.

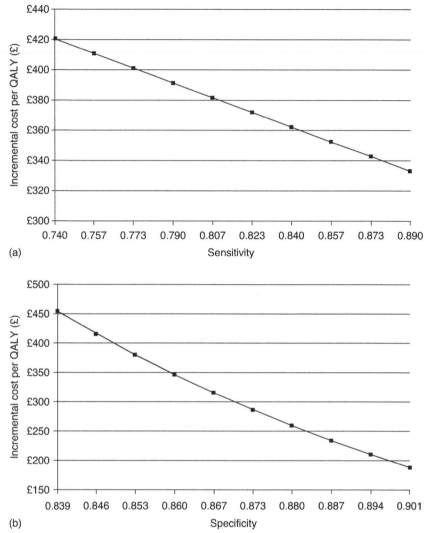

Fig. 8.8 a) One-way sensitivity analysis of parameter input probability that test results return a positive result when the disease is present, i.e. test sensitivity. b) One-way sensitivity analysis of parameter input probability that test results return a negative result when the disease is absent, i.e. test specificity.

The implicit assumption when using decision tree models is that they are suited to diseases where events occur over a discrete short time period. The developer needs to explicitly define the time period over which the events occur, as there is no implicit time variable within a decision tree; the passage of time is accounted for by the outcome measures or pay-offs. This means that implementing time dependency into a decision tree model can be difficult. This applies not only to estimating the final outcomes in terms of adjusting the quality of life for the appropriate survival time, but also to ensuring the appropriate discounting of both the costs and outcomes.

A related limitation is that when decision trees are used to model diseases with lengthy prognoses or events that are likely to recur over time (e.g. chronic diseases), the structure of a decision tree only allows for one-way progression of the patient through the model, and does not permit movement back and forth between disease states. In principle this could be addressed by adding additional branches and extending the time horizon. However, the model can quickly become complex and unmanageable. Other modelling techniques such as Markov modelling, as we shall see in Chapter 9, are superior for handling repeated events. Finally, it should be noted that decision trees can often be used as a submodel in a larger model. For example, a decision tree could be built to identify the number of cases detected by a screening programme, and a Markov model could then be built to model future costs and effects following detection.

References

Ades, A.E. (2003). A chain of evidence with mixed comparisons: models for multi-parameter synthesis and consistency of evidence. *Statistics in Medicine*, **22**, 2995–3016.

Ades, A.E. and Cliffe, S. (2002). Markov chain Monte Carlo estimation of a multiparameter decision model: consistency of evidence and the accurate assessment of uncertainty. *Medical Decision Making*, **22**, 359–71.

Ades, A.E. and Sutton, A. (2006). Multiparameter evidence synthesis in epidemiology and medical decision-making: current approaches. *Journal of the Royal Statistical Society*, **169**, 5–35.

Ades, A.E., Sculpher, M., Sutton, A., *et al.* (2006). Bayesian methods for evidence synthesis in cost-effectiveness analysis. *Pharmacoeconomics*, **24**, 1–19.

Akehurst, R., Anderson, P., and Brazier, J. (2000) Decision analytic modelling in the economic evaluation of health technologies: a consensus statement. Consensus Conference on Guidelines on Economic Modelling in Health Technology Assessment. *Pharmacoeconomics*, **17**, 443–4.

Barton, P., Bryan, S., and Robinson, S. (2004). Modelling in the economic evaluation of health care: selecting the appropriate approach. *Journal of Health Services Research and Policy*, **9**, 110–18.

Bravo, V.Y., Palmer, S., Asseburg, C., *et al.* (2007). Is primary angioplasty cost effective in the UK? Results of a comprehensive decision analysis. *Heart*, **93**, 1238–43.

Brennan, A., Chick, S.E., and Davies, R. (2006). A taxonomy of model structures for economic evaluation of health technologies. *Health Economics*, **15**, 1295–1310.

Briggs, A.H. (2000). Handling uncertainty in cost-effectiveness models. *Pharmacoeconomics*, **17**, 479–500.

Brisson, M. and Edmunds, W.J. (2003). Economic evaluation of vaccination programs: the impact of herd-immunity. *Medical Decision Making*, **23**, 76–82.

Caro, J. J. (2005). Pharmacoeconomic analyses using discrete event simulation. *Pharmacoeconomics*, **23**, 323–32.

Chilcott, J., Brennan, A., Booth, A., Karnon, J., and Tappenden, P. (2003). The role of modelling in prioritising and planning clinical trials. *Health Technology Assessment*, **7**, 1–125.

CISNET (2010). Available online at: http://cisnet.cancer.gov/

Clarke, P.M., Gray, A.M., Briggs, A., *et al.* (2004). A model to estimate the lifetime health outcomes of patients with type 2 diabetes: the United Kingdom Prospective Diabetes Study (UKPDS) Outcomes Model (UKPDS no. 68), *Diabetologia*, **47**, 1747–59.

Claxton, K., Neumann, P.J., Araki, S., and Weinstein, M.C. (2001). Bayesian value-of-information analysis: an application to a policy model of Alzheimer's disease. *International Journal of Technology Assessment in Health Care*, **17**, 38–55.

Claxton, K., Ginnelly, L., Sculpher, M., Philips, Z., and Palmer, S. (2004). A pilot study on the use of decision theory and value of information analysis as part of the NHS Health Technology Assessment programme, *Health Technology Assessment*, **8**, 1–103.

Cochrane Collaboration (2008). *Cochrane Handbook for Systematic Reviews of Interventions* Version 5.0.1.

Cooper, N.J., Sutton, A.J., Abrams, K.R., Turner, D., and Wailoo, A. (2004). Comprehensive decision analytical modelling in economic evaluation: a Bayesian approach. *Health Economics*, **13**, 203–26.

Cooper, N., Coyle, D., Abrams, K., Mugford, M., and Sutton, A. (2005). Use of evidence in decision models: an appraisal of health technology assessments in the UK since 1997. *Journal of Health Services Research and Policy*, **10**, 245–50.

Cooper, K., Brailsford, S.C., and Davies, R. (2007). Choice of modelling technique for evaluating health care interventions. *Journal of the Operational Research Society*, **58**, 168–76.

Draisma, G., Etzioni, R., Tsodikov, A., *et al.* (2009). Lead time and overdiagnosis in prostate-specific antigen screening: importance of methods and context. *Journal of the National Cancer Institute*, **101**, 374–83.

Eddy, D. (1985). Technology assessment: the role of mathematical modelling. In: Mosteller, F. (ed.) *Assessing Medical Technologies*, pp.144–60. National Academy Press, Washington, DC.

Edmunds, W.J., Medley, G.F., and Nokes, D.J. (1999). Evaluating the cost-effectiveness of vaccination programmes: a dynamic perspective. *Statistics in Medicine*, **18**, 3263–82.

Fryback, D.G., Chinnis, J.O., Jr, and Ulvila, J.W. (2001a). Bayesian cost-effectiveness analysis: an example using the GUSTO trial. *International Journal of Technology Assessment in Health Care*, **17**, 83–97.

Fryback, D.G., Stout, N.K., and Rosenberg, M.A. (2001b). An elementary introduction to Bayesian computing using WinBUGS. *International Journal of Technology Assessment in Health Care*, **17**, 98–113.

Gerard, K., Johnston, K., and Brown, J. (1999). The role of a pre-scored multi-attribute health classification measure in validating condition-specific health state descriptions. *Health Economics*, **8**, 685–99.

Ginnelly, L., Claxton, K., Sculpher, M.J., and Golder, S. (2005). Using value of information analysis to inform publicly funded research priorities. *Applied Health Economics and Health Policy*, **4**, 37–46.

Golder, S., Glanville, J., and Ginnelly, L. (2005). Populating decision-analytic models: the feasibility and efficiency of database searching for individual parameters. *International Journal of Technology Assessment in Health Care*, **21**, 305–11.

Griffin, S., Bojke, L., Main, C., and Palmer, S. (2006). Incorporating direct and indirect evidence using Bayesian methods: an applied case study in ovarian cancer. *Value in Health*, **9**, 123–31.

Halpern, M.T., McKenna, M., and Hutton, J. (1998). Modeling in economic evaluation: an unavoidable fact of life. *Health Economics*, **7**, 741–2.

Hunink, M.G.M., Glaziou, P.P., Siegell, J.E., *et al.* (2001). *Decision Making in Health and Medicine. Integrating Evidence and Values.* Cambridge University Press.

Iglesias, C.P. and Claxton, K. (2006). Comprehensive decision-analytic model and Bayesian value-of-information analysis: pentoxifylline in the treatment of chronic venous leg ulcers. *Pharmacoeconomics*, **24**, 465–78.

Karnon, J. (2003). Alternative decision modelling techniques for the evaluation of health care technologies: Markov processes versus discrete event simulation. *Health Economics*, **12**, 837–48.

Karnon, J. and Brown, J. (1998) Selecting a decision model for economic evaluation: a case study and review, *Health Care Management Science*, **1**, 133–40.

Karnon, J., Brennan, A., and Akehurst, R. (2007). A critique and impact analysis of decision modeling assumptions. *Medical Decision Making*, **27**, 491–9.

Kennedy, M.C. and O'Hagan, A. (2001). Bayesian calibration of computer models. *Journal of the Royal Statistical Society, Series B (Statistical Methodology)*, **63**, 425–64.

Kim, L.G., Thompson, S.G., Briggs, A.H., Buxton, M.J., and Campbell, H.E. (2007). How cost-effective is screening for abdominal aortic aneurysms? *Journal of Medical Screening*, **14**, 46–52.

Leal, J., Wordsworth, S., Legood, R., and Blair, E. (2007). Eliciting expert opinion for economic models: an applied example. *Value in Health*, **10**, 195–203.

Lu, G. and Ades, A.E. (2004). Combination of direct and indirect evidence in mixed treatment comparisons. *Statistics in Medicine*, **23**, 3105–24.

McCabe, C. and Dixon, S. (2000). Testing the validity of cost-effectiveness models. *Pharmacoeconomics*, **17**, 501–13.

Matchar, D.B., Samsa, G.P., Matthews, J.R., *et al.* (1997). The Stroke Prevention Policy Model: linking evidence and clinical decisions. *Annals of Internal Medicine*, **127**, 704–11.

Mihaylova, B., Briggs, A., Armitage, J., Parish, S., Gray, A., and Collins, R. (2006). Lifetime cost effectiveness of simvastatin in a range of risk groups and age groups derived from a randomised trial of 20,536 people. *British Medical Journal*, **333**, 1145.

Mount Hood (2007). Computer modeling of diabetes and its complications: a report on the Fourth Mount Hood Challenge Meeting. *Diabetes Care*, **30**, 1638–46.

Mueller, E., Maxion-Bergemann, S., Gultyaev, D., *et al.* (2006). Development and validation of the Economic Assessment of Glycemic Control and Long-Term Effects of diabetes (EAGLE) model. *Diabetes Technology and Therapeutics*, **8**, 219–36.

NHS Centre for Reviews and Dissemination (2001). *Undertaking Systematic Reviews of Research on Effectiveness: CRD's Guidance for Those Carrying Out or Commissioning Reviews.* Report no.4, NHS Centre for Reviews and Dissemination, University of York.

NICE (2008). *Guide to the Methods of Technology Appraisal.* National Institute for Health and Clinical Excellence, London.

Nuijten, M.J. (1998). The selection of data sources for use in modelling studies. *Pharmacoeconomics*, **13**, 305–16.

Parmigiani, G., Samsa, G.P., Ancukiewicz, M., Lipscomb, J., Hasselblad, V., and Matchar, D.B. (1997). Assessing uncertainty in cost-effectiveness analyses: application to a complex decision model. *Medical Decision Making*, **17**, 390–401.

Petitti, D.B. (2000). *Meta-analysis, Decision Analysis and Cost-Effectiveness Analysis, Methods for Quantitative Synthesis in Medicine* (2nd edn). Oxford University Press.

Philips, Z., Ginnelly, L., Sculpher, M., *et al.* (2004). Review of guidelines for good practice in decision-analytic modelling in health technology assessment, *Health Technology Assessment*, **8**, 1–158.

Philips, Z., Bojke, L., Sculpher, M., Claxton, K., and Golder, S. (2006). Good practice guidelines for decision-analytic modelling in health technology assessment: a review and consolidation of quality assessment, *Pharmacoeconomics*, **24**, 355–71.

Raiffa, H. (1968). *Decision Analysis: Introductory Readings on Choices Under Uncertainty*. Addison Wesley, Reading, MA.

Sculpher, M., Fenwick, E., and Claxton, K. (2000). Assessing quality in decision analytic cost-effectiveness models: a suggested framework and example of application, *Pharmacoeconomics*, **17**, 461–77.

Sculpher, M.J., Claxton, K., Drummond, M., and McCabe, C. (2006). Whither trial-based economic evaluation for health care decision making? *Health Economics*, **15**, 677–87.

Sonnenberg, F.A., Roberts, M.S., Tsevat, J., Wong, J B., Barry, M., and Kent, D.L. (1994). Toward a peer review process for medical decision analysis models, *Medical Care*, **32** (Suppl.), JS52–64.

Soto, J. (2002). Health economic evaluations using decision analytic modeling: principles and practices. Utilization of a checklist to their development and appraisal. *International Journal of Technology Assessment in Health Care*, **18**, 94–111.

Sox, H.C., Blatt, M.A., Higgins, M.C., and Marton, K.L. (1998). *Medical Decision Making*. Butterworths, Stoneham, MA.

Stout, N.K., Knudsen, A.B., Kong, C.K., McMahon, P.M., and Gazelle, G.S. (2009). Calibration methods used in cancer simulation models and suggested reporting guidelines. *Pharmacoeconomics*, **27**, 533–45.

Sutton, A.J. and Abrams, K.R. (2001). Bayesian methods in meta-analysis and evidence synthesis. *Statistical Methods in Medical Research*, **10**, 277–303.

Sutton, A.J., Abrams, K., Jones, D.R., Sheldon, T.A., and Song, F. (2000). *Methods for Meta-analysis in Medical Research*. John Wiley, Chichester.

van Houwelingen, H.C. (2000). Validation, calibration, revision and combination of prognostic survival models, *Statistics in Medicine*, **19**, 3401–15.

van Houwelingen, H.C. and Thorogood, J. (1995). Construction, validation and updating of a prognostic model for kidney graft survival. *Statistics in Medicine*, **14**, 1999–2008.

Weinstein, M.C., Toy, E.L., Sandberg, E.A., *et al.* (2001). Modeling for health care and other policy decisions: uses, roles, and validity. *Value in Health*, **4**, 348–61.

Weinstein, M.C., O'Brien, B., Hornberger, J., *et al.* (2003). Principles of good practice for decision analytic modeling in health-care evaluation: report of the ISPOR Task Force on Good Research Practices—Modeling Studies. *Value in Health*, **6**, 9–17.

Welton, N. and Ades, A.E. (2005). Estimation of Markov chain transition probabilities and rates from fully and partially observed data: uncertainty propagation, evidence synthesis, and model calibration. *Medical Decision Making*, **25**, 633–45.

Constructing and analysing a decision tree model

Overview

The purpose of this exercise is to build a decision tree model and to familiarize yourself with the steps and techniques involved. Although this is a simple example, the process will make you think about the fundamentals involved in decision tree modelling, structuring a tree, inputting probabilities and payoffs, analysing the tree in terms of calculating expected values and cost-effectiveness, and exploring uncertainty. The step-by-step guide will take you through a number of stages of developing and analysing the model. The exercise can be undertaken using either DATA TreeAge Pro or MS Excel. The worked solutions can be found at www.herc.ox.ac.uk/books/applied.

Exercise instructions

You have been asked to assess the cost-effectiveness of two proposed alternatives to routine practice in the follow-up of patients who have had treatment for colorectal cancer. The alternatives are (1) a primary-care-based follow-up approach and (2) a hospital-based follow-up approach. Each strategy has two possible outcomes: early or late detection of cancer recurrence. The probabilities related to the possible outcomes for these alternative options are as follows. In primary care the probability of early detection is 0.4 and in the hospital strategy it is 0.45; in routine practice the rate of patients found to have early stage recurrence in one year is 43 out of 100 patients. The probability of early detection after follow-up in the primary care setting is represented by an uncertain probability value ranging from 0.36 to 0.44. The payoffs in the model are in terms of costs and outcomes (life-years). For each strategy, early detection is associated with a life expectancy of 7 years and late detection with a life expectancy of 1.5 years. In terms of costs, the primary-care-based strategy has a cost of £3900 for early detection and £12,800 for late detection. The hospital-based approach has a cost of £6200 for early detection and £14,400 for late detection. Routine practice has a cost of £3030 for early detection and £12,020 for late detection.

♦ Using the information outlined below structure the decision tree. The decision tree can be constructed using either Excel or TreeAge Pro. Enter the relevant probabilities and payoffs.

- You have been given a rate of early detection of recurrence for the patients who receive routine practice follow-up. This needs to be converted to a probability (the process involved is outlined in Chapter 9, section 9.1.3).

- Calculate the incremental cost-effectiveness of the alternative follow-up options.

- Explore the impact on the results of the uncertain parameter for the probability of early detection with primary-care-based follow-up.

Step-by-step guide: TreeAge Pro

Step 1

The first step is to tell TreeAge Pro that you are going to develop a decision tree model by selecting:

- **File> New > Tree>OK**

Then it is important to set up the preferences for the model.

- Select: **Edit>preferences**
- Select: **Calculation method** in the category box, and then select **Method: cost-effectiveness** in the drop-down menu.
- Set '**Payoff 1**' for cost and '**Payoff 2**' for effectiveness.
- Then set the numerical formats: initially it is often best to set cost and effectiveness payoffs and expected values at three decimal points.
- Select currency for costs: this should be set to the currency of the country setting (usually default, e.g. pounds in the UK).
- Select custom suffix for effectiveness. If you intend to measure effectiveness in life years gained, you can enter LYG as the tag for a custom suffix, or if the outcome measure is in quality-adjusted life-years the custom suffix can be entered as QALYs.

You have now set up your initial preferences for the purpose of this exercise. However, it is also possible to alter the way your decision tree is displayed in TreeAge Pro by changing the display preferences such as the font, tree layout, node text, etc.

In the exercise there are two proposed alternatives to routine practice in the follow-up of patients who have had treatment for colorectal cancer:

- a primary-care-based approach
- a hospital-based approach.

Therefore the next step is to structure the decision tree (Figure 8E.1 shows the final structure). The three alternative follow-up strategies need to be entered into the decision tree; primary care, hospital care, and routine practice. All emanate from a decision node. Label each arm, by clicking above the arm and entering text.

- The starting point of the tree will be a decision node, for example where different treatment choices are made.

- To enter branches, select the node you wish the branch to emanate from by left-clicking once on it, then double-click and two branches will be created (this is a default that can be altered in **Edit>Preferences>Tree Display**). If you want to add additional branches, double-click again, or use the menu **Options>Add branch**.

- You can control whether added branches are placed at the top or the bottom of existing branches by going to **Edit>Preferences>Tree Display**.
- Label each branch by clicking above the branch and directly entering text. Each follow-up strategy has two possible outcomes: early detection or late detection of recurrence. Enter two branches emanating from the chance node for the first option (routine practice) and label them 'early detection' and 'late detection'.
- Label each branch by clicking above the branch and directly entering text.

Instead of repeating this process for the primary care and hospital care branches, it is possible to use the copy and paste functions. Cutting, copying, and pasting is done with the **Options** and **Edit** menus.

- To copy and paste the 'early detection' and 'late detection' branches from the routine practice strategy and paste to the primary care and hospital care branches, select the routine practice branch by clicking once on it, use **Options>Select sub-tree**, then **Edit>Copy sub-tree**, and then select the branch and node to which you want to copy. In this exercise click once on the primary care branch and use **Edit>Paste...sub-tree**. This process is then repeated for the hospital care branch.
  - To delete an individual branch, use **Options>Delete branch**.
  - To cut a sub-tree, use **Options>Select sub-tree**, then **Edit>Cut sub-tree**.
  - To copy a sub-tree, use **Options>Select sub-tree**, then **Edit>Copy sub-tree**, then select the node to which you want to copy and use **Edit>Paste... sub-tree**.

Before inserting the probabilities you need to convert the rate of early detection of recurrence for the patients who receive routine practice follow-up to a probability. In routine practice the rate of patients who are found to have early detection of recurrence in one year is 43 out of 100 patients. Therefore the probability is $P = 1 - \exp(-0.43*1) = 0.35$.

Now it is possible to insert the probabilities under each arm. In primary care the probability of early detection is 0.4, in the hospital strategy it is 0.45, and in routine practice it is 0.35. It is possible to enter these directly by clicking under the branch labelled early or late detection for each strategy and typing the relevant values in directly.

However, it would be better to create separate variables for all the probabilities to be used in the model and use these variable names to define the associated probabilities of early detection for each alternative strategy. The probability of late detection can then be entered as 1 – this variable or #.

- Select: **Values>Variables and Tables**. Make sure the **Variables List** box is selected, select **New variable**.
- Starting with the probability of early detection for routine practice, **Name** the variable and give it a **Description** in the basic properties box. **Name**: RPed, **Description**: probability of routine practice early detection.
- Define it numerically at root as 0.35 by selecting **Define numerically (at root)** and typing in the **Value** box 0.35. Select **OK** to close the dialogue box.

This process can be repeated for the probabilities related to early detection in the primary care strategy (PCed) and early detection in the hospital care strategy (HCed). The variable names that you have just created are displayed in the **Variables and Tables** dialogue box. This can now be closed by selecting **Close**.

◆ Use the variables that you have just created to enter the probabilities into the decision tree. Click below the branch for early detection of the routine practice strategy and select from the toolbar menu **Values>Insert variable** and choose the appropriate variable to insert (RPed), (alternatively you can click on the **•••** under each branch and from the **Formula Editor** dialogue box select **variables** and select the appropriate variable >**OK**). Either process is then repeated for the primary care and hospital care strategies.

◆ The probabilities of late detection are therefore the residuals. Use (1 − RPed) for routine care, (1 − PCed) for primary care, and (1 − HCed) for the hospital care follow-up strategy or alternatively use the hash symbol (#). These can be entered directly below the appropriate branch.

You can now enter the costs and outcomes for each arm.

◆ You need to convert each end node to a terminal node. Select the branch for which you want to change the node **Options>change node type>terminal node**. An **Enter Payoff** dialogue box will appear. Here you need to enter the appropriate cost and effects for the strategy selected.

  • There are six node types. In this exercise you will use three: decision nodes, chance nodes, and terminal nodes.

  • These can be changed from the button bar or from the menu **Options>Change node type**.

  • A decision node (represented by a square) will be the starting point of the tree, for example where different treatment choices are made.

  • Chance nodes (represented by a circle) will be used where probabilistic events occur, such as success and failure of treatment.

  • Terminal nodes (represented by a triangle) will be used at the end of the tree, where the decision process terminates and payoffs occur.

◆ In each strategy, early detection is associated with a life expectancy of 7 years, and late detection with a life expectancy of 1.5 years.

◆ The primary-care-based strategy has a cost of £3900 for early detection and £12,800 for late detection. The hospital-based approach has a cost of £6200 for early detection and £14,400 for late detection. Routine practice has a cost of £3030 for early detection and £12,020 for late detection.

◆ Finally ensure that the sum of probabilities at each chance node equals 1. Select the decision node and select **Analysis>Verify probabilities** (needs to be done after converting to terminal nodes).

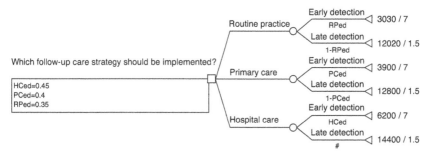

Fig. 8E.1 Structure of the decision tree for comparing the cost-effectiveness of alternative strategies of follow-up care for colorectal cancer patients.

Step 2

Now that you have set up the structure of the decision tree you are ready to look at some results.

+ Select the decision node, then go to **Analysis>Cost-effectiveness.**

+ Select **Effectiveness on the x-axis**; this is the convention used by health economists.

+ The first information presented will be the three options plotted on the north-east quadrant of the cost-effectiveness plane (Figure 8E.2).

+ It is possible to export this information and graphic directly to Excel by selecting the **Excel chart** button.

+ Alternatively you can look at the text report by selecting the **Actions** button. A dialogue box will appear inviting you to select the baseline strategy; the default in

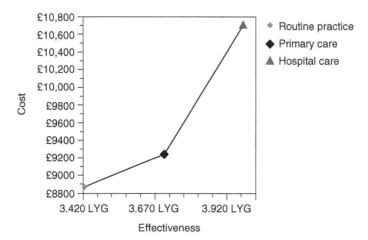

Fig. 8E.2 Incremental cost-effectiveness of the three follow-up strategies plotted on the cost-effectiveness plane.

Table 8E.1 Results from the text report in TreeAge Pro

Strategy	Cost (C)	Incremental cost	Effective-ness (E)	Incremental effective-ness	C/E	ICER
Routine care	£8873.5		3.425		£2590.803	
Primary care	£9240	£366.5	3.7	0.275	£2497.297	£1332.727
Hospital care	£10,710	£1470	3.975	0.275	£2694.34	£5345.455

TreeAge Pro is the least costly strategy. You can use this default. Select **Continue**. The text report will then be displayed (Table 8E.1).

◆ This first table in the report is the standard cost-effectiveness analysis table, showing the options in order of increasing cost, with their average and incremental cost and effectiveness values, as well as incremental cost-effectiveness ratios.

◆ The second table shows incremental cost and effectiveness calculated between the baseline option specified in the text report set-up dialogue box (default is the least costly option) and every other option.

Step 3

Now you are asked to consider a one-way sensitivity analysis to assess whether the results are robust to the likelihood that the primary care follow-up strategy has a higher or lower rate of early detection than currently assumed. In order to undertake the sensitivity analysis you will use the variable that you created for the probability of primary care early detection (PCed).

◆ Select **Values>Variables and Tables>** select the variable name 'PCed'

◆ Select **Edit Properties>** and under **Properties for sensitivity analysis**

◆ Set a low value at 0.36 and the high value at 0.44.

◆ Then close the dialogue box by selecting **OK**. And close the **Variables and Tables** dialogue box by selecting **Close**.

(NB. If you had originally entered the probabilities directly it is now important to modify the tree. For the primary care probability arm, in place of the value 0.4, go to **Values>Insert variable**, and select PCed from the drop-down menu. Then modify the late detection arm for primary care, to 1-PCed or #)

◆ Now select the decision node and then select **Analysis >Sensitivity analysis > One-way**.

◆ In the sensitivity analysis dialogue box change the choice of **variable** to PCed using the drop-down menu.

◆ It is worth increasing the **Number of intervals** option to get a fuller range of results: here, set it to 8. Select **OK**.

◆ You will now be offered a range of options for comparison: **Text report** or **Graph**. It is usually best to view the text report to get a clear idea of what is going on.

- You will then be asked whether you want to eliminate strategies based on extended dominance. It is up to you whether you want to view the text report with these included or eliminated.

- To obtain a graphical representation of the sensitivity analysis select **Graph**. This will give you a range of options to choose from, one of which is **Cost-effectiveness** (**animated**).

- If you operate the **animate** button you can see the graphics for each value of the variable.

Step-by-step guide: Excel

Step 1

Open the file *Template Exercise 8 Excel version* and start with the <**Parameters**> worksheet. The cells to be completed throughout the exercise are highlighted in a number of colour-codes.

Using the information provided in the exercise instructions, input the appropriate values in column C of the <**Parameters**> worksheet. Remember to change the rate of early detection under routine follow-up care into a probability (see TreeAge step-by-step guide).

It is useful to 'name' the cells for these values, so that the values can be referred to as their shortened 'name' when used elsewhere in the workbook. In order to name the cells highlight the range of cells B2:C16 and on the toolbar select **Formulas, Create from selection**. This will produce a **Create Names** dialogue box. Highlight the box **Left column** and click **OK**. Now when you highlight one of the values in Column C you will notice in the **name box** in Excel that instead of the cell reference its name corresponding to that shown in column B appears.

Once all the input parameters have been entered, open the worksheet <**Decision model**>. The structure of the decision tree has been provided for you. In the exercise there are two proposed alternatives to routine practice in the follow-up of patients who have had treatment for colorectal cancer:

- a primary-care-based approach
- a hospital-based approach.

The three alternative follow-up strategies—primary care, hospital care, and routine practice—need to be entered into the decision tree. All emanate from a decision node. Label each branch by entering text above the branch.

Each follow-up strategy has two possible outcomes: early or late detection of recurrence. Label the two branches emanating from the chance node for the first option (routine practice), 'early detection' and 'late detection' (label above the branch). This can be repeated for the primary care and hospital care branches.

Now it is possible to insert the probabilities under each arm in the light blue cells. In primary care the probability of early detection is 0.4, in the hospital strategy it is 0.45, and in routine practice it is 0.35. It is good practice to link these to the values set out in the <**Parameters**> worksheet. You can either write in their corresponding shortened names in the light blue cells under the appropriate branches (e.g. the probability of early detection with primary care follow-up (PCed)) or highlight the cell where you want the value to appear and type '=' and go to the <**Parameters**> worksheet and choose the appropriate value in column C. The probabilities of late detection are therefore the residuals. Use (1 – RPed) for the routine care follow-up strategy, (1 – PCed) for the primary care follow-up strategy, and (1 – HCed) for the hospital care follow-up strategy.

You can now enter the costs and outcomes for each arm. Again using the shortened names to link to the values in column C of the <**Parameters**> sheet, fill in the cost and outcomes payoffs in columns M and N of the <**Decision model**> sheet.

Step 2

Now that you have set up the parameters and structure of the decision tree you need to obtain the results. First, you need to calculate the expected costs and outcomes for each alternative follow-up option. In the <**Decision Model**> sheet enter the expected costs and outcomes in the light yellow and green cells under the branches in the decision tree. An explanation of how to calculate these expected values is given in section 8.5.5. These expected values can be put into the appropriate cells on the <**Results**> sheet and used to calculate the incremental costs and effects and incremental cost-effectiveness ratios (ICERs). The expected cost and effect results can then be plotted on the worksheet <**Graph – ICER**>.

Step 3

You can now continue to use your baseline results to conduct a simple one-way sensitivity analysis. You are asked to consider a one-way sensitivity analysis to assess whether the results are robust to the likelihood that the primary care follow-up strategy has a higher or lower rate of early detection than currently assumed. In order to undertake the sensitivity analysis you will use the variable that you created for the probability of primary care early detection (PCed).

Begin setting up your one-way sensitivity analysis by creating a 'what-if table' by using the **Data table** function in Excel. In the <**Parameters**> worksheet under the header **sensitivity analysis**, fill in cells B25 and B26 with the corresponding ICERs for primary and hospital care (making sure that these are linked to the ICERs in the <**Results**> worksheet). The cells C24:K24 contain the plausible range of values (0.36–0.44) for the probability of early detection in primary care (PCed). Select the table you have created (B24:K26); in the Excel menu choose >**Data**>**What-If Analysis Data Table**…, and a dialogue box will appear. As your data in the table are in rows, you need to choose **Row input cell**, use the baseline value for PCed (use the cell reference C3) and choose **OK**. The table will now display the corresponding ICER values for primary and hospital care for each plausible probability ranging from 0.36 to 0.44. You can then graph these results in the worksheet <**Graph of sensitivity analysis**>.

Chapter 9

Decision analytic modelling:
Markov models

In this chapter the focus will be on providing a theoretical and practical example of cost-effectiveness analysis in health care using Markov modelling. The use of Markov models for the purpose of economic evaluation is discussed using a worked example, with a guide to the steps that a researcher has to undertake in order to construct, analyse, and evaluate such a model.

9.1 Markov models: what are they?

Markov models analyse uncertain processes over time. They are suited to decisions where the timing of events is important and when events may happen more than once, and therefore they are appropriate where the strategies being evaluated are of a sequential or repetitive nature. Whereas decision trees model uncertain events at chance nodes, Markov models differ in modelling uncertain events as transitions between health states. In particular, Markov models are suited to modelling long-term outcomes, where costs and effects are spread over a long period of time. Therefore Markov models are particularly suited to chronic diseases or situations where events are likely to recur over time (Sonnenberg and Beck 1993; Briggs *et al.* 1998)

Over the past decade there has been an increase in the use of Markov models for conducting economic evaluations in a health-care setting. Examples include studies where it was necessary to extrapolate beyond the trial results (Johannesson *et al.* 1997; Karnon *et al.* 2006), studies where modelling the disease progression is imperative, such as in Alzheimer's disease or epilepsy (Fenn and Gray 1999; Hawkins *et al.* 2005), studies where the disease may present with recurrent events, such as cancer interventions (Legood *et al.* 2006; Moeremans and Annemans 2008), and studies assessing the cost-effectiveness of disease management (Palmer *et al.* 2005; Steuten *et al.* 2007).

A Markov model comprises a finite set of health states in which an individual can be found. The states are such that in any given time interval, the individual will be in only one health state. All individuals in a particular health state have identical characteristics. The number and nature of the states are governed by the decision problem. Unlike decision trees, where fixed time periods are used, Markov models are concerned with transitions during a series of cycles consisting of short time intervals. The model is run for several cycles, and patients move between states or remain in the same state between cycles (issues determining the appropriate cycle length are discussed in section 9.1.4). Movements between states are defined by transition probabilities which can be time dependent or constant over time. All individuals within a given health state are assumed to be identical, and this leads to a limitation of Markov models in that the transition probabilities only depend on the current health state and not on past health states—this is known as the Markovian assumption (section 9.1.3). Rewards (analogous to payoffs in decision trees), such as costs, life-years, or quality-adjusted life-years (QALYs), are assigned to each health state and earned at the end of each cycle.

The following well-defined steps are involved in building and analysing a Markov model:

- structure the model by defining the states and allowable transitions
- identify the starting probabilities, i.e. the initial distribution of patients within the states
- determine the transition probabilities
- decide on a cycle length
- set the stopping rule
- determine rewards
- implement discounting if required
- analyse and evaluate the model
- explore uncertainty.

Each step will be discussed in detail throughout the rest of this chapter:

9.1.1 Defining states and allowable transitions

The first step is to identify the Markov states required to answer the research question posed. They should represent clinically and economically important events, such as alive, well, dead, disease stage, or treatment status. They should be clearly defined according to notions of disease. The states should be mutually exclusive, so that an individual cannot be in more than one state at any time, and exhaustive in the sense that all possibilities are covered, none overlap, and their probabilities sum to 1. Figure 9.1 uses a state-transition diagram to depict the model that will be used as an example in this chapter.

In this illustrative hypothetical example, there are three states: well, recurrence of breast cancer, and dead. The Markov model is used to evaluate the decision as to whether to implement a treatment intervention for those patients who have had breast cancer in the past, with the expectation that doing so may reduce the number of recurrences. By convention, each state is represented by an oval or circle. The arrows represent the transitions between the three states. It is possible to remain in a particular state for more than one cycle of the model, represented by arrows pointing back into the state from which it begins. In section 9.2.2 we show how it is also possible to represent returning to a state after leaving it. Movements between states are governed by transition probabilities (see section 9.1.3).

For the Markov process to end, there must be at least one state that cannot be left, and such states are called 'absorbing states'. (Note, however, that it is possible to run non-absorbing models that reach a point of equilibrium after a certain number of cycles.) The process of moving between states continues until a patient enters an

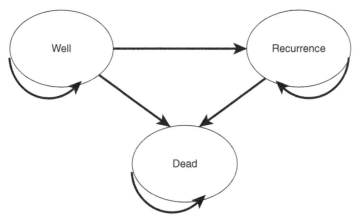

Fig. 9.1 Markov state transition diagram depicting states and allowable transitions.

absorbing state such as the state 'Dead' in this particular example. Here the dead state may occur after a patient has been in the 'Well' state, as a result of all-cause mortality, or after a patient has been in the 'Recurrence' state, as a result of disease-specific or all-cause mortality. Despite having two routes into the dead state, it is not necessary to have more than one dead state because, by convention, the cost and utility associated with being in the dead state is zero.

Figure 9.2 shows that in this model it is possible to move as follows:

♦ from 'Well' to 'Recurrence'; from 'Well' to 'Dead' (from other causes); remain in the 'Well' state

♦ from 'Recurrence' to 'Dead' (from disease and other causes); remain in 'Recurrence' state.

However, more than one dead state can be used if it is considered useful to keep track of the causes of death. Therefore the state 'Dead' in this example could be split into two Markov states: 'Dead from disease' and 'Dead from other causes' (see Figure 9.6).

9.1.2 Identify the starting probabilities, i.e. the initial distribution of patients within the states

A separate set of starting probabilities is required to describe the initial distribution of the population being modelled—the Markov cohort—across the states immediately before the process begins. This distribution is determined by the analyst. For example, it may be that all patients start in the same state (this is equivalent to setting the starting probabilities to 1). An alternative is to have different proportions in different states at the start of the modelling process. The proportions can be determined from published studies. In the example (Figure 9.2) all of the cohort start in the 'Well' state and therefore a starting probability of 1 is assigned to this state; the states 'Recurrence' and 'Dead' are assigned a starting probability of zero. In subsequent cycles, the distribution of patients among the states will of course depend on their distribution in the previous cycle and the transition probabilities between the states.

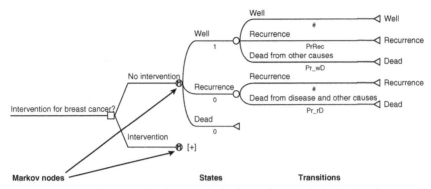

Fig. 9.2 Example of one arm (no-intervention) of a Markov model in TreeAge Pro.

9.1.3 **Determine transition probabilities**

Transition probabilities determine how patients move from state to state. The set of transition probabilities for each state must sum to 1 (i.e. are mutually exhaustive).

Transition matrix

Transition probabilities can be represented in the form of a transition matrix (Tables 9.1 and 9.2). By convention, the rows of the transition matrix represent the state an individual is in at the beginning of the period/cycle (t). The columns represent the state an individual is in at the beginning of the next period/cycle ($t + 1$). Therefore each element in the matrix depicts the probability of a move from the row state to the column state. In the breast cancer example, the probability PrRec of moving from the 'Well' state to the 'Recurrence' state is 0.3, while the probability Pr_wD of moving from the 'Well' state to the 'Dead' state is 0.1. The probability Pr_rD of transiting from the 'Recurrence' state to the 'Dead' state is 0.2. In practice some of the transitions may not occur and thus are set to zero. For example, in this model transitions from 'Recurrence' back to 'Well' are not possible and so this is set at zero. In addition, since the sum of the row probabilities must equal 1 (because everyone must go somewhere), if we know all but one of the row probabilities, we can infer the remaining probability as the residual (represented by # in TreeAge Pro). Hence the probability of remaining in the 'Well' state is the residual # or 1 – (0.3+0.1) and the probability of remaining in

Table 9.1 Transition matrix depicting allowable transitions and transition probabilities for the no-intervention arm

		To $t + 1$		
		Well	**Recurrence**	**Dead**
From t	**Well**	1 – (0.3 + 0.1) or #	0.3 (PrRec)	0.1 (Pr_wD)
	Recurrence	0	1 – (0.2) or #	0.2 (Pr_rD)
	Dead	0	0	1

Table 9.2 Transition matrix depicting allowable transitions and transition probabilities for the intervention arm

		To $t + 1$		
		Well	**Recurrence**	**Dead**
From t	**Well**	$1 - [(0.3 \times RR) + 0.1]$ or #	$0.3(PrRec) \times RR$	0.1 (Pr_wD)
	Recurrence	0	$1 - (0.2)$ or #	0.2 (Pr_rD)
	Dead	0	0	1

the 'Recurrence' state is $1 - 0.2$ or #. The transition probability from an absorbing state to an absorbing state is always one ('Dead' to 'Dead' = 1).

In the transition matrix depicted in Table 9.1, three probabilities are required:

- probability of moving from 'Well' to 'Recurrence' (PrRec) is 0.3
- probability of moving from 'Well' to 'Dead' (Pr_wD) is 0.1
- probability of moving from 'Recurrence' to 'Dead' (Pr_rD) is 0.2.

As the purpose of the intervention in this example is to reduce the risk of recurrence, i.e. to reduce the proportion of the cohort moving from the 'Well' state to the 'Recurrence' state, a relative risk associated with the intervention needs to be incorporated into the transition matrix to adjust the baseline risk of this transition from the 'Well' to 'Recurrence' state. The relative risk (RR) is 66%. Table 9.2 displays the transition matrix for the intervention arm with the baseline risk adjustment in the 'Well' to 'Recurrence' transition. To adjust this baseline risk, PrRec needs to be multiplied by the relative risk of disease progression.

In some cases the measure of treatment effectiveness is reported in the form of odds ratios or hazard ratios. Care is required when applying these measures directly to the baseline risk/probabilities of the non-intervention arm of the model. It is necessary to ensure consistency between the measure of treatment effect and the baseline risk. Hence, odds ratios should be converted into relative risks or, alternatively, the baseline risk should be converted into odds, multiplied by the odds ratio, and converted back to risk. The same applies to hazard ratios; despite being broadly equivalent to a relative risk, they differ by being a ratio of rates and not probabilities. Hence, hazard ratios should be either converted to a probability or applied to a baseline rate with the outcome being converted back to a probability (see section on rates and probabilities).

Rates and probabilities

Transition probabilities can be identified from a variety of data sources such as published reports of a clinical trial, or from epidemiological studies or administrative data. Ideally, where a number of sources are available, evidence synthesis methods (described in Chapter 8, section 8.3.4) can be undertaken. If disease-specific or all-cause mortality data are required, nationally published life-tables can be used. In the past, researchers have erroneously used probabilities interchangeably with rates. Therefore a note of caution is required. Rates differ from probabilities in that rates are:

- represented by the potential for an event at any point in time.
- instantaneous.
- can vary from zero to infinity.
- cannot be measured directly—a rate is inferred from a population over time (e.g. the number of events per number of patients per unit of time).
- instantaneous rates can be added and subtracted within a given time interval.

In contrast, probabilities are:

- represented by the likelihood of an event happening in a given time period.
- their value is bounded from zero to one.
- the relationship with time depends on the underlying rate, so one cannot divide or multiply probabilities to change the time period.

Rates can be useful for converting to a probability, assuming that an event occurs at a constant rate r over a time period t:

$$P = 1 - e^{-rt}$$

where e is the base of natural logarithm. In Excel, this formula is expressed as

$$P = 1 - \exp(-rt)$$

where exp is the base of natural logarithm.

Similarly, it is possible to rearrange the above equation to convert probabilities to rates to exploit their mathematical features. This is useful when it is necessary to add or subtract rates or when changing the cycle length in a Markov model (see section 9.5):

$$r = (1/t)\ln(1 - P)$$

which in Excel is

$$r = - [\ln (1 - P)]/t.$$

Markovian assumption

The Markovian assumption is that all patients in a given health state are homogenous regardless of past health states or how long they have been in that particular state. Hence the transitions in any given cycle may depend on time from the start of the model but not on what has happened prior to that cycle—this is known as the Markovian assumption. Therefore the Markov model has no memory of what has occurred in previous cycles. For instance, in the worked example the probability of dying from breast cancer is independent of the number of recurrences in the past and is also independent of how long the person spent in the 'Well' state before moving to the 'Recurrent' state. We shall see in section 9.2.4 how this Markovian assumption can be overcome.

Markov chain and Markov process

The Markov model may be governed by transitions that are either constant or time dependent. In a Markov chain, transition probabilities remain constant over time.

This means that the transition probabilities are assumed to occur with equal probability across all cycles of the model. This assumption is often inappropriate, and use of time-dependent probabilities may be required. When the transition probabilities vary from cycle to cycle (i.e. are 'time dependent') this is defined as a Markov process. This occurs when the probabilities are an increasing, or decreasing, function of time. An example of a transition probability that is time dependent would be the all-cause probability of death, which increases with age (i.e. the risk of death is time dependent). This can easily be derived from life-tables. Models may consist of both constant and time-dependent probabilities. Time dependency is discussed in greater detail in section 9.2.3.

9.1.4 Determine the cycle length

The time horizon of the analysis is split into equal components, such as weeks, months, or years. These are known as 'cycles'. A cycle represents the minimum amount of time that any individual will spend in a state before the possibility of transition to another state. Defining the appropriate cycle length for a Markov model should reflect the underlying natural history of the disease. It may depend on the frequency of events: for example, 1 year may be an appropriate cycle length for conditions with low frequencies of clinical events. Similarly, 1 year may be appropriate if the model is set up to reflect the entire lifespan of a patient. Shorter periods (cycle lengths) may be more suitable for acute illnesses or where the model reflects shorter time horizons; these could be six-monthly, monthly, or even daily. The cycle length will also depend on the nature of the study question and the availability of the data required to populate the model. The cycle length has implications for the nature of the probabilities and rewards used in the model. For example, a 1 year cycle requires annual transition probabilities, annual costs, and annual values for outcomes. Generally, the length of the cycle remains fixed for the duration of the model, but it is possible to adjust the cycle length throughout the model. If this is the case, the corresponding input parameters will also have to change accordingly: for example, if the model is set up to start with a cycle length representing six-monthly periods over the first 10 years, and then annually thereafter, the corresponding costs, utilities, and probabilities will have to reflect these six-month and annual time periods.

The literature contains examples of Markov models using a wide range of cycle lengths. In the economic evaluation of screening for abdominal aortic aneurysms (the MASS study) the cycle length was selected to reflect clinical evidence on the length of time over which an individual was known to change disease states, but also took into account computational considerations. This was represented by a cycle length of 3 months (Kim *et al.* 2007). However, in a cost-effectiveness study comparing total knee replacement using computer-assisted surgery with that using a conventional manual method (Dong and Buxton 2006), a cycle length of 1 month was chosen; hence the transition probabilities between states were all expressed as 1 month probabilities. Similarly, in a study comparing the cost-effectiveness of treatment for gastro-oesophageal reflux disease (GORD), a 1 month cycle with 1 month transition probabilities, costs, and outcomes was used (Bojke *et al.* 2007). In the breast cancer example used here, a 1 year cycle length has been implemented.

9.1.5 **Set the stopping rule**

A decision has to be made over what time period the model should be run. If the model includes an absorbing state, the model can run until all of the cohort end up in that state. The model may be structured so that the proportion of the cohort reaching this state may never reach 100%, and so it may be necessary to force the model to stop after a specified number of cycles or when the proportion of the original cohort still changing states has fallen to a very low level. Many disease models can be run for the estimated remaining life expectancy of the cohort. In the breast cancer example, because the starting age of the cohort is 55 with an annual cycle length, an assumption can be made that if the model is run for a further 55 cycles, almost all of the cohort would have reached the 'Dead' state. Alternatively, a decision can be made as to whether running the model for a specified period of time, such as 15 years, may be sufficient and will include all the likely scenarios.

9.1.6 **Determine the rewards**

Markov models are run through a series of cycles, and the rewards (costs and outcomes) are accrued within each cycle and accumulate throughout the life-cycle of the model. There are several types of reward: State rewards (defined as 'Incremental' in TreeAge) are the values of the costs or outcomes assigned to a Markov health state. This reflects the value of being in that state during a given cycle. Transition rewards are accrued when there is a cost or outcome related to the individual transiting to a new state. Transition rewards are useful if there is no need for the reward to be of a recurring nature. In the breast cancer example a transition cost is incurred by the transition from the 'Recurrence' state to the 'Dead' state. The cost has not been assigned to the 'Dead' state as this would be incurred for every cycle in the model, whereas if the cost (e.g. the cost of palliative care) is assigned to the actual time of transition between the two states, it will only be incurred once when the patient moves from one state to the other.

One-time rewards occur at the beginning or end of the model. For example, a one-time reward is usually entered for cycle zero (the first cycle in the model). A one-time reward may also be required for the final cycle. These one-time rewards are also used in TreeAge to adjust for the timing of the transition. These adjustments, termed half-cycle corrections, are dealt with in section 9.2.1.

Rewards may be costs and life-years or QALYs. Costs are attached to individual health states to reflect the cost of remaining in that health state for one cycle. Utility values can be attached to each state reflecting the severity of the state. A utility is assigned to each state to represent the relative value of occupying it for one cycle. Attaching weights that represent quality of life on a standard 0–1 scale to the Markov states will generate a QALY score when summed over a large number of model cycles. Costs and outcomes can also be attached to the transitions, to represent the costs and outcomes associated with making the transition from one state to another.

As already mentioned, the period of reward should correspond to the cycle length. For example, a 1 year cycle requires annual costs and annual utilities. In the example used in this chapter, the cycle length corresponds to 1 year. The corresponding incremental cost rewards required are as follows:

- cost of 1 year in the 'Well' state (C_well) = £350
- cost of 1 year in the 'Recurrence' state (C_rec) = £3190
- cost related to palliative care before disease-specific death (C_death) = £1400
- cost related to intervention (C_Int) = £46.

The utility incremental rewards are:

- utility related to being in the 'Well' state for 1 year (U_well) = 0.89
- utility related to being in the 'Recurrence' state for 1 year (U_rec) = 0.5.

The utility rewards are entered alongside life-year estimates to derive QALYs. If life-years are the outcome of interest, a state reward of one life-year can be assigned to both the 'Well' and 'Recurrence' states.

9.1.7 Discounting

Costs and outcomes can be discounted as if they have occurred at the midpoint of the cycle. Markov models allow the discounting of costs and outcomes at the point in time that they occur. If the cycle length is assumed to be 1 year, this can be achieved automatically by feeding the cycle number in years into the standard discounting formula (see Chapter 6). To undertake discounting, the formula used is:

$$C_p = \frac{Cf_1}{(1+r)} + \frac{Cf_2}{(1+r)^2} + \frac{Cf_3}{(1+r)^3} \ldots\ldots + \frac{Cf_n}{(1+r)^n}$$

where C_p is the present value of costs (or outcomes), Cf_n is the future cost (or outcome) at year n, and r is the rate of discount.

9.1.8 Analysis and evaluation of the Markov model

Cohort analysis

Cohort simulation commences with a hypothetical cohort who are distributed among the possible model states according to the starting probabilities. The simulation then follows the transition of the cohort among the states from one cycle to the next depending on the transition probabilities. This simply involves multiplying the proportion of the cohort ending in one state by the relevant transition probabilities attached to that state in order to calculate the proportion starting in the next state. Figure 9.3 depicts this diagrammatically: the first column in the diagram shows that all patients start in the 'Well' state. The middle columns show the distribution of the cohort part way through the analysis. The final column (cycle k) shows the final distribution at the end of the process, with the entire cohort in the 'Dead' state (the absorbing state in this example).

Figure 9.4 presents a numerical illustration. Here the cohort size is 10,000, but this is subjective and the starting cohort size has no impact on the final answer. The cohort is distributed among the possible states: 'Well', 'Recurrence', and 'Dead'. In this example

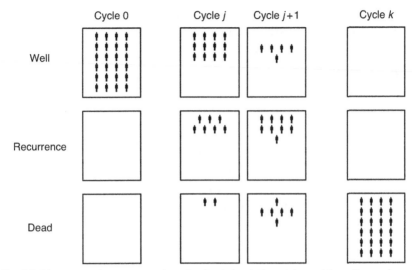

Fig. 9.3 Diagrammatic representation of cohort simulation. Adapted from Sonnenberg and Beck (1993). Reprinted by permission of SAGE Publications.

the cohort of 10,000 all start in the 'Well' state. This illustrative model is a simple Markov chain, i.e. there are no time-dependent transition probabilities and no backward transitions are allowed.

The transition probabilities for the no-intervention arm imply that there is a 0.6 chance that the patient who is well will remain in the 'Well' state for the next cycle,

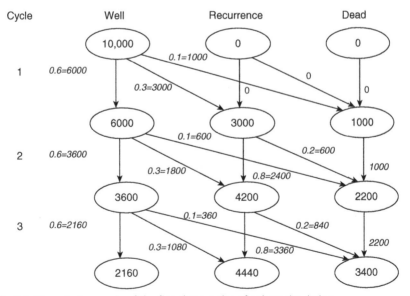

Fig. 9.4 Numerical example of the first three cycles of cohort simulation.

a 0.3 chance that they will progress to the recurrent state, and a 0.1 chance that they will die. For those in the 'Recurrence' state there is a 0.8 chance that they will remain in that state in the next cycle and a 0.2 chance that they will die. Hence we would expect 6000 patients (0.6 × 10,000) in the 'Well' state, 3000 patients (0.3 × 10,000) in the 'Recurrence' state, and 1000 (0.1 × 10,000) in the 'Dead' state after the first cycle. In the second cycle there are 3600 (6000 × 0.6) in the 'Well' state, 4200 ((6000 × 0.3) + (3000 × 0.8)) in the 'Recurrence' state, and 2200 (1000 + (6000 × 0.1) + (3000 × 0.2)) in the 'Dead' state. This continues until all the patients are in the absorbing state (dead). Notice that because it is assumed that the transition probabilities attached to each state are mutually exhaustive (i.e. sum to 1), the sum of the proportion of the cohorts in each state will sum to the original cohort size (here 10,000) in each cycle.

This cohort simulation aids the calculation of expected costs and outcomes, as described in Chapter 8, and involves summing the costs and outcomes of all consequences weighted by the probability of the consequence. This entails multiplying the rewards of each state by the proportion of the cohort in the state for each cycle and then summing these expected cycle costs and outcomes (referred to as stage cost and stage effect in TreeAge Pro) across all cycles. Table 9.3 provides a Markov trace for the first 34 cycles (out of 55 cycles) of the cohort analysis for the no-intervention arm.

Here we have started with a cohort of 100,000. The undiscounted expected cycle costs are calculated as follows.

- Cycle 1: {(60,000 × £350) + (30,000 × £3190) + [(0.2 × 30,000) × £1400]}/100,000 = £1251
- Cycle 2: {(36000 × £350) + (42,000 × £3190) + [(0.2 × 42000) × £1400]}/100,000 = £1583.4
- Cycle 3: {(21600 × £350)+(44400 × £3190)+[(0.2 × 44400) × £1400]}/100,000 = £1616.3.

The total expected cost for the intervention arm (across all 55 cycles in the model) is £13,537.

Expected outcomes in terms of life expectancy can be calculated by summing the proportion of live patients in each cycle ('Well' and 'Recurrence' states) and then summing across all cycles in the model. In the example:

- Cycle 1: (60,000 + 30,000)/100,000 = 0.9
- Cycle 2: (36,000 + 42,000)/100,000 = 0.78
- Cycle 3: (21,600 + 44,400)/100,000 = 0.66.

The resulting total expected life expectancy (across all 55 cycles in the model) is 5.25 years.

Expected outcomes in terms of QALYs involves summing the utilities for each state weighted by the proportion of the cohort in that state for each cycle and then adding these expected cycle QALYs across all cycles:

- Cycle 1: [(60,000 × 0.89) + (30,000 × 0.5)]/100,000 = 0.684
- Cycle 2: [(36,000 × 0.89) + (42,000 × 0.5)]/100,000 = 0.530
- Cycle 3: [(21,600 × 0.89) + (44,400 × 0.5)]/100,000 = 0.414.

The resulting total expected QALYs (across all 55 cycles in the model) is 3.2.

Table 9.3 Markov trace of model: no-intervention arm

Cycle	Well	Recurrence	Dead	Cycle cost	Cycle life-years	Cycle QALY	Cum. cost	Cum. life-years	Cum. QALYs
0	100,000	0	0	0.0	0.000	0.000	0	0.000	0.000
1	60,000	30,000	10,000	1251.0*	0.90†	0.684‡	1251	0.900	0.684
2	36,000	42,000	22,000	1583.4	0.780	0.530	2834.4	1.680	1.214
3	21,600	44,400	34,000	1616.3	0.660	0.414	4450.68	2.340	1.629
4	12,960	42,000	45,040	1502.8	0.550	0.325	5953.44	2.890	1.954
5	7776	37,488	54,736	1328.0	0.453	0.257	7281.49	3.342	2.211
6	4665.6	32,323.2	63,011.2	1137.9	0.370	0.203	8419.434	3.712	2.414
7	2799.4	27,258.2	69,942.4	955.7	0.301	0.161	9375.093	4.013	2.575
8	1679.6	22,646.4	75,674.0	791.7	0.243	0.128	10,166.8	4.256	2.703
9	1007.8	18,621.0	80,371.2	649.7	0.196	0.102	10,816.48	4.452	2.805
10	604.7	15,199.1	84,196.2	529.5	0.158	0.081	11,346	4.610	2.887
11	362.8	12,340.7	87,296.5	429.5	0.127	0.065	11,775.5	4.737	2.952
12	217.7	9981.4	89,800.9	347.1	0.102	0.052	12,122.61	4.839	3.003
13	130.6	8050.4	91,819.0	279.8	0.082	0.041	12,402.42	4.921	3.045
14	78.4	6479.5	93,442.1	225.1	0.066	0.033	12,627.53	4.987	3.078
15	47.0	5207.1	94,745.9	180.9	0.053	0.026	12,808.39	5.039	3.104
16	28.2	4179.8	95,792.0	145.1	0.042	0.021	12,953.52	5.081	3.125

(continued)

17	16.9	3352.3	96,630.8	116.4	0.034	0.017	13,069.91	5.115	3.142
18	10.2	2686.9	97,302.9	93.3	0.027	0.014	13,163.18	5.142	3.156
19	6.1	2152.6	97,841.3	74.7	0.022	0.011	13,237.9	5.164	3.167
20	3.7	1723.9	98,272.4	59.8	0.017	0.009	13,297.73	5.181	3.175
21	2.2	1380.2	98,617.6	47.9	0.014	0.007	13,345.63	5.195	3.182
22	1.3	1104.8	98,893.9	38.3	0.011	0.006	13,383.97	5.206	3.188
23	0.8	884.3	99,115.0	30.7	0.009	0.004	13,414.66	5.215	3.192
24	0.5	707.6	99,291.9	24.6	0.007	0.004	13,439.21	5.222	3.196
25	0.3	566.3	99,433.5	19.7	0.006	0.003	13,458.86	5.227	3.199
26	0.2	453.1	99,546.7	15.7	0.005	0.002	13,474.59	5.232	3.201
27	0.1	362.5	99,637.4	12.6	0.004	0.002	13,487.17	5.235	3.203
28	0.1	290.1	99,709.9	10.1	0.003	0.001	13,497.23	5.238	3.204
29	0.0	232.1	99,767.9	8.1	0.002	0.001	13,505.29	5.241	3.205
30	0.0	185.7	99,814.3	6.4	0.002	0.001	13,511.73	5.243	3.206
31	0.0	148.5	99,851.5	5.2	0.001	0.001	13,516.88	5.244	3.207
32	0.0	118.8	99,881.2	4.1	0.001	0.001	13,521.01	5.245	3.208
33	0.0	95.1	99,904.9	3.3	0.001	0.000	13,524.3	5.246	3.208
34	0.0	76.1	99,923.9	2.6	0.000	0.000	13,526.94	5.246	3.208

*{(60,000×£350) + (30,000×£3190) + [(0.2×30,000)×£1400)]}/100,000 = £1251 (undiscounted) 1251/[(1+0.035)^1]= £1208.70 (discounted at 3.5%).

†(60,000 + 30,000/100,000 = 0.9 (undiscounted) 0.9/[(1+0.035)^1] = 0.85 (discounted at 3.5%).

‡(60,000×0.89+(30,000×0.50)/100,000 = 0.68 (undiscounted) 0.68/[(1+0.035)^1]= 0.65 (discounted at 3.5%).

Cost-effectiveness

The aim of the cohort simulation is to provide the expected costs and expected outcomes for both the intervention arm and no-intervention arm. The same process as detailed above would also be undertaken for the intervention arm of the model, but would involve incorporating the relative risk (RR) related to the effectiveness of the intervention and intervention cost.

From these simulations it is possible to calculate the incremental cost-effectiveness ratio of implementing an intervention for breast cancer patients aimed at reducing the number of subsequent breast cancer recurrences compared with no intervention. The model can be checked for consistency and validity using the methods outlined in Chapter 8, section 8.3.6. In addition, the underlying uncertainty in the model can be addressed. The theory and methods that can be used will be described in Chapter 10.

9.2 Adapting the simple Markov model

We can now look at techniques that can be implemented when undertaking a Markov modelling exercise to increase its applicability to the disease or intervention in question. This section also illustrates that using different software platforms for model building may lead to slightly different results, something that the analyst should be aware of. Here this issue is illustrated using TreeAge Pro and Microsoft Excel as different software programmes to build and analyse the Markov models.

9.2.1 Half-cycle corrections

There are additional issues concerning cycle length. The assumption is that transitions only occur once in each cycle, and computer-based Markov models usually model these to occur at a discrete point in time at either the beginning or end of a cycle. In reality transitions may occur at any time within a cycle, and counting cohort membership at either the beginning or end of each cycle leads to bias in the form of overestimation or underestimation, respectively, of the cohort within a state during that cycle. Therefore half-cycle corrections can be used to compensate for the timing of the transition, making the assumption that, on average, state transitions occur halfway through the cycle, hence reflecting the continuous nature of the timing of transitions within a cycle.

Sonnenberg and Beck (1993) provide a useful explanation of the half-cycle correction, and more recently Naimark et al. (2008) have provided two pedagogical approaches to the half-cycle correction. They also note that the important principle with the half-cycle correction is not when the transitions occur, but when state membership (i.e. the proportion of the cohort in that state) is counted. The longer the cycle length, the more important it may be to use half-cycle corrections. For example, if the cycle length were 5 years, rather than 1 year, it may be particularly important to use half-cycle corrections. In the breast cancer example, it can be seen from Table 9.3 that in cycle zero there are 100,000 patients in the 'Well' state, and in cycle 1 there are 60,000 patients in the 'Well' state, 30,000 in the 'Recurrence' state, and 10,000 in the 'Dead' state. The transition takes place at the beginning of the cycle and the state membership is counted at the end of the cycle, resulting in an underestimation of state membership.

Half-cycle correction can be undertaken either by a process of adding the state membership at time t to the state membership at time $t + 1$, multiplying by the relevant cost or outcome, and dividing the result by 2 (Table 9.4), or alternatively as in Table 9.5 by adding 0.5 to the total estimated life expectancy and/or half of a cycle's worth of incremental utility/cost to the total cumulative utility/cost for each state in the model. If we do not simulate the whole life expectancy of a cohort (i.e. the model does not reach full absorption), we need to make an additional correction for members of the cohort who are still alive at the end of the simulation. To do this this, we subtract a half-cycle from the survivors in the final accounting. This method is used by TreeAge Pro.

One should be aware that both these methods will lead to the same cumulative cost and outcome results if left undiscounted, but they will differ when discounting is performed. For example, once costs and outcomes are discounted at 3.5%, the half-cycle correction using the method set out in Table 9.4 results in a cumulative cost of £11,372.33, whereas using the method set out in Table 9.5 the cumulative cost is £11,194.36. Similarly, the Table 9.4 approach results in life-years and QALYs of 4.582 and 3.010 respectively, compared with 4.465 and 2.935 using the Table 9.5 method. These differences are summarized in Table 9.6.

The importance of the half-cycle correction depends on the length of the overall time horizon and the cycle length. Differences arising from the methods used are something that the analyst should be aware of, but in the context of cost-effectiveness modelling, where the differences in costs and outcomes are the focus, the use of different half-cycle correction methods is unlikely to make a great deal of difference.

9.2.2 Allowing forward and backward progression in the model

In the example shown in Figure 9.1 all transitions were forward transitions. However, it is possible to build backward transitions into the model, as shown in Figure 9.5 (black dashed line from 'Recurrence' state to the 'Well' state) and Figure 9.6. This enables the analyst to capture repetitive events within the disease process or treatment pathways.

In this particular example it is highly likely that a proportion of patients who have a recurrence of breast cancer are treated successfully and return to the 'Well' state, and it is not unheard of for some breast cancer patients to have more than one recurrence over their lifetime. Markov models provide an ideal analytical framework for capturing this repetitive nature of some diseases or treatments. It is important to remember that, because of the rule that Markov states must be mutually exhaustive (defined such that all possibilities are covered and none overlap and their probabilities must sum to 1), all the probabilities in rows in a transition matrix sum to 1. The transition matrix (Table 9.7) shows that there is a probability of 0.2 of moving from the 'Recurrence' state to the 'Dead' state in the next cycle, a probability of 0.1 of moving from the 'Recurrence' state back to the 'Well' state in the next cycle, and, because of the rule of mutually exhaustive states, a probability of $1 - (0.2 + 0.1)$ of remaining in the 'Recurrence' state.

Table 9.4 Half-cycle correction: no intervention arm (using the process of adding the state membership at time t to the state membership at time $t + 1$, multiplying by the relevant cost or outcome, and halving the result)

Cycle	Well	Recurrence	Dead	Cycle cost	Cycle life-years	Cycle QALY	Cum. cost	Cum. life-years	Cum. QALYs
0	100,000	0	0						
1	60,000	30,000	10,000	758.50	0.950	0.787	758.50	0.950	0.787
2	36,000	42,000	22,000	1400.40*	0.840†	0.607‡	2158.90	1.790	1.394
3	21,600	44,400	34,000	1596.48	0.720	0.472	3755.38	2.510	1.867
4	12,960	42,000	45,040	1562.88	0.605	0.370	5318.26	3.115	2.236
5	7776	37,488	54,736	1421.72	0.501	0.291	6739.98	3.616	2.527
6	4665.6	32,323.2	63,011.2	1240.23	0.411	0.230	7980.21	4.027	2.757
7	2799.4	27,258.2	69,942.4	1053.89	0.335	0.182	9034.10	4.362	2.939
8	1679.6	22,646.4	75,674.0	880.14	0.272	0.145	9914.24	4.634	3.084
9	1007.8	18,621.0	80,371.2	726.33	0.220	0.115	10,640.57	4.854	3.199
10	604.7	15,199.1	84,196.2	594.39	0.177	0.092	11,234.96	5.031	3.291
11	362.8	12,340.7	87,296.5	483.51	0.143	0.073	11,718.47	5.174	3.364
12	217.7	9981.4	89,800.9	391.61	0.115	0.058	12,110.08	5.288	3.422
13	130.6	8050.4	91,819.0	316.17	0.092	0.047	12,426.25	5.380	3.469
14	78.4	6479.5	93,442.1	254.66	0.074	0.037	12,680.91	5.454	3.506
15	47.0	5207.1	94,745.9	204.76	0.059	0.030	12,885.67	5.513	3.536

(continued)

16	28.2	4179.8	95,792.0	164.43	0.047	0.024	13,050.10	5.560	3.560
17	16.9	3352.3	96,630.8	131.92	0.038	0.019	13,182.02	5.598	3.579
18	10.2	2686.9	97,302.9	105.76	0.030	0.015	13,287.78	5.629	3.594
19	6.1	2152.6	97,841.3	84.74	0.024	0.012	13,372.52	5.653	3.606
20	3.7	1723.9	98,272.4	67.87	0.019	0.010	13,440.40	5.672	3.616
21	2.2	1380.2	98,617.6	54.35	0.016	0.008	13,494.75	5.688	3.624
22	1.3	1104.8	98,893.9	43.51	0.012	0.006	13,538.25	5.700	3.630
23	0.8	884.3	99,115.0	34.82	0.010	0.005	13,573.08	5.710	3.635
24	0.5	707.6	99,291.9	27.87	0.008	0.004	13,600.95	5.718	3.639
25	0.3	566.3	99,433.5	22.30	0.006	0.003	13,623.25	5.725	3.642
26	0.2	453.1	99,546.7	17.84	0.005	0.003	13,641.09	5.730	3.645
27	0.1	362.5	99,637.4	14.28	0.004	0.002	13,655.37	5.734	3.647
28	0.1	290.1	99,709.9	11.42	0.003	0.002	13,666.79	5.737	3.648
29	0.0	232.1	99,767.9	9.14	0.003	0.001	13,675.93	5.740	3.650
30	0.0	185.7	99,814.3	7.31	0.002	0.001	13,683.25	5.742	3.651
31	0.0	148.5	99,851.5	5.85	0.002	0.001	13,689.10	5.743	3.652
32	0.0	118.8	99,881.2	4.68	0.001	0.001	13,693.78	5.745	3.652
33	0.0	95.1	99,904.9	3.74	0.001	0.001	13,697.52	5.746	3.653
34	0.0	76.1	99,923.9	3.00	0.001	0.000	13,700.52	5.747	3.653

$*\{[(60,000+36,000)\times£350)\times0.5] + [(30,000+42,000)\times£3190]\times0.5 + [(0.2\times30,000)\times£1400)]\}/100,000 = £1400.4.$

$†[(60,000+36,000+(22,000-10,000)]\times0.5]/100,000 = 0.84.$

$‡\{(60,000+36,000)\times0.89]\times0.5 + [(30,000 + 42,000)\times0.5]\times0.5/100,000\} = 0.607.$

Table 9.5 Half-cycle correction using the methods utilized in TreeAge Pro

Cycle	Well	Recurrence	Dead	Cycle cost	Cycle life-years	Cycle QALY	Cum Cost	Cum. life-years	Cum. QALYs
0	100,000	0	0	175*	0.500†	0.445‡	175	0.500	0.445
1	60,000	30,000	10,000	1251	0.900	0.684	1426	1.400	1.129
2	36,000	42,000	22,000	1583.4	0.780	0.530	3009.4	2.180	1.659
3	21,600	44,400	34,000	1616.28	0.660	0.414	4625.68	2.840	2.074
4	12,960	42,000	45,040	1502.76	0.550	0.325	6128.44	3.390	2.399
5	7776	37,488	54,736	1328.05	0.453	0.257	7456.49	3.842	2.656
6	4665.6	32,323.2	63,011.2	1137.94	0.370	0.203	8594.434	4.212	2.859
7	2799.4	27,258.2	69,942.4	955.659	0.301	0.161	9550.093	4.513	3.020
8	1679.6	22,646.4	75,674.0	791.709	0.243	0.128	10,341.8	4.756	3.148
9	1007.8	18,621.0	80,371.2	649.676	0.196	0.102	10,991.48	4.952	3.250
10	604.7	15,199.1	84,196.2	529.526	0.158	0.081	11,521	5.110	3.332
11	362.8	12,340.7	87,296.5	429.492	0.127	0.065	11,950.5	5.237	3.397
12	217.7	9981.4	89,800.9	347.117	0.102	0.052	12,297.61	5.339	3.448
13	130.6	8050.4	91,819.0	279.807	0.082	0.041	12,577.42	5.421	3.490
14	78.4	6479.5	93,442.1	225.114	0.066	0.033	12,802.53	5.487	3.523
15	47.0	5207.1	94,745.9	180.852	0.053	0.026	12,983.39	5.539	3.549
16	28.2	4179.8	95,792.0	145.138	0.042	0.021	13,128.52	5.581	3.570
17	16.9	3352.3	96,630.8	116.384	0.034	0.017	13,244.91	5.615	3.587

(continued)

18	10.2	2686.9	97,302.9	93.2719	0.027	0.014	13,338.18	5.642	3.601
19	6.1	2152.6	97,841.3	74.7161	0.022	0.011	13,412.9	5.664	3.612
20	3.7	1723.9	98,272.4	59.8321	0.017	0.009	13,472.73	5.681	3.620
21	2.2	1380.2	98,617.6	47.9011	0.014	0.007	13,520.63	5.695	3.627
22	1.3	1104.8	98,893.9	38.3422	0.011	0.006	13,558.97	5.706	3.633
23	0.8	884.3	99,115.0	30.6866	0.009	0.004	13,589.66	5.715	3.637
24	0.5	707.6	99,291.9	24.5569	0.007	0.004	13,614.21	5.722	3.641
25	0.3	566.3	99,433.5	19.6501	0.006	0.003	13,633.86	5.727	3.644
26	0.2	453.1	99,546.7	15.7229	0.005	0.002	13,649.59	5.732	3.646
27	0.1	362.5	99,637.4	12.5799	0.004	0.002	13,662.17	5.735	3.648
28	0.1	290.1	99,709.9	10.065	0.003	0.001	13,672.23	5.738	3.649
29	0.0	232.1	99,767.9	8.05256	0.002	0.001	13,680.29	5.741	3.650
30	0.0	185.7	99,814.3	6.4424	0.002	0.001	13,686.73	5.743	3.651
31	0.0	148.5	99,851.5	5.15414	0.001	0.001	13,691.88	5.744	3.652
32	0.0	118.8	99,881.2	4.12344	0.001	0.001	13,696.01	5.745	3.653
33	0.0	95.1	99,904.9	3.29883	0.001	0.000	13,699.3	5.746	3.653
34	0.0002	76.1	99,923.9	1.21§	0.000¶	0.000**	13,700.52	5.747	3.653

* [(100,000×£350)×0.5]/100,000 = £175.
† (100,000×0.5)/100,000 = 0.5.
‡ (100,000×0.89)/100,000 = 0.445.
§ {[(0.00286×£350) + (76.1×£3190)]×0.5}/100,000 = £1.21.
¶ [(0.00286 + 76.1)×0.5]/100,000 = 0.00038.
** {[(0.00286×0.89)+(76.1×0.5)]×0.5}/10,000 = 0.00019

Table 9.6 Comparison of Markov trace with half-cycle correction and discounting

Stage	Table 9.4 method			Table 9.5 method (TreeAge Pro method)		
	Discount cost	Discount life-year	Discount QALY	Discount cost	Discount life-year	Discount QALY
0				175.00	0.500	0.445
1	758.50	0.950	0.787	1208.70	0.849	0.645
2	1353.04	0.792	0.573	1478.12	0.694	0.472
3	1490.33	0.641	0.420	1457.79	0.554	0.348
4	1409.63	0.508	0.310	1309.57	0.435	0.258
5	1238.95	0.397	0.230	1118.18	0.338	0.192
6	1044.24	0.307	0.172	925.72	0.261	0.143
7	857.34	0.236	0.128	751.14	0.200	0.107
8	691.78	0.181	0.096	601.23	0.153	0.080
9	551.58	0.138	0.072	476.69	0.116	0.060
10	436.12	0.105	0.054	375.39	0.088	0.045
11	342.77	0.080	0.041	294.18	0.067	0.034
12	268.23	0.060	0.031	229.72	0.051	0.026
13	209.23	0.046	0.023	178.91	0.038	0.019
14	162.83	0.035	0.017	139.07	0.029	0.015
15	126.50	0.026	0.013	107.95	0.022	0.011
16	98.15	0.020	0.010	83.70	0.017	0.008
17	76.08	0.015	0.007	64.85	0.013	0.006
18	58.93	0.011	0.006	50.21	0.009	0.005
19	45.62	0.009	0.004	38.86	0.007	0.004
20	35.31	0.006	0.003	30.07	0.005	0.003
21	27.31	0.005	0.002	23.26	0.004	0.002
22	21.13	0.004	0.002	17.99	0.003	0.002
23	16.34	0.003	0.001	13.91	0.002	0.001
24	12.63	0.002	0.001	10.75	0.002	0.001
25	9.77	0.002	0.001	8.31	0.001	0.001
26	7.55	0.001	0.001	6.43	0.001	0.000
27	5.84	0.001	0.000	4.97	0.001	0.000
28	4.51	0.001	0.000	3.84	0.001	0.000

Table 9.6 (continued) Comparison of Markov trace with half-cycle correction and discounting

Stage	Table 9.4 method			Table 9.5 method (TreeAge Pro method)		
	Discount cost	Discount life-year	Discount QALY	Discount cost	Discount life-year	Discount QALY
29	3.49	0.001	0.000	2.97	0.000	0.000
30	2.70	0.000	0.000	2.30	0.000	0.000
31	2.08	0.000	0.000	1.77	0.000	0.000
32	1.61	0.000	0.000	1.37	0.000	0.000
33	1.25	0.000	0.000	1.06	0.000	0.000
34	0.96	0.000	0.000	0.38	0.000	0.000
Total	£11,372.33	4.582	3.010	£11,194.36	4.463	2.935

9.2.3 Introducing time-dependent transition probabilities into the model

In the simple example used in this chapter, one assumption so far has been that the transition probabilities within the model did not vary over time. However, in most models the evidence is likely to show a temporal trend of increasing or decreasing probabilities.

There are two general types of time dependency that impact on transition probabilities. One is where it is a function of the number of cycles that have elapsed since the start of the model, i.e. how long the cohort has been modelled. This is the case where a transition probability is linked to age. This is straightforward to implement if the assumption holds that all patients within the cohort start at the same age, and this

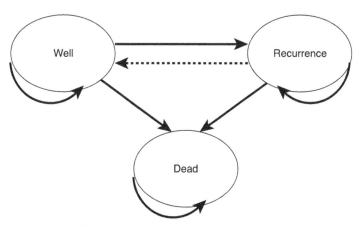

Fig. 9.5 Markov state diagram depicting states and allowable transitions.

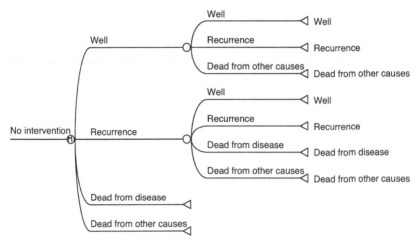

Fig. 9.6 Markov model depicting allowable transitions.

should be explicitly stated. A simple way of introducing this is to use a look-up table in Excel to change the probabilities of transitions depending on age. In the breast cancer example, rather than assuming that all-cause mortality Pr_wD is constant over the lifetime of the model, it could be based on age-specific all-cause mortality data from nationally provided life-tables. With the assumption that everyone in the cohort starts the model aged 55, the annual age-related values of Pr_wD up to age 64 are outlined in Table 9.8.

The second type of time dependency, which is more difficult to implement, relates to the amount of time a patient has remained in a state. In the breast cancer example the likelihood is that the probability of cancer-related mortality would increase according to the amount of time a patient remains in the 'Recurrence' state but, because of the Markovian assumption (see section 9.1.3), the model cannot keep track of when the patient enters this state or how long they remain there. However, transitions from the 'Well' state to the other states in the model can be modelled as time dependent based on the time spent in the 'Well' state (assuming that all the cohort start in the 'Well' state at the start of the model, and also assuming that no returns to the 'Well' state were allowed). In the example, it is easy to track the time spent by patients in the 'Well' state and use the time-dependent transition probabilities in the same way as was

Table 9.7 Transition matrix depicting allowable transitions (forwards and backwards) and transition probabilities

		To $t + 1$		
		Well	**Recurrence**	**Dead**
From t	**Well**	1 − (0.3+0.1) or #	0.3 (PrRec)	0.1 (Pr_wD)
	Recurrence	0.1	1 − (0.1+0.2) or #	0.2 (Pr_rD)
	Dead	0	0	1

Table 9.8 Time-dependent values for transition probability Pr_wD

Cycle	1	2	3	4	5	6	7	8	9	10
Age	55	56	57	58	59	60	61	62	63	64
Pr_wD	0.014	0.018	0.022	0.026	0.030	0.034	0.038	0.042	0.046	0.050

undertaken for age in Table 9.8. The reader is referred to Chapter 3 in *Decision Modelling for Health Economic Evaluation* (Briggs *et al.* 2006) for a discussion on using survival analysis to inform time-dependent transition probabilities.

9.2.4 Overcoming the Markovian assumption: temporary and tunnel states

Temporary states may be useful where the model involves a one-time cost or temporary change in utility. These one-off events can be incorporated by adding a new temporary state to the model which patients can stay in for only one cycle, i.e. transitions from this state are to other states and not to itself.

Temporary states can also be used in succession to overcome the Markovian lack of memory limitation. In the example shown in Figure 9.1, it might be assumed that the members of the cohort who remain in the 'Recurrence' state for more than two cycles differ from those who remain for just one or two cycles. As set up in Figure 9.5, it is impossible to differentiate between those experiencing just one or two cycles of recurrence from those experiencing more than two cycles of recurrence. Furthermore, all patients in a given health state are assumed homogenous, regardless of past health states or how long they have been in that particular state.

If it is necessary to incorporate some aspect of memory in the model, this can be achieved by creating new states (known as tunnel states). These are a series of temporary states that must be visited in a fixed sequence, with each one leading to the next, each representing differing transition probabilities, costs, and outcomes.

A reasonable assumption with the breast cancer example is that the annual probability of death and annual costs and quality of life values are different for each of the first 2 years following the recurrence of breast cancer. Thereafter the annual probability of death, and cost, remains constant. Figure 9.7 shows the addition of two temporary states ('rec 1' and 'rec 2') into the model which represent the first 2 years following recurrence. Transitions to and from these states can only be made in this sequence and no patient is allowed to stay for more than one cycle, hence the term 'tunnel states'.

9.2.5 Patient-level simulation models

Although Markov models can be adapted to capture 'memory', they are not ideally suited to this. When the analyst requires memory to be an inherent part of their model, or when the model requires a lot of states to be incorporated, it may be more appropriate to use patient-level simulation models (also referred to as individual patient sampling or microsimulations). Rather than modelling the progression of a cohort, these model individual patients. However, these models typically require a greater amount of evidence and have a greater computational burden, especially when assessing

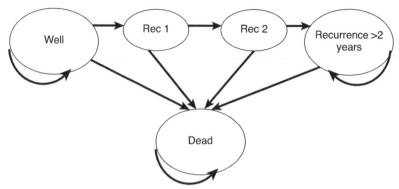

Fig. 9.7 Diagrammatic representation of tunnel states.

parameter and decision uncertainty. A number of detailed reviews and examples of patient-level simulation are available (Karnon 2003; Barton *et al.* 2004; Clarke *et al.* 2004; Brennan *et al.* 2006; Cooper *et al.* 2007).

9.3 **Summary**

In this chapter we have set out the methods required to construct a Markov model in order to undertake a cost-effectiveness analysis of a health-care intervention, accompanied by a guide to the practical steps that a researcher has to undertake in order to construct, analyse, and evaluate such a model. The following exercise provides a detailed step-by-step guide on how to construct a Markov model in Excel and TreeAge. This treatment of modelling is extended in Chapter 10 by examining ways of handling and propagating uncertainty in the model.

References

Barton, P., Bryan, S., and Robinson, S. (2004). Modelling in the economic evaluation of health care: selecting the appropriate approach. *Journal of Health Services Research and Policy*, **9**, 110–18.

Bojke, L., Hornby, E., and Sculpher, M. (2007). A comparison of the cost effectiveness of pharmacotherapy or surgery (laparoscopic fundoplication) in the treatment of GORD. *Pharmacoeconomics*, **25**, 829–41.

Brennan, A., Chick, S.E., and Davies, R. (2006). A taxonomy of model structures for economic evaluation of health technologies. *Health Economics*, **15**, 1295–1310.

Briggs, A. and Sculpher, M. (1998). An introduction to Markov modelling for economic evaluation. *Pharmacoeconomics*, **13**, 397–409.

Briggs, A., Sculpher, M., Britton, A., Murray, D., and Fitzpatrick, R. (1998). The costs and benefits of primary total hip replacement. How likely are new prostheses to be cost-effective? *International Journal of Technology Assessment in Health Care*, **14**, 743–61.

Briggs, A.H., Sculpher, M., and Claxton, K. (2006). *Decision Modelling for Health Economic Evaluation*. Oxford University Press.

Clarke, P.M., Gray, A.M., Briggs, A., *et al.* (2004). A model to estimate the lifetime health outcomes of patients with type 2 diabetes: the United Kingdom Prospective Diabetes Study (UKPDS) Outcomes Model (UKPDS no. 68). *Diabetologia*, **47**, 1747–59.

Cooper, K., Brailsford, S.C., and Davies, R. (2007). Choice of modelling technique for evaluating health care interventions. *Journal of the Operational Research Society*, **58**, 168–76.

Dong, H. and Buxton, M. (2006). Early assessment of the likely cost-effectiveness of a new technology: a Markov model with probabilistic sensitivity analysis of computer-assisted total knee replacement. *International Journal of Technology Assessment in Health Care*, **22**, 191–202.

Fenn, P. and Gray, A. (1999). Estimating long-term cost savings from treatment of Alzheimer's disease: a modelling approach. *Pharmacoeconomics*, **16**, 165–74.

Hawkins, N., Epstein, D., Drummond, M., *et al.* (2005). Assessing the cost-effectiveness of new pharmaceuticals in epilepsy in adults: the results of a probabilistic decision model. *Medical Decision Making*, **25**, 493–510.

Johannesson, M., Jonsson, B., Kjekshus, J., Olsson, A.G., Pedersen, T.R., and Wedel, H. (1997). Cost effectiveness of simvastatin treatment to lower cholesterol levels in patients with coronary heart disease: Scandinavian Simvastatin Survival Study Group. *New England Journal of Medicine*, **336**, 332–6.

Karnon, J. (2003). Alternative decision modelling techniques for the evaluation of health care technologies: Markov processes versus discrete event simulation. *Health Economics*, **12**, 837–48.

Karnon, J., Bakhai, A., Brennan, A., *et al.* (2006). A cost-utility analysis of clopidogrel in patients with non-ST-segment-elevation acute coronary syndromes in the UK. *International Journal of Cardiology*, **109**, 307–16.

Kim, L.G., Thompson, S.G., Briggs, A.H., Buxton, M.J., and Campbell, H.E. (2007). How cost-effective is screening for abdominal aortic aneurysms? *Journal of Medical Screening*, **14**, 46–52.

Legood, R., Gray, A., Wolstenholme, J., and Moss, S. (2006). Lifetime effects, costs, and cost effectiveness of testing for human papillomavirus to manage low grade cytological abnormalities: results of the NHS pilot studies. *British Medical Journal*, **332**, 79–85.

Moeremans, K. and Annemans, L. (2008). Cost-effectiveness of anastrozole compared to tamoxifen in hormone receptor-positive early breast cancer: analysis based on the ATAC trial. *International Journal of Gynecological Cancer*, **16**, 576–8.

Naimark, D.M., Bott, M., and Krahn, M. (2008). The half-cycle correction explained: two alternative pedagogical approaches. *Medical Decision Making*, **28**, 706–12.

Palmer, S., Sculpher, M., Philips, Z., *et al.* (2005). Management of non-ST-elevation acute coronary syndromes: how cost-effective are glycoprotein IIb/IIIA antagonists in the UK National Health Service? *International Journal of Cardiology*, **100**, 229–40.

Sonnenberg, F.A. and Beck, J.R. (1993). Markov models in medical decision making: a practical guide. *Medical Decision Making*, **13**, 322–38.

Steuten, L., Palmer, S., Vrijhoef, B., van Merode, F., Spreeuwenberg, C., and Severens, H. (2007). Cost-utility of a disease management program for patients with asthma. *International Journal of Technology Assessment in Health Care*, **23**, 184–91.

Constructing and analysing a Markov model

Overview

The purpose of this exercise is to build a Markov model and to familiarize yourself with the steps and techniques involved. Although this is a simple example, the process will get you to think about the basics involved in Markov modelling: deciding on the structure of the model by defining the states and allowable transitions, identifying the starting probabilities, determining the transition probabilities, deciding on a cycle length, setting the stopping rule, determining rewards, implementing discounting, and analysing and evaluating the model. Alongside these steps the exercise includes the use of time-dependent transition probabilities, half-cycle corrections, and backward transitions. The step-by-step guide will take you through a number of stages of developing and analysing the model. Worked solutions are also available at www.herc.ox.ac.uk/books/applied. The exercise is adapted from a model developed by Briggs and Sculpher (1998).

Exercise instructions

A Markov model of disease progression is presented in Figure 9E.1. It consists of four states, represented by ovals, to characterize a chronic disease. Possible transitions between states are shown by arrows:

- asymptomatic disease (a patient has the disease, but is not showing any ill effects)
- progressive disease (a patient is showing symptoms of disease)
- dead from the disease
- death from other causes.

A drug has become available that may reduce the likelihood of disease progression (only for those in the asymptomatic state). We want to know the cost-effectiveness of this drug. The exercise asks you to build a Markov model comparing the costs and outcomes of two options: (i) no drug therapy and (ii) drug therapy. Table 9E.1 gives the parameters of the model.

What are the possible transitions?

Before trying to build the model, familiarize yourself with the possible transitions.

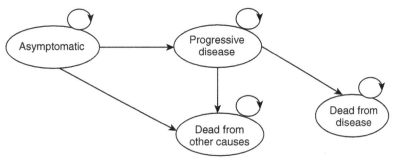

Fig. 9E.1 Markov state diagram.

Table 9E.1 Parameter values for the Markov model of disease progression

Name	Value	Description
Costs		
cAsymp	500	State cost of one cycle in the asymptomatic disease state
cProg	3000	State cost of one cycle in the progressive disease state
cDrug	1000	State cost of drug for one cycle
cDeath	1000	Transition cost associated with transition to the "dead from disease" state following the progressive disease state
Quality-of-life adjustments		
uAsymp	0.95	Quality-of-life weight for one cycle in the asymptomatic disease state
uProg	0.75	Quality-of-life weight for one cycle in the progressive disease state
Transition probabilities		
tpProg	0.01	Coefficient of increase for probability of entering the progressive disease state, i.e. transition probability increases by 0.01 with each added year
tpDcm	0.15	Probability of dying from the disease during the progressive disease state
natDeath	0.0138	Other-cause mortality for age 55–64
	0.0379	Other-cause mortality for age 65–74
	0.0912	Other-cause mortality for age 75–84
	0.1958	Other-cause mortality for age 85+
Other parameters		
eff	50%	Relative risk of disease progression from using the drug
ini_age	55	Initial age at which patients are deemed to start the model
oDR	3.5%	Discount rate for outcomes
cDR	3.5%	Discount rate for costs

◆ Record the transition probabilities that have to be estimated in the transition matrix in Table 9E.2. Put a tick where a transition is allowed and a cross where it is not allowed. This will help you to think through the structure of the model.

◆ Consider the nature of the transition probabilities required. First, look at Table 9E.1. This gives you the names and descriptions of the transition probabilities. Write each transition probability next to where you have put the ticks in the transition matrix. Identify which transitions are going to be residual probabilities (mark as #). (Remember that you need to know three of the four values for each row in the matrix.)

Build the basic Markov model in TreeAge Pro

◆ This requires entering two branches after the decision node (one for the no-drug option and one for the drug option).

◆ Insert a Markov node for each of the no-drug and drug options.

◆ Add branches to represent the states and transitions according to the transition matrix shown in Table 9E.2.

◆ Set up the calculation method you want to use. Go to the decision node (Select **Edit > Preferences > Calculation Method > Methods: Cost-Effectiveness, payoff 1** for costs, **payoff 2** for effectiveness, **payoff 3** for effectiveness. Choose **Numeric Format** to enter the units for each payoff, i.e. 1 = currency units, 2 = QALYs, 3 = life-years).

◆ It might be useful to view what you are doing, i.e. what information you are entering into your model. Select **Edit > Preferences > Variables/Markov Info**, select **Show definitions**, and ensure that boxes **Expand node to fit variables** and **Show Markov information** are both checked.

◆ Hint: It might be best to build one arm first (structure, rewards, probabilities, etc.) and check that this is working. Then copy and paste to the other arm and make appropriate changes.

For more details see the step-by-step guide.

Table 9E.2 Transition matrix

State (From)	(To) Asymptomatic	Progressive disease	Dead (from disease)	Dead (other causes)
Asymptomatic				
Progressive disease				
Dead (from disease)				
Dead (other causes)				

Enter rewards

The rewards (costs and quality of life adjustments) for the model are given in the table of parameter values.

- Create variables for the costs and quality-of-life adjustments.
- Create separate variables for the discount rate for costs and outcomes.
- Enter the state (incremental) rewards, (1 for costs, 2 for utilities, 3 for life-years).
- Make sure you allow for a half-cycle correction.
- Enter the transition reward.
- Ensure that you discount the rewards appropriately (see the step-by-step guide).

For more details see the step-by-step guide.

Enter probabilities

- The probabilities for the model are given in Table 9E.1.
- Enter the set of starting probabilities (all patients are assumed to start in the asymptomatic disease state).
- Create variables for transition to progression and transition to death following progression (tpProg and tpDcm) and enter the transitions in the model.
- Note that the tpProg variable is a coefficient of increase. Therefore it has to be linked with the number of cycles (see step-by-step guide).
- Create a table using the other-cause mortality data. Name the table natDeath (see step-by-step guide).
- Enter the transitions to other-cause death and link to age: natDeath[age].
- Enter the effectiveness parameter in the drug arm.

For more details see the step-by-step guide.

Analyse the Markov model

- Terminate each arm of the Markov model using the command _stage>45.
- Use the **Analysis> Cost-effectiveness** command. Keep effectiveness on the *x*-axis and then explore the findings using >**Graph** >**Text report**. Use 'no-drug therapy' as your baseline. You should find:
  - the cost for the no-drug arm is £12,082 and the cost for the drug intervention is £20,865 (cost difference of £8,783)
  - the QALYs for the no-drug arm are 9.69 and the QALYs for the drug intervention are 10.95 (QALY difference of 1.26)
  - therefore the incremental cost-effectiveness ratio is £6970 (£8783/1.26).

Note that TreeAge defaults to provide results in thousands (i.e. £12K). To generate exact results you will need to use the **Analysis > Cost-effectiveness** command. When you obtain the graph you will need to convert the axis format by using >**Options**>**axes** and changing the format of the *x*-axis, the *y*-axis, and CE ratios to **Show numbers exactly**.

- If you remove the half-cycle-correction the results are as follows:
  - the cost for the no-drug arm is £11,832 and the cost for the drug intervention is £20,115 (cost difference of £8283)
  - the QALYs for the no-drug arm are 9.22 and the QALYs for the drug intervention are 10.48 (QALY difference of 1.26)
  - therefore the incremental cost-effectiveness ratio is £6573 (£8283/1.26).

For more details see the step-by-step guide.

Cohort (expected value) analysis

To obtain more detailed information about the Markov model, select the Markov node (**drug/nodrug**) > **Analysis**> **Markov Cohort** (**full detail**) or (**Quick**) (see step-by-step guide).

Step-by-step guide: TreeAge Pro

What are the possible transitions?

Familiarize yourself with the possible transitions as described above.

Building the basic Markov model in TreeAge Pro

To build a Markov model in TreeAge, first enter two branches from the decision node that automatically appears when you build a new tree in TreeAge (**Options** > **Add branch***). Alternatively right click on a branch and go to **Branch (es)** > **Add branch**.

Enter text above each branch to indicate the no-drug option and the drug option. In order for TreeAge to know that you want to build a Markov model, you need to change the chance nodes to Markov nodes (**Options** > **Change node type**> **Markov node**). The Markov node signifies the entrance to the Markov model.

After the 'Drug' Markov node, add branches to reflect the four possible Markov health states and enter their names above the respective branch ('Asymptomatic', 'Progressive disease', 'Dead from disease' and 'Dead from other causes'). Now, add branches after the Markov health states to represent the allowable transitions between states and name them. Finally, change the chance nodes at the end of the branches to terminal nodes (**Options** > **Change node type**> **Terminal node**) and select the state to which a patient will move.

Now, you could do the same for 'No-drug' Markov node or you could copy and paste the structure from the 'Drug' arm. For this, click on the 'Drug' Markov node, select all branches (**Options**>**Select Subtree**), and copy them (**Edit**>**Copy Subtree**). Now, select the 'No-drug' Markov node and paste the copied structure (**Edit**>**Paste Subtree**). In the following sections you will learn how to enter rewards and probabilities in your model. One way of building the model is to use the approach just described, i.e. complete one arm of the model, populate it with probabilities and rewards, and once it is finished copy and paste it to the other arm of the model. Then change the inputs that differ between the two arms, such as drug effectiveness and costs, and analyse the Markov model.

The basic structure of your model should be as shown in Figure 9E.2.

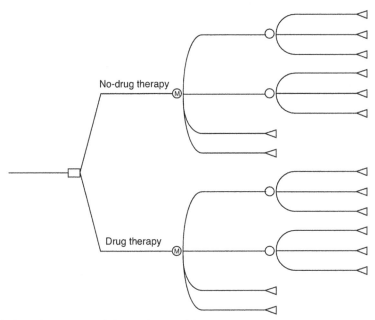

Fig. 9E.2 Basic structure of the Markov model.

Set up the calculation method you want to use, go to the decision node and select **Edit > Preferences > Calculation Method >** from the drop-down menu. Select **Cost-effectiveness, payoff 1** for costs**, payoff 2** for effectiveness**, payoff 3** for effectiveness. To set the units for each payoff (i.e. 1 = costs, 2 = QALYs, 3 = life-years), click on **Numeric Format**. For costs select **Currency units**; for effects choose **Custom suffix** and type in QALYs. Change the payoff value to 3 and repeat this process for life-years.

It might be useful to view what you are doing, i.e. what information you are entering into your model. Select **Edit > Preferences > Variables/Markov Info**, select **Show definitions**, and ensure that boxes **Expand node to fit variables** and **Show Markov information** are both checked.

Enter rewards

Create variables for the rewards (costs and quality-of-life adjustments) using **Values > Variables and Tables** (make sure **Variable list** is highlighted) > **New Variable** command. Use the variable names given in Table 9E.1. Select the check-box > **Define numerically** and enter values.

Create separate variables for the discount rate for costs (cDR) and outcomes (oDR).

Entering incremental rewards

◆ Click on the state you want to add a reward to and go to **Values> Markov State Information**. Assign rewards for costs (1), utilities (2), and life expectancy (3) in turn.

These different rewards can be selected by clicking on the drop-down menu next to the **Rewards** box. For this model, rewards should be entered into the middle row (incremental), which represents the rewards that are accrued in every cycle. For example:

- cost rewards for the asymptomatic state: cAsymp/$((1+cDR)^\wedge$_stage) (NB: remember to include the cost of the drug in the drug arm of the model)
- QALY rewards for the asymptomatic state: uAsymp/$((1+oDR)^\wedge$_stage)
- life-years for the asymptomatic state: 1/$((1+oDR)^\wedge$_stage)

(NOTE: _stage is TreeAge's in-built function referring to cycle number and this can be entered by either typing it in manually or selecting it from the Keywords drop-down. Furthermore, if you are planning on using a cycle length other than annual, you will need to adjust your annual discount rates for that particular period).

- Click on the **Half-cycle correct** box to allow for a half-cycle correction (note that rewards now appear in the initial and final rewards boxes.

NB. In TreeAge instead of using the formula above for discounting you can use a built-in discounting function Discount(). It takes three parameters: value, rate, and time. For example the formula Discount (Casymp;3.5%; _stage) will yield the same result as the formula set out above.

Entering transition rewards

Click on the branch of interest, then select **Values> Markov Transition Rewards**. We want to enter the cost of transition to 'Dead from disease' after progressive disease. In the box enter formula cDeath/$((1+cDR)^\wedge$_stage)

Enter probabilities

Entering starting probabilities

As already mentioned, we assume that the whole cohort enters the model at time zero in the asymptomatic state. Enter 1, 0, 0, and 0 as raw numbers below the branches for the four health states (just after the Markov node and immediately below the Markov information box).

Transitions to progressive disease and death following progression

Create variable names for tpProg and tpDcm and enter their values (**Values > Variables and Tables > New Variable,** then enter the value). Enter the variable names underneath the branches for the transitions. For residual probabilities enter #.

Note that tpProg is a coefficient of increase and therefore has to be linked to the number of cycles. Since _stage is TreeAge's built-in function referring to number of cycles, the probability can be entered as tpProg*(_stage +1). This means that as the model runs over an increasing number of years, the transition probability will increase by the coefficient of increase with each additional year.

Transitions to death from other causes

For transitions to death from other causes, where the probability of death varies with age, the probabilities can be stored in a separate table in TreeAge, indexed by cycle number and age.

- Create a variable for the initial age of the patient. In **Values** > **Variables and Tables** > **New Variable**, define ini_age as 55.

- Create a variable for age in the same way, but set the value to age = ini_age +_stage. To do this go to **Values** > **Variables and Tables**> **New variable**>. Under **Name** enter 'age' > **OK**. In the Variables and Tables box click on **Define variable** > **Default for tree** and then enter ini_age+_stage.

- Create a table by going to **Value** > **Variables and Tables**. Ensure that the **Tables List** button at the top of the window is highlighted. Click on **New table**> from the list. Name the table (in this case, natDeath). Select the look-up method for missing row indexes as 'truncation' (this ensures that the table returns the correct values for index numbers greater than or equal to the index and is useful here because we are using age bands). Then click **OK** to return to the **Variables and Tables** box. Press **Open table**> **Edit table** and in the **Add table entry** box enter the other-cause mortality data. The index should be 55 and the value should be 0.0138. Click on **OK** and then click on **More** to add the rest.

- To link the natDeath table you have just created to the model, enter natDeath[age] underneath the 'Dead other causes' branches.

- Create the effectiveness parameter (eff) as a variable and then enter it in the drug arm, asymptomatic state underneath the 'Progressive disease' branch.

Once you have both arms fully built you can start analysing the Markov model.

Analyse the Markov model

Terminate each arm of the Markov model using the following command. Click on the branch just before the Markov node and go to **Values** > **Markov Termination**. In the **Terminate if** box enter _stage>45. Do this for each arm of the model.

Analyse the model

Go to the decision node and select **Analysis** > **Cost-effectiveness** command. The results should be (see: www.herc.ox.ac.uk/books/applied):

- the cost for the no-drug intervention is £12,082 and the cost for the drug intervention is £20,865 (cost difference £8783).

- the QALYs for the no-drug intervention are 9.69 and the QALYs for the drug intervention are 10.95 (QALY difference of 1.26).

- therefore the incremental cost-effectiveness ratio is £6970 (£8783/1.26).

If you were to remove the half-cycle correction the results would be:

- the cost for the no-drug intervention is £11,832 and the cost for the drug intervention is £20,115 (cost difference £8283)

- the QALYs for the no-drug intervention are 9.22 and the QALYs for the drug intervention are 10.48 (QALY difference of 1.26)

- therefore the incremental cost-effectiveness ratio is £6573 (£8283/1.26).

Cohort (expected value) analysis

Select the Markov node (**drug/nodrug**) > **Analysis**> **Markov Cohort** (**full detail**) or (**Quick**). The full detail analysis will allow you to obtain the Markov trace whereas the Quick analysis will provide you with a summary report. It is worth trying both. Have a look at the various options under **Graph** or **Excel graph**. For example, select **Graph**>**State probabilities** to see the percentage of individuals in different states over time.

Step-by-step guide: Excel

The purpose of this exercise is to replicate the TreeAge Markov model in Excel.

Open the Excel file *Exercise* and click on 'Yes' to enable the macros. To check if you have macros enabled in Excel 2007, click on the **Start** button, then **Excel Options**>**Trust Centre**>**Trust Centre Settings**>**Macro Settings**, and select **Enable all macros**. If your macro settings are usually set to a lower security level, please ensure that this setting is changed back after you have completed this exercise.

The first worksheet in the workbook, <**Diagram**>, has the structure of the Markov model that you will build. Unlike the TreeAge model, this Excel version is built across a number of worksheets with separate sheets for the parameters of the model <**Parameters**>, for each of the Markov model arms of the model <**No drug**>/<**Drug**>, for the final analysis results <**Analysis**>, and for the probabilistic sensitivity analysis sheets <**PSA**>.

In terms of structure, the model consists of four states that characterize a chronic disease:

- ◆ asymptomatic disease (a patient has acquired the disease, but is not suffering any ill effects)
- ◆ progressive disease (a patient is showing symptoms of disease)
- ◆ dead from the disease
- ◆ dead from other causes.

The states are represented by the ovals and possible transitions between these states are shown by arrows. State costs are shown in red while transition costs are shown in pink. Transition probabilities between states are shown in blue and the utilities of each state are shown in green. All the cells for you to complete in the exercise are shaded green.

Overview of steps to complete the exercise

- ◆ Preparing parameters and naming cells
- ◆ Building a Markov model for no-drug therapy
- ◆ Adapting the model for new-drug therapy
- ◆ Estimating cost-effectiveness (deterministically)
- ◆ Half-cycle correction

Preparing parameters and naming cells

First you have to prepare the <**Parameters**> worksheet to allow the use of parameter names throughout the rest of this exercise. You will find that the discount rates and initial age at which patients are deemed to start the model are already included in the worksheet. In this section, you will enter the transition probabilities, state and transition costs, and state utilities, and name the parameters of your model. Take some time to read the descriptions of each variable.

To begin with, focus on just four columns: 'Name', 'Live value' 'Deterministic', and 'Description'. The 'Live value' column is useful as it enables an easy switch between deterministic and probabilistic analysis. It contains an IF(...) statement that enables the switch between 'deterministic' (column C) and 'probabilistic' (column D) values depending on what you enter in cell D5. At present, you should have a value of 0 in cell D5. It may be useful at this stage to look up the IF statement syntax in the Excel help file.

1 Enter the cost rewards for each of the model states in cells C12:C15. Hence, for cAsymp you should enter 500 in cell C12, and so on.

2 Enter the utility rewards for asymptomatic and progressive states in cells C19:C20.

3 Enter the transition probabilities for disease progression and death from disease in cells C25:C26.

4 Enter the time dependent probabilities for death from other causes in cells B27:B30.

5 Enter the relative risk of disease progression from the drug (eff) in cell C33. Using names instead of cell references will help you to build the model and prevent mistakes.

6 Highlight the 'Name' and 'Live value' of the asymptomatic cost parameter (i.e. highlight cells A12:B12) and choose **Insert>Name>Create** from the menu bar. Now check 'Left column' and click OK on the pop-up box.

In Excel 2007, highlight the 'Name' and 'Live value' of the asymptomatic cost parameter (i.e. highlight cells A12:B12), select **Formulas>Create From Selection**, ensure that 'Left Column' is selected, and click 'OK'. Check whether the name has been set up successfully by selecting cell B12. If everything is correct, you should read 'cAsymp' in the 'Name box' at the top left of the screen above the workbook. Now, name all othe remaining parameters down to row 38.

Building a Markov model for no drug therapy

Open the <**No Drug**> worksheet. You should first model death from other causes (natDeath, column C) using the time-dependent variables that you named in the <**Parameters**> worksheet. You can do this by using the IF(...) statement in Excel.

1 Use the IF(...) statement to choose between natdeath55, natdeath65, natdeath75, and natdeath85 based on the age of the patient at each point in time (ini_ age+cycle).

:=IF(ini_age+A6<55,"error",IF(ini_age+A6>=85,natDeath85,IF(ini_age+A6>=75,natDeath75,IF(ini_age+A6>=65,natDeath65,IF(ini_age+A6>=55,natDeath55,"error")))))

Next, you will build a Markov trace that will show the number of patients that are in any one state at any one time. Columns E to H represent the four main states of the model: column E represents the asymptomatic state, column H represents deaths from other causes, and column I provides a check (the sum across E to H must equal the size of the original cohort). Now, familiarize yourself with the possible transitions between model states.

2 Make sure that you understand the transition matrix shown in Table 9E.3

3 Use the transition matrix to populate the Markov model. Start with row 7, and once you have this row correct copy it down to the other rows. It is good practice to complete all states as in the transition matrix and then sum across the states (in column I) to make sure that the total is equal to the size of the original cohort (i.e. 1000). Do not set up one state as the residual of the remaining states.

4 In column K, calculate the life-years for each cycle of the model. You just need to add the number of patients in the asymptomatic and progressive states per cycle.

5 In column L, calculate the QALYs by cycle. You should multiply the state utilities by the number of patients in each state per cycle.

6 In columns M and N, calculate the life years and QALYs appropriately discounted. The discount factor is $1/[(1+\text{discount rate})\wedge\text{cycle}]$.

7 In column P, calculate the state costs for each cycle of the model. Again, multiply the number of patients in each state by the state costs.

8 In column Q, calculate the transition cost from the progressive state to dead from disease. We assume that these costs occur in the beginning of the cycle.

9 In column R, sum the state and transition costs. This will help you to estimate the total discounted costs in column S. The discount factor is $1/[(1+\text{discount rate})\wedge\text{cycle}]$.

Table 9E.3 Transition matrix for no drug therapy

State	(To)			
(From)	Asymptomatic	Progressive disease	Dead (from disease)	Dead (other causes)
Asymptomatic	1 − tpProg*cycle − natDeath	tpProg*cycle		natDeath
Progressive disease		1 − tpDcm −natDeath	tpDcm	natDeath
Dead (from disease)			1	
Dead (other causes)				1

Table 9E.4 Transition matrix for drug therapy

State	(To)			
(From)	Asymptomatic	Progressive disease	Dead (from disease)	Dead (other causes)
Asymptomatic	1 – tpProg*cycle* eff –natDeath	tpProg*cycle*eff		natDeath
Progressive disease		1 – tpDcm – natDeath	tpDcm	natDeath
Dead (from disease)			1	
Dead (other causes)				1

10 In row 54, sum the columns to obtain the total effects and costs of the entire cohort. Finally, in row 55, divide the totals by 1000 to obtain per patient predictions of life expectancy, QALYs, and cost for this arm of the model.

Adapting the model for new drug therapy

Select the left-hand highest corner cell (i.e. grey cell above 1 and to the left of A), right-click on the selected cell, and chose 'Copy'. Open the <**Drug**> worksheet, right-click on cell A1, and select 'Paste'. You now have an exact duplicate model of the 'No-drug' arm. This is to avoid repeating building the model arm again from scratch.

1 Change cells A1 and G3 to 'Drug therapy'.

There are only two differences between the 'No-drug' and 'Drug' arms of the model. First, you have to introduce the drug treatment effect in preventing disease progression. Secondly, you have to incorporate the costs of the drug therapy.

2 Use the transition matrix shown in Table 9E.4 to make your changes to this arm of the model. Start with row 7, and once you have this row correct copy it down to the other rows.

Estimating cost-effectiveness (deterministically)

You have now successfully replicated the TreeAge model in Excel. Now, select the <**Analysis**> worksheet to estimate the cost-effectiveness of drug therapy compared with no-drug therapy.

1 Link the cells for costs, life-years, and QALYs with the total discounted values per patient of the two different treatment arms (<**Drug**> and <**No drug**>).

2 In cells D11:F11, calculate the difference in cost, life years, and QALYs between the two arms.

3 In cells D14:E14, calculate ICERs using life-years and then QALYs as the measure of health benefit.

Half-cycle correction

In both arms of the model, we assumed that transitions between model states occur at the beginning of the cycle with the number of patients in each state being counted at the end of the cycle. However, the transitions could occur at any point in time during each cycle. One possibility is that on average transitions happen halfway through the cycle. Hence, our 1000 patients would transit from the asymptomatic to the progressive/dead from other causes states halfway through cycle 1 rather than at the beginning. Each of these patients would then contribute an additional half-cycle to the estimated life expectancy of 13.7 years. Therfore we should add this 0.5 to total life expectancy as well as adjusting the quality-adjusted life-expectancy (QALE) and lifetime costs. QALE and costs should be adjusted by adding half the expected utility and costs of the individuals at the beginning of cycle 1, i.e. 1000 individuals in the asymptomatic state and no individuals in the remaining states, to the estimated lifetime QALYs and costs.

Remember that we are adjusting our estimates in this way because we assume that the transitions occur at the beginning of the cycle while we count the number of people in each state at the end of the cycle.

You will find the half-cycle correction made for you in columns V to AD in the <Drug> and <No Drug> worksheets. Take some time to look at row 6 of these columns.

Chapter 10

Representing uncertainty in decision analytic models

The aim of this chapter is to provide an introductory overview of theory, methods, and techniques that can be used by analysts to represent uncertainty in their cost-effectiveness models. The chapter provides a guide to the terminology used in representing uncertainty and variability. It outlines the analytical methods that can be used to deal with uncertainty and variability and provides detail on the theory and practice of incorporating probabilistic sensitivity analysis into models. More detailed reviews of the theory and practical examples of handling uncertainty alongside model development can be found in a companion to this handbook (Briggs *et al.* 2006).

10.1 Defining uncertainty

What is meant by 'uncertainty'? It is widely recognized that uncertainty is inherent within all economic evaluation models and consequently needs to be addressed appropriately so that decision-makers have confidence in the model's results. Before looking at methods to deal with uncertainty, it is important to clarify what is meant by the term. Over the past two decades health economists have strived to define what is meant by uncertainty, commencing with the development of a taxonomy of uncertainty in economic evaluation alongside trials by Briggs *et al.* (1994), closely followed by a different taxonomy developed by Manning and colleagues for the US Panel on Cost-effectiveness (Gold *et al.* 1996). Briggs (2000, 2001) then transferred the definitions to model-based economic evaluations. The terminology and definitions used varied throughout the literature, but were consolidated by Briggs *et al.* (2006) and are now being used more consistently by analysts. A key feature of this literature is the distinction between variability, heterogeneity, and uncertainty.

We can think of variability as the variation or randomness we observe when recording information on resource use or outcomes within a homogenous sample of patients. This has sometimes been referred to in the past as first-order uncertainty or stochastic uncertainty, and can be defined as the random chance that identical patients will experience different outcomes. Variability is reflected in the standard deviations associated with the mean value.

Heterogeneity relates to observed differences between patients which can, in part, be explained. For example, the hospital costs arising as a result of a myocardial infarction may differ between young and old patients because older patients typically spend longer in hospital. There will still be variability between patients within each of these subgroups in terms of whether or not they will experience a particular outcome over time. However, there is no uncertainty here as the baseline characteristics will be known with certainty. It has been argued that heterogeneity is not a source of uncertainty as it relates to differences that can in principle be explained (Briggs *et al.* 2006). Sculpher (2008) has pointed out that subgroup differences in cost-effectiveness can be a result of differing types of heterogeneity which could be related to the treatment, the underlying disease, unrelated to the disease, unrelated to the patient (e.g. costs and effects may vary systematically by hospital/clinician), or related to patient preference.

Structural uncertainty is something rather different, although it is also important. Structural uncertainty concerns the decisions and assumptions we make about the structure of the model, such as the inclusion of relevant states, the links between the states, the way the intervention and disease pathway are modelled, and so on. These decisions and assumptions are taken under conditions of uncertainty, which have been grouped into four general themes: inclusion of relevant comparators, inclusion of relevant events, alternative statistical estimation methods, and clinical uncertainty (Bojke *et al.* 2009).

Parameter uncertainty relates to the precision in the parameter (input) estimates for the model: for example, transition and event probabilities, costs, utilities, and treatment effects. The uncertainty around the mean estimates of these parameter estimates needs to be reflected in the cost-effectiveness results. In the past this has sometimes been referred to as second-order uncertainty.

10.2 Dealing with uncertainty, heterogeneity, and variability

Table 10.1 outlines how the analyst can deal with variability, heterogeneity, and different forms of uncertainty in model-based analyses. Koerkamp *et al.* (2010) have used an example of modelling the cost-effectiveness of imaging tests for patients with chest pain to highlight the practicalities involved in these methods.

10.2.1 Dealing with variability

Variability within decision models, especially cohort models, is largely a by-product of the modelling process rather than an attempt to capture a real-world phenomenon, and so the analytical concern is to take steps to eliminate variability from the results. For example, Figure 10.1 depicts the state transitions of a single person until death in

Table 10.1 Dealing with uncertainty, heterogeneity, and variability

Type	Analytical method
Variability	Reflected in standard deviations, microsimulation
Heterogeneity	Subgroup analysis
Structural uncertainty	One-way sensitivity analysis/scenario analysis, model averaging, parameterization, model discrepancy
Parameter uncertainty	Probabilistic sensitivity analysis

Data from Briggs (2001).

a Monte Carlo microsimulation. Monte Carlo microsimulation determines the pathways of a large number of individual patients with identical initial characteristics. Patients traverse the model one by one, and at each transition phase the next state is determined by the transition matrix and the output of a random number generator. This is the Monte Carlo part of the process, in which the parameter value is compared with the random number to determine if the event/transition is deemed to have occurred in that model run.

Therefore the path followed by individual patients with the same initial characteristics will differ because of random variation. In Figure 10.1, the patient spends three cycles in the well state, followed by two cycles in the recurrence state before moving to the dead state in cycle 6. However, because this pathway has been determined partly on the basis of random numbers, an identical patient going through the model a second time would not necessarily follow the same path; he/she might stay in the well state until cycle 6, or transition to the recurrence state in cycle 2 and die in cycle 3.

After a large number of iterations the central tendency or expected value of survival and costs can be observed, and this will be the primary interest of the analyst. Indeed, a rule of thumb would be that a sufficient number of simulations should be performed to reach a stable estimate of these mean values (Briggs 2000). The different pathways are not in themselves informative; they are simply the means by which a distribution of cost and outcome values can be built up and the central tendency identified. However, there may be interest in knowing more about the distribution of pathways

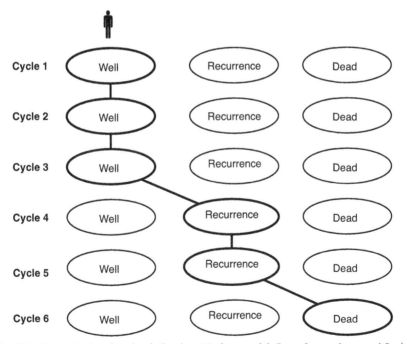

Fig. 10.1 Monte Carlo microsimulation in a Markov model. From Sonnenberg and Beck (1993). Reprinted by permission of SAGE Publications.

through a microsimulation model, and in TreeAge Pro it is possible to use tracker variables to record information about an individual's history through the model.

10.2.2 Dealing with heterogeneity

A decision model provides a flexible framework to deal with assumptions about heterogeneity. Heterogeneity can be due to either variations between subgroups in baseline characteristics, such as age, sex, social class, disease severity, or subgroup variability in both baseline characteristics and relative treatment effects. A model can be rerun for different subgroups, or an overall measure of cost-effectiveness across an entire population can be estimated along with a summary of the variability due to patient heterogeneity. In models, heterogeneity can be incorporated by making model parameters functions of other parameters: for example, basic transition probabilities might be a function of age or disease severity. The approach adopted by Mihaylova et al. 2005, 2006), when considering the cost-effectiveness of 40 mg simvastatin daily continued for life in people of different ages with differing risks of vascular disease, was to estimate the relative effect of treatment on the risk of major vascular events and then apply the relative risk reduction to the absolute baseline risk levels in different groups. This method avoided the danger of spurious differences in treatment effects in subgroups due to the play of chance. Bayesian methods can also be used for simultaneous investigation of patient heterogeneity and parameter uncertainty (Spiegelhalter and Best 2003).

10.2.3 Dealing with structural uncertainty

Structural uncertainty is an under-researched area of uncertainty, but may contribute to even greater uncertainty than parameter uncertainty. Bojke et al. (2009) conducted a review of recent Health Technology Assessment reports to identify current approaches used to characterize structural uncertainty in decision analytic models, with a focus on analytical rather than qualitative methods. They found that the most common method used was simply to produce alternative scenarios, each based on a specification representing alternative assumptions and judgements about the structure of the model. They then conducted a second literature review from which they identified and applied two methods that could be used to characterize structural uncertainty. The first was model (or scenario) averaging, where the set of plausible models is weighted by some measure of model adequacy. The second was parameterization of other sources of uncertainty, where the source of structural uncertainty is represented directly in the analysis by including additional uncertain parameters in the model, this being analogous to model averaging but on individual model inputs or sets of inputs.

Strong et al. (2009), as well as identifying model averaging as an approach for dealing with structural uncertainty, suggested a 'model discrepancy' approach (as described by Kennedy and O'Hagan 2001), in which the focus is on quantifying judgements about the difference between the model output and the 'true' value of the target that is being modelled, i.e. reality. They argue that both approaches run into problems when used alongside health economic decision models and propose a development of the discrepancy modelling approach whereby a model is first decomposed into a series of sub-units, revealing a set of intermediate parameters that may make it easier to quantify the discrepancy between the modelled value and reality (compared with doing this for the final model output) (Strong *et al.* 2009).

An economic evaluation conducted to assess the cost-effectiveness of routine vaccination of 12-year-old UK schoolgirls against human papillomavirus infection used a hybrid of the model-averaging method to account for structural uncertainty. A 'large' number (2700 possible scenarios for high-risk papillomavirus types and 900 scenarios for low-risk types) of possible model structures were parameterized to match epidemiological data. The approach involved an exhaustive search for possible structures, then fitting available data to the models, followed by sampling from the distribution of economic parameters (Choi *et al.* 2009; Jit *et al.* 2008, 2010).

10.2.4 Dealing with parameter uncertainty

In order that results from decision analytic models be used by policy-makers it is necessary to reflect how the inherent uncertainty in parameter estimates impacts on the final results and to be able to convey this in a meaningful way. Until fairly recently this was undertaken by performing a simple sensitivity analysis (one-way and multi-way) but, because of limitations with that method, probabilistic sensitivity analysis has now become the standard. The focus of the remainder of this chapter is on how to deal with parameter uncertainty.

10.3 Sensitivity analysis

Sensitivity analysis involves varying parameter estimates across a range and seeing how this impacts on the model's results. Briggs and colleagues have described the various methods of sensitivity analysis available to the analyst (Briggs *et al.* 1994; Briggs 1999; Briggs and Gray 1999a,b). The simplest form is a one-way analysis where each parameter estimate is varied independently and singly to observe the impact on the model results. The range over which each parameter is varied can be from highest to lowest if a range of estimates is available, or 95% confidence limits if reported, or simply a 'plausible' range which could be arbitrary (e.g. 20% more and less than the baseline value). One-way sensitivity analysis can give some insight into the factors influencing the results, and may provide a validity check to assess what happens when particular variables take extreme values. However, it is likely to grossly underestimate overall uncertainty, and ignores correlation between parameters.

The more refined approach of multi-way sensitivity analysis can also be used, where more than one parameter estimate is varied. This is sometimes described as a scenario analysis: for example, setting all main parameters simultaneously at their highest or lowest bounds will give estimates for optimistic or pessimistic scenarios. However, deciding which mix of parameters to vary in combination, and how they should relate to each other, can become a complicated matter of design. Also, because uncertainty propagates itself throughout all the parameters in the model, one-way and multi-way sensitivity analyses need to be conducted on a sequential basis. Other forms of sensitivity analysis include threshold analysis, where the critical value of parameter(s) above or below which the conclusion of a study will change is identified.

These deterministic approaches to representing uncertainty have been criticized as being partial (Briggs *et al.* 2002). They fail to take account of the joint parameter uncertainty and correlation between parameters, and rather than providing the decision-maker with a useful indication of the likelihood of a result, they simply provide a range of results associated with varying one or more input estimates. They are also dependent on the arbitrary choices of the analyst. However, they can be useful when used alongside probabilistic sensitivity analysis, discussed in the next section, by helping to identify which model parameters are critical in driving a decision (Andronis *et al.* 2009).

10.4 **Probabilistic sensitivity analysis**

Probabilistic sensitivity analysis (PSA) started to be used in health economic decision analyses in the mid 1980s (Doubilet *et al.* 1983; Critchfield and Willard 1986; Critchfield *et al.* 1986). Since then it has increasingly been used to explore the implications of parameter uncertainty for the results of cost-effectiveness analyses, and has now become embedded as part of standard practice, either when conducting an economic evaluation with patient-specific data or when using a decision analytic model.

PSA permits the joint uncertainty across all the parameters in the model to be assessed at the same time. It involves sampling model parameter values from distributions imposed on variables in the model. A probability distribution identifies the probability of a variable value falling within a particular interval. These distributions should represent uncertainty around the mean estimate (i.e. standard error of the mean) and not the variation around it (i.e. standard deviation). The types of distribution imposed are dependent on the nature of the input parameters. In fact, decision analytic models for the purpose of economic evaluation tend to use homogenous types of input parameters, namely costs, life-years, QALYs, probabilities, and relative treatment effects, and consequently the number of distributions that are frequently used, such as the beta, gamma, and log-normal distributions, is relatively small. These are discussed in more detail in section 10.4.2 and in Briggs *et al.* (2006). Uncertainty is then propagated through the model by randomly selecting values from these distributions for each model parameter using Monte Carlo simulation (see section 10.4.3).

10.4.1 **Data sources for parameter estimation**

There are three basic sources of data for estimating parameters: primary data, secondary data, and expert opinion. Where primary data on the parameter of interest are available, it may be possible to fit a distribution using standard statistical methods. This will often involve using parametric assumptions relating to the data that are available, as if the estimation of that parameter were the sole focus of the study. Where the analyst has patient-level data available, but does not wish to make parametric assumptions, the non-parametric bootstrapping approach can be employed.

However, it is often the case that analysts do not have primary data, but rather have obtained evidence on the likely value of the parameter of interest in the form of summary statistics drawn from reviews of the relevant literature. In such a situation, fitting the parameter is less straightforward. Nevertheless, a distributional form can be assumed based on that typically associated with that type of data.

In the absence of individual patient data, the analyst relies on the authors of primary data studies having reported appropriate summary statistics. Of course, secondary data sources may not be individual studies, but rather meta-analyses of a number of primary studies. In many ways this is the ideal source of data, as the synthesis of data on a particular analysis has already been performed. Where the analyst uncovers multiple primary studies on a particular parameter, it may be necessary for them to perform their own meta-analysis.

The lowest ranked source of data for estimating parameters is expert opinion. However, it is often necessary to include expert opinion when it becomes clear that no data sources are available for the particular parameter of interest for the model (O'Hagan *et al.* 2006; Leal *et al.* 2007).

10.4.2 Choosing distributions for parameters

A brief summary of the choice of distributions for parameters in decision models is given in this chapter. The reader is referred to the exercise in this chapter for a practical application, and to the companion to this handbook for a more detailed explanation with a practical guide to fitting the distributions (Briggs *et al.* 2006).

It is important that the choice of distribution reflects the nature of the data. For example, probability parameters such as transition probabilities can only take values between 0 and 1, and probabilities relating to mutually exclusive events must sum to 1. It is important that these rules are maintained even when random variation is introduced by fitting and sampling on the distributions. A beta distribution is a continuous probability distribution defined on the interval [0,1] and can be used to reflect the probability of two mutually exclusive events. If more than two events occur, a Dirichlet distribution can be used (Briggs *et al.* 2003).

Distributions used to reflect the uncertainty in costs are the gamma distribution, which is constrained on the interval $[0,+\infty]$, or the log-normal distribution. Both have the ability to reflect the skew often present in cost data.

Distributions which reflect the uncertainty in utilities must match the slightly unusual range, with the value of 1 at the upper end reflecting the best possible health state, zero reflecting death, and a negative number (which could be bounded or unbounded depending on the instrument) at the lower end reflecting the worst possible health state. If the utilities in the model are likely to be far from zero and positive, a pragmatic approach is to use the beta distribution. When states are close to or worse than death, it may be best to use a transformation to utility decrements or disutilities, where these are constrained on the interval $[0,+\infty]$ using a gamma distribution. Finally, treatment effects in models tend to be incorporated using relative risks. The uncertainty in this parameter distribution can be dealt with using the log-normal distribution as this reflects the ratio nature of a relative risk.

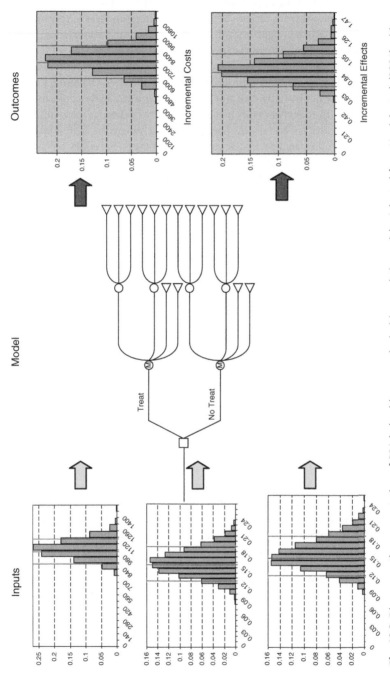

Fig. 10.2 Diagrammatic representation of PSA in health economic decision analytic models. Adapted from Hunink *et al.* (2001) with permission.

10.4.3 **Incorporating parameter uncertainty in the model**

Uncertainty is propagated through the model by randomly selecting values from the chosen distributions for each model parameter using Monte Carlo simulation. The model is then run repeatedly for each combination of parameter estimates, and the resulting cost and effect pairs are recorded. At the end of the Monte Carlo simulations, the cost and effect pairs are used to estimate the 95% confidence range around the results, as discussed in Chapter 11. Figure 10.2 presents a diagrammatic representation of this process. The uncertainty of the parameter inputs are modelled with their corresponding distributions; for each run of the Monte Carlo simulation a random value from each input parameter is picked from its distribution. Each iteration will result in one set of outcomes in terms of incremental costs and effects. By repeating this process a large number of times the outcomes will be represented by a distribution of the incremental costs and effects. A commonly used number of iterations is 1000, but this could be more or less depending on the degree of uncertainty in the model and the computational requirements.

Where correlation between parameters exists, joint distributions should be used and independence should not be assumed. A more detailed explanation of the process of drawing values from the distributions and correlating parameters can be found elsewhere (Briggs *et al.* 2006) and a practical example using two different software platforms (TreeAge Pro and Excel) is given at the end of this chapter. More recently, Bayesian Monte Carlo synthesis methods have been advocated as they permit more data to be incorporated into the model and therefore increase parameter precision (Ades *et al.* 2006). This approach is linked to the discussion on comprehensive decision analytic models in Chapter 8.

It is also possible to undertake PSA alongside patient simulation models, although structuring the model as a microsimulation and using PSA will inflate the analysis times considerably (Griffin *et al.* 2006; Barton *et al.* 2008;). PSA can also be combined with dynamic models (Brisson and Edmunds 2006; Duintjer Tebbens *et al.* 2008; Jit *et al.* 2008, 2009).

10.4.4 **Presenting the results from a PSA**

Once a PSA has been undertaken, the results can be presented in terms of incremental cost-effectiveness ratios (ICERs) with confidence intervals, or as incremental net benefits using a cost-effectiveness acceptability curve complemented by the scatter plot of the simulations of the cost-effect pairs on the cost-effectiveness plane. More details on how cost-effectiveness results should be presented and reported are given in Chapter 11.

10.5 **Summary**

A brief overview of the theory, methods, and techniques that can be used by analysts to represent uncertainty in their cost-effectiveness models has been presented in this chapter. The terminology and methods for dealing with variability, heterogeneity, and uncertainty have been outlined, and details on the theory and practice of incorporating probabilistic sensitivity analysis into models have been described. The exercise related to this chapter provides a detailed practical example of how to incorporate PSA in a Markov model. More comprehensive reviews of the theory and practical examples of handling uncertainty alongside model development can be found in a companion to this handbook (Briggs *et al.* 2006).

References

Ades, A.E., Claxton, K., and Sculpher, M. (2006). Evidence synthesis, parameter correlation and probabilistic sensitivity analysis. *Health Economics*, **15**, 373–81.

Andronis, L., Barton, P., and Bryan, S. (2009). Sensitivity analysis in economic evaluation: an audit of NICE current practice and a review of its use and value in decision-making. *Health Technology Assessment*, **13**, iii, ix–xi, 1–61.

Barton, P.M., Moayyedi, P., Talley, N.J., Vakil, N.B., and Delaney, B.C. (2008). A second-order simulation model of the cost-effectiveness of managing dyspepsia in the United States. *Medical Decision Making*, **28**, 44–55.

Bojke, L., Claxton, K., Sculpher, M., and Palmer, S. (2009). Characterizing structural uncertainty in decision analytic models: a review and application of methods. *Value in Health*, **12**, 739–749.

Briggs, A. (1999). Economics notes: handling uncertainty in economic evaluation. *British Medical Journal*, **319**, 120.

Briggs, A.H. (2000). Handling uncertainty in cost-effectiveness models. *Pharmacoeconomics*, **17**, 479–500.

Briggs, A.H.(2001). Handling uncertainty in economic evaluation. In: Drummond, M. and McGuire, A. (eds). *Economic Evaluation in Health Care: Merging Theory with Practice*. Oxford University Press.

Briggs, A.H. and Gray, A.M. (1999a). Handling uncertainty in economic evaluations of healthcare interventions. *British Medical Journal*, **319**, 635–8.

Briggs, A.H. and Gray, A.M. (1999b). Handling uncertainty when performing economic evaluation of healthcare interventions. *Health Technology Assessment*, **3**, 1–134.

Briggs, A., Sculpher, M., and Buxton, M. (1994). Uncertainty in the economic evaluation of health care technologies: the role of sensitivity analysis. *Health Economics*, **3**, 95–104.

Briggs, A.H., Goeree, R., Blackhouse, G., and O'Brien, B.J. (2002). Probabilistic analysis of cost-effectiveness models: choosing between treatment strategies for gastroesophageal reflux disease. *Medical Decision-Making*, **22**, 290–308.

Briggs, A.H., Ades, A.E., and Price, M.J. (2003). Probabilistic sensitivity analysis for decision trees with multiple branches: use of the Dirichlet distribution in a Bayesian framework. *Medical Decision Making*, **23**, 341–50.

Briggs, A.H., Sculpher, M., and Claxton, K. (2006) *Decision Modelling for Health Economic Evaluation*. Oxford University Press.

Brisson, M. and Edmunds, W.J. (2006). Impact of model, methodological, and parameter uncertainty in the economic analysis of vaccination programs. *Medical Decision Making*, **26**, 434–46.

Choi, Y.H., Jit, M., Cox, A., Garnett, G.P., and Edmunds, W.J. (2009). Transmission dynamic modelling of the impact of human papillomavirus vaccination in the United Kingdom, *Vaccine*, **28**, 4091–4102.

Critchfield, G.C. and Willard, K.E. (1986). Probabilistic analysis of decision trees using Monte Carlo simulation. *Medical Decision Making*, **6**, 85–92.

Critchfield, G.C., Willard, K.E., and Connelly, D.P. (1986). Probabilistic sensitivity analysis methods for general decision models. *Computers and Biomedical Research*, **19**, 254–65.

Doubilet, P., McNeil, B.J., and Weinstein, M.C. (1983). Optimal strategies for the diagnosis and treatment of coronary artery disease: analysis using a microcomputer. *Medical Decision Making*, **3**, 23–28.

Duintjer Tebbens, R.J., Thompson, K.M., Hunink, M.G., *et al.* (2008). Uncertainty and sensitivity analyses of a dynamic economic evaluation model for vaccination programs. *Medical Decision Making*, **28**, 182–200.

Gold, M.R., Siegel, J.E., Russel, L.B., and Weinstein, M.C. (1996). *Cost-effectiveness in Health and Medicine*. Oxford University Press, New York.

Griffin, S., Claxton, K., Hawkins, N., and Sculpher, M. (2006). Probabilistic analysis and computationally expensive models: necessary and required? *Value in Health*, **9**, 244–52.

Hunink, M.G., Glasziou, P.P., Siegel, J.E., *et al.* (2001). *Decision Making in Health and Medicine. Integrating Evidence and Value*. Cambridge University Press.

Jit, M., Choi, Y.H., and Edmunds, W.J. (2008). Economic evaluation of human papillomavirus vaccination in the United Kingdom. *British Medical Journal*, **337**, a769.

Jit, M., Gay, N., Soldan, K., Choi, Y.H., and Edmunds, W.J. (2010). Estimating progression rates for human papillomavirus infection from epidemiological data. *Medical Decision Making*, **30**, 84–98.

Kennedy, M.C. and O'Hagan, A. (2001). Bayesian calibration of computer models. *Journal of the Royal Statistical Society. Series B, Statistical Methodology*, **63**, 425–64.

Koerkamp, B.G., Weinstein, M.C., Stijnen, T., Heijenbrok-Kal, M.H., and Hunink, M.G. (2010). Uncertainty and patient heterogeneity in medical decision models. *Medical Decision Making*, **30**, 194–205.

Leal, J., Wordsworth, S., Legood, R., and Blair, E. (2007). Eliciting expert opinion for economic models: an applied example. *Value in Health*, **10**, 195–203.

Mihaylova, B., Briggs, A., Armitage, J., Parish, S., Gray, A., and Collins, R. (2005). Cost-effectiveness of simvastatin in people at different levels of vascular disease risk: economic analysis of a randomised trial in 20,536 individuals. *Lancet*, **365**, 1779–85.

Mihaylova, B., Briggs, A., Armitage, J., Parish, S., Gray, A., and Collins, R. (2006). Lifetime cost effectiveness of simvastatin in a range of risk groups and age groups derived from a randomised trial of 20,536 people. *British Medical Journal*, **333**, 1145.

O'Hagan, A., Buck, C.E., Daneshkhah, A., *et al.* (2006). *Uncertain Judgements: Eliciting Experts' Probabilities*. John Wiley, Chichester.

Sculpher, M. (2008). Subgroups and heterogeneity in cost-effectiveness analysis. *Pharmacoeconomics*, **26**, 799–806.

Sonnenberg, F.A. and Beck, J.R. (1993). Markov models in medical decision making: a practical guide. *Medical Decision Making*, **13**, 322–38.

Spiegelhalter, D.J. and Best, N.G. (2003). Bayesian approaches to multiple sources of evidence and uncertainty in complex cost-effectiveness modelling. *Statistics in Medicine*, **22**, 3687–709.

Strong, M., Pilgrim, H., Oakley, J., and Chilcott, J. (2009). *Structural Uncertainty in Health Economic Decision Models*. ScHARR Occasional Paper, School of Health and Related Research, University of Sheffield.

Exercise

Using PSA to assess uncertainty

Overview

The purpose of this exercise is to build on the Markov model used in Chapter 9 and to familiarize yourself with the steps and techniques involved in undertaking probabilistic sensitivity analysis. Although this is a simple example, the process will get you to think about the processes involved in PSA, choosing distributions for the model parameters, setting up the parameters so that the appropriate data can be used for the PSA, fitting distributions to the parameters, and undertaking a probabilistic cost-effectiveness analysis. The exercise follows on from the exercise in Chapter 9 and uses the Markov model that was developed there. A step-by-step guide that will take you through the stages of undertaking a PSA in a Markov model, first using TreeAge Pro and then replicating this using Excel, is also provided. Fully worked solutions can be found at www.herc.ox.ac.uk/books/applied.

Exercise instructions

A   For the PSA use the data already set out in the Excel file *<Parameters for PSA>* which can be obtained at www.herc.ox.ac.uk/books/applied. Take some time to look at how the alpha and beta/lambdas were obtained for the distributions and look at the distribution check to ensure that we are making reasonable assumptions about the data. Table 10E.1 contains all the statistics you need to make the model probabilistic.

B   Once you have checked that you understand how the alpha and beta/lambdas were obtained for the distributions, and checked the distributions to ensure that reasonable assumptions about the data have been made, you now need to use this information to create distribution variables in TreeAge Pro using the Markov model developed in Chapter 9 (TreeAge file *<PSA Markov model>* at www.herc. ox.ac.uk/books/applied).

C   Use the distributions to parameterize the input variables in the model.

D   Undertake the PSA and present and report your results.

Step-by-step guide: TreeAge Pro

Preparing parameters for probabilistic parameter analysis

Follow the steps set out in A above to check that you understand how the alpha and beta/lambdas were obtained for the distributions, and check the distributions to ensure reasonable assumptions about the data have been made.

Table 10E.1 Statistics of model parameters

Parameter	Mean	Standard error	95% CI	Distribution
cAsymp	500	127.6		Gamma
cProg	3000	510.2		Gamma
cDrug	1000	102.0		Gamma
uAsymp	0.95	0.026		Beta
uProg	0.75	0.077		Beta
tpProg	0.01	0.003	0.005–0.015	Log-normal
tpDcm	0.15	0.026		Beta
Eff	0.5	0.051	0.4–0.6	Log-normal

Gamma distribution

Uncertainty surrounding the cost parameters is modelled using a gamma distribution which is constrained on the interval $[0,+\infty]$. We used the method of moments approach to estimate the hyperparameters of the gamma distribution (alpha and beta), where

$$\text{alpha} = (\text{mean}^2)/(\text{se}^2)$$
$$\text{beta} = (\text{se}^2)/(\text{mean})$$

and se is the standard error of the mean. The GAMMAINV(RAND(), alpha, beta) function in column D was used to generate a random draw from each distribution.

It should be noted that in TreeAge Pro 1/beta = lambda, so by way of example for the parameter cAsymp:

$$\text{alpha} = (500^2)/(127.6^2) = 15.37$$
$$\text{beta} = (127.6^2)/500 = 32.54$$
$$\text{lambda} = 1/32.54 = 0.030783.$$

Beta distribution

The state utilities and the transition probability 'tpDcm' are modelled using a beta distribution, which is constrained on the interval $[0,1]$. Again, you will use the method of moments approach to estimate the hyperparameters of the beta distribution (alpha and beta), where

$$(\text{alpha} + \text{beta}) = [\text{mean}*(1-\text{mean})/(\text{se}^2)] - 1$$
$$\text{alpha} = \text{mean}*(\text{alpha} + \text{beta})$$

and se is the standard error of the mean. We used the BETAINV(RAND(), alpha, beta) function in column D to generate a random draw from each distribution.

Log-normal distribution

The effectiveness of drug and the coefficient of increase 'tpProg' are modelled using a log-normal distribution, which assumes the parameters to be normally distributed in the log scale and is very useful for modelling uncertainty in ratios. Hence, log-transform (natural log) the mean and 95% CI of the effectiveness parameter to give −0.69 (−0.91 to −0.51) on the log scale, and calculate the SE on the log scale:

$$(-0.51 \text{ to } -0.91)/(1.96*2) = 0.10.$$

We generate a normally distributed random variable with mean −0.69 and SE 0.10 (NORMINV(RAND(), −0.69, 0.10)) and exponentiate the resulting variable. The same approach was used for the parameter 'tpProg'.

Create distribution variables

Open the TreeAge file <*PSA Markov model*> at www.herc.ox.ac.uk/books/applied to obtain the Markov model that you developed in Chapter 9. Now go to **Values>Distributions>New>** and choose a distribution that fits your data. (Hint: for beta distributions make sure that you check the 'real number parameters' box and use alphas and betas. For the log-normal distribution use ln (mean value) and SE of ln (mean value)). Type in the corresponding alpha/beta/lambda/ln mean, etc. Click **OK.** In the **Distribution Properties** window, name the distribution and describe it. (Hint: it is useful to use a name that can be linked to the parameter for which you are going to use that distribution, e.g. c_Death, c_Asymp, u_Prog, tp_Dcm, etc.) Note when using gamma distributions that you will need to convert the lambda value given in the Excel sheet to use it in TreeAge as 1/lambda (from Excel). This is because TreeAge uses a different formula for its distributions.

When you open **Values> Distributions**, a list of all the new distribution variables that you have just created will appear. If you click on one of them you will notice that a summary will be given below the box with their distribution and expected value. It is useful to check these expected values to ensure that they are in line with the original values used.

Parameterize the input variables in the model using distribution variables

We are now going to use these distributions in the model. Right click on the root node > **Define Variable**. Choose from your variables one that you want to parameterize, e.g. cAsymp, and in place of the value 500 >**insert distribution >choose appropriate distribution variable (c_Asymp) > Use > OK**. Repeat this process for all the parameters that you wish to have distributions around.

Undertake a probabilistic cost-effectiveness analysis

To undertake the PSA select **Analysis> Monte Carlo simulation > Sampling (Probabilistic analysis)**. You can either sample all or choose which distributions to sample and decide on the number of samples (expected value calculations) you want to undertake. Select **Begin**. Look at the different features: Stats Reports, Graphs>CE scatterplot/Acceptability curves, Excel charts, etc.

Replicating the model in Excel

The purpose of this exercise is to replicate the TreeAge Markov model in Excel.

Open the Excel file **PSA Exercise** at www.herc.ox.ac.uk/books/applied and click on 'Yes' to enable the macros. To check if you have macros enabled in Excel, click on the 'Start' button, then **Excel Options>Trust Centre>Trust Centre Settings>Macro Settings** and select **Enable all macros**. If your macro settings are usually set to a lower security level, please ensure that this setting is changed back after you have completed this exercise.

The first worksheet in the workbook, <**Diagram**>, has the structure of the Markov model that you will build. Unlike the TreeAge model, this Excel version is built across a number of worksheets with separate sheets for the parameters of the model <**Parameters**>, for each of the Markov model arms of the model <**No drug**>/<**Drug**>, for the final analysis results <**Analysis**>, and for the probabilistic analysis sheets <**PSA**>.

The model structure consists of four states that characterize a chronic disease:

♦ asymptomatic disease (a patient has acquired the disease, but is not suffering any ill effects)

♦ progressive disease (a patient is showing symptoms of disease)

♦ dead from the disease

♦ dead from other causes.

The states are represented by the ovals and possible transitions between these states are shown by the arrows. State costs are shown in red and transition costs are shown in pink. Transition probabilities between states are shown in blue and the utilities of each state are shown in green. All the cells for you to complete in the exercise are coloured green. You are asked to:

A. prepare the parameters for probabilistic sensitivity analysis
B. estimate the cost-effectiveness (probabilistic).

Step-by-step guide: Excel

Preparing parameters for probabilistic sensitivity analysis

Open <**Parameters**> worksheet at www.herc.ox.ac.uk/books/applied and enter the value 1 in cell D5. You will see that most 'live value' cells now become blank. The model parameters of initial age, discount rates, and death from other causes were left deterministic. Table 10E.2 has all the statistics you need to make the model probabilistic and you will find them set out for you in the worksheet.

A.1 Uncertainty surrounding the cost parameters is modelled using a gamma distribution which is constrained on the interval $[0,+\infty]$. You should use the method of moments approach to estimate the hyper parameters of the gamma distribution (alpha and beta), where:

$$alpha = (mean^2)/(se^2)$$
$$beta = (se^2)/(mean)$$

and se is the standard error of the mean. Use the GAMMAINV(rand(), alpha, beta) function in column D to generate a random draw from each distribution. At this stage it may be useful to look up the function in the Excel help file.

Table 10E.2 Statistics of model parameters

Parameter	Mean	Standard error	95% CI	Distribution
cAsymp	500	127.6		Gamma
cProg	3000	510.2		Gamma
cDrug	1000	102.0		Gamma
cDeath	795	255.1		Gamma
uAsymp	0.95	0.026		Beta
uProg	0.75	0.077		Beta
tpProg	0.01	0.003	0.005-0.015	Log-normal
tpDcm	0.15	0.026		Beta
Eff	0.5	0.051	0.4-0.6	Log-normal

A.2 State utilities and the transition probability 'tpDcm' are modelled using a beta distribution, which is constrained on the interval [0,1]. Again, you should use the method of moments approach to estimate the hyperparameters of the beta distribution (alpha and beta), where:

$$\text{(alpha + beta)} = [\text{mean}^*(1\text{-mean})/(\text{se}^\wedge 2)] - 1$$
$$\text{alpha} = \text{mean}^*(\text{alpha + beta})$$

and se is the standard error of the mean. Use the BETAINV(rand(), alpha, beta) function in column D to generate a random draw from each distribution.

A.3 The effectiveness of drug, 'Eff', and the coefficient of increase 'tpProg' are modelled using a log-normal distribution, which assumes that the parameters are normally distributed in the log scale and is very useful for modelling uncertainty in ratios. Hence, log transform the mean and 95%CI of the effectiveness parameter to give –0.69 (–0.91 to –0.51) on the log scale. Calculate the SE on log scale: (-0.51 to -0.91)/(1.96*2) = 0.10. Enter the mean of logs in cell G33 and the standard error on log scale in cell H33. In cell D33, generate a normally distributed random variable with mean –0.69 and SE 0.10 (NORMINV(rand(), -0.69, 0.10)) and exponentiate the resulting variable.

Now, use the same approach to model uncertainty around the parameter 'tpProg'.

Estimating cost-effectiveness (probabilistic)

Open the <**PSA**> worksheet and take some time to look at the contents of the worksheet. The purpose of PSA is to model the uncertainty of the model parameters using probability distributions of their values. For each run of the model, a value of each parameter is taken at random from its probability distribution. Then costs and effects are estimated for each run using the randomly collected values of all parameter distributions. If we perform a large number of runs or trials (e.g. 1000), we obtain a distribution of costs and effects that represents the uncertainty in the results of the model conditional on the distributions of the parameter values and the structure and assumptions of the model.

B.1 Cells B3:J3 are labelled with the parameter names. The aim is to record the parameter values as well as the overall cost and effect results (cells B4:Q4) for each round of simulations. Now, link the cell under the parameter name with the relevant probabilistic parameter, using either the name of the parameter or the 'live value' in the <**Parameters**> worksheet. Link the cells under the cost and effect labels with the respective cells in the <**Analysis**> worksheet. Cells B4:Q4 should update to new parameters when the <F9> key is pressed if you have correctly entered 1 in cell D5. We have built a macro for you that should repeatedly copy cells B4:Q4 into the 1000 rows below. This will enable you to estimate the mean costs and effects of the 1000 probabilistic trials for each arm of the model (see cells L1007:Q1007) and the respective ICERs.

B.2 Open <**Analysis**> and click on the **Run probabilistic sensitivity analysis** button to perform the 1000 simulations. Once the simulations are finished, link cells K9:L10 in the <**Analysis**> worksheet with cells L1007:Q1007 in the <**PSA**> worksheet.

B.3 Estimate the ICERs using both life-years and QALYs as the measure of health benefit.

B.4 Open <**CEA curve**> to see the cost-effectiveness acceptability curve.

Chapter 11

Presenting cost-effectiveness results

This chapter reviews and demonstrates appropriate ways of presenting cost-effectiveness results, with particular reference to stochastic results from clinical trials in which data on effects and resource use have been collected for each patient. It begins with a brief discussion of the different types of uncertainty that can arise in economic evaluation, followed by a discussion of the methods that can be employed to handle the different forms of uncertainty: either statistical analysis or sensitivity analysis. The main methods of estimating confidence intervals for incremental cost-effectiveness ratios and the use of cost-effectiveness acceptability curves to summarize uncertainty are described. The net-benefit framework is also set out, and its advantages and limitations discussed.

11.1 Types of uncertainty in stochastic analyses

Chapter 10 differentiated between variability, heterogeneity, and uncertainty in the context of model-based economic evaluation. In a stochastic analysis, such as an evaluation alongside a clinical trial collecting patient-level information on costs and outcomes, we need a slightly different typology, as shown in Table 11.1.

Instead of variability arising from the modelling process, a stochastic analysis will typically confront uncertainty due to sampling variation, and standard methods of statistical analysis can be deployed to obtain estimates of mean costs and effects in two (or more) treatment arms and the variance around these means. However, as we shall see, these estimates have to be combined in some way to obtain an estimate of the incremental cost-effectiveness ratio, and particular statistical methods may be required to do this.

As even the longest clinical trials normally cease follow-up before all events of interest to economists have been observed, some form of extrapolation is likely to be required to link intermediate and final endpoints and allow for censored outcome and cost information (as we have seen in Chapters 4 and 7). Developing a model for this purpose will raise the issues of parameter uncertainty and structural or model uncertainty discussed in Chapter 10, but may also require statistical methods to estimate parameters from the patient-level data and assess goodness of fit.

As noted in Chapter 10, heterogeneity may be an issue, as particular groups which are different with respect to observed or unobserved characteristics, such as age, sex, prior disease history, or ethnicity, may differ systematically in their baseline risk, their treatment costs, or the benefit they receive from an intervention. In general it will not

Table 11.1 Uncertainty, heterogeneity, and variability in stochastic analyses

Type	Analytical method
Sampling variation	Statistical analysis
Extrapolation	Statistical analysis
	Sensitivity analysis
Heterogeneity	Statistical analysis
Methodological uncertainty	Reference case
	Sensitivity analysis

Data from Briggs and O'Brien (2001) with permission.

be appropriate to simply divide a population into different subgroups to calculate cost-effectiveness, as sample size will be reduced, the power to detect significant differences between groups will fall, and increasing the number of statistical tests conducted will increase the risk of identifying apparently significant differences that have arisen purely as a result of the play of chance, or of failing to identify genuine differences because of lack of power.

Methodological uncertainty affects stochastic as well as modelling-based analyses, reflecting the absence of complete consensus among health economists over the most appropriate methods to use. This could encompass the choice of discount rate, the range of costs to include, or the methods employed to place valuations on health states. Typically these have been handled by means of sensitivity analyses or scenario analyses in which the discount rate or valuation method is varied to assess the effect on the results. However, a major step forward in dealing with such uncertainty is the use of a reference case or set of specified methods to which all analysts could adhere, supplemented if necessary by other analyses employing other methods and assumptions. The reference case approach was a key recommendation of the US Panel on cost-effectiveness (Gold *et al.* 1996) and has been embraced by NICE in its guidelines for economic evaluations conducted to inform their decision-making process (NICE 2008).

11.2 Mean cost and effect estimates

Let us begin by briefly outlining an example of an economic evaluation alongside a randomized clinical trial, and introduce some (hypothetical) data that will form the basis of the worked examples for this section. At this stage, we will make the assumption (which will be relaxed later in the chapter) that the point estimate of cost-effectiveness and the associated uncertainty are contained within the north-east quadrant of the cost-effectiveness plane.

In a clinical trial there are (usually) two groups: a treatment group and a control group. A randomization procedure for allocating patients to these two groups should ensure that they are independent, similar at baseline, and differ only with respect to the therapy to which they have been allocated. In an economic analysis alongside a trial, the opportunity exists to collect patient-level data for both effects and resource use.

Therefore we will have a two-item vector with a cost observation and effect observation for each patient in the trial, as shown in Figure 11.1.

Costs and effects will then be averaged across all patients in the control or the treatment group to obtain mean cost $\bar{C}$ and mean effect $\bar{E}$ for each arm of the trial. Within each group it is likely that costs and effects are correlated, as these come from the same patients. As the control and treatment groups are independent, there should be no covariance of costs or effects between the groups. Differences in mean costs and mean effects between the two groups can then be calculated, as can the standard errors around these differences and any correlation or covariance between **incremental** cost and **incremental** effect.

Table 11.2 gives the summary statistics for a dataset of this type from a trial containing 150 patients in each group. The mean cost and effect in each group are reported, along with standard deviations and standard errors. Mean differences in cost and effect are also reported, along with the standard errors for the difference in costs and the difference in effects. Recall the difference between the standard deviation, a measure of the variability or dispersion of the observations, and the standard error, a measure of uncertainty around the value of the parameter of interest, in this case the mean. This can be thought of as analogous to the distinction made in Chapter 10 between first-order uncertainty (chance or random variability) and second-order uncertainty (uncertainty or variation in the parameter value). Hence the differences between the

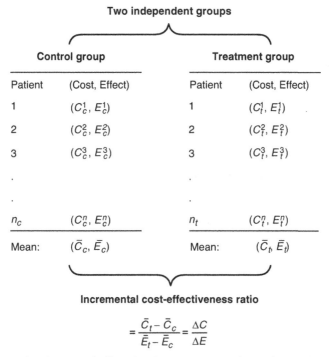

Fig. 11.1 Stochastic cost and effect data in a two-arm randomized controlled trial.

Table 11.2 Summary statistics for example dataset

	Control group (C) (n = 150)		Treatment group (T) (n = 150)		Difference (T – C)	
	Cost (£)	Effect (QALYs)	Cost (£)	Effect (QALYs)	Cost (£)	Effect (QALYs)
Mean	4000	7.50	5000	7.80	1000	0.3
Standard deviation	1763	0.78	2340	0.94	–	–
Standard error	144	0.06	191	0.08	239	0.10
Correlation	0		0		0	

means have no standard deviation since differences are calculated rather than observed.

It is possible to calculate a standard error for the differences in mean cost and mean effect, which will give some idea of how different these differences might be if another sample was drawn; in turn, the standard error will allow us to calculate confidence intervals. For costs, for example, the standard error of the difference $(se(\Delta\bar{C}))$ will be given by the square root of the standard deviation squared in costs in the control group (s_C^2) divided by sample size (n_C) plus the standard deviation squared in costs in the treatment group (s_T^2) divided by sample size (n_T):

$$se(\Delta\bar{C}) = \sqrt{\frac{s_C^2}{n_C} + \frac{s_T^2}{n_T}}$$

Using this formula, we can say that the point estimate for the incremental cost-effectiveness ratio of the comparison in Table 11.2 is given by $\Delta\bar{C}/\Delta\bar{E}$, which is £1000/0.3 QALYs, or £3333 per QALY gained. We can also say that the cost difference of £1000 has a 95% confidence interval from £531 to £1469, and the effect difference has a confidence interval from 0.11 to 0.5. What is required next is some method of estimating the uncertainty around the cost-effectiveness estimate, for example in the form of a confidence interval.

11.3 **Confidence limits for cost-effectiveness ratios**

11.3.1 **The confidence box**

One intuitively attractive way of addressing the uncertainty around the incremental cost-effectiveness ratio is to combine the upper and lower limits of the confidence intervals for the effect and cost difference (O'Brien *et al.* 1994). In Figure11.2 the information presented in Table 11.2 has been plotted on the cost-effectiveness plane. The mean difference in cost and effect between the control and treatment groups is shown by the white circle, and the 95% confidence intervals (approximated by the mean ± 1.96 × standard error) around the cost difference and the effect difference are shown by the I bars.

The shaded area shows a 'confidence box' defined by the upper and lower limits of the cost and effect differences. As Figure 11.2 shows, a lower confidence limit could then be estimated as the lower limit on the confidence interval for incremental costs divided by the upper limit on the confidence interval for incremental effects i.e. the most optimistic combination of costs and effects. This would give an ICER of £1068 per QALY gained, well below the mean estimate of £3333. Similarly, the upper confidence limit could be derived from the most pessimistic combination of costs and effects, i.e. by dividing the upper limit on the cost difference with the lower limit on the effect difference, giving an ICER of £13,652 per QALY gained.

This gives a first approximation to the degree of uncertainty around the mean ICER, but the results are not 95% confidence limits. The ICER is by definition a combination of a cost estimate and an effect estimate, so it is necessary to represent accurately the **joint uncertainty** surrounding costs and effects. The likelihood of both the incremental cost and the incremental effect lying inside the confidence interval defined by the box method will not be $(1 - 0.05)$, but $(1 - 0.05) \times (1 - 0.05)$ or approximately 90% (Briggs and Fenn 1998). Moreover, while we have assumed no covariance between cost and effect differences here, in practice the existence of positive or negative covariance would render the box method even less precise, and so it is not recommended.

11.3.2 **Confidence ellipses**

An alternative approach, set out by van Hout *et al.* (1994), is to approximate the 95% confidence interval of the ICER by calculating a surface in the shape of an ellipse on the cost-effectiveness plane that would cover 95% of the integrated probability, assuming that the cost and effect differences on the numerator and denominator of the ratio

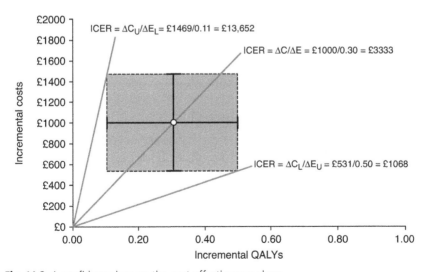

Fig. 11.2 A confidence box on the cost-effectiveness plane.

follow a joint normal distribution. Once this ellipse has been calculated, the upper and lower ICERs corresponding to the ellipse, i.e. the lines of tangency to the ellipse from the origin, can be used as an interval covering at least 95% of the probability distribution.

Figure 11.3 shows the 95% ellipse for the information in Table 11.2, with the confidence box and its intervals left on the figure to allow comparison. It is evident that the upper and lower tangents to the ellipse do not correspond to the upper and lower limits from the box method, illustrating the point made in section 11.3.1 that a box formed from the separately defined 95% confidence intervals of cost and effect will not precisely define the joint uncertainty surrounding costs and effects. As noted above, the difference would be greater if incremental costs and effects were correlated. This is shown in Figure 11.4, which is formed using the same estimates of the cost and effect difference, but assuming either negative or positive covariance.

The degree of correlation between costs and effects in these examples (−0.6 and +0.6, respectively) is far greater than might normally be encountered in a real dataset, but serves to illustrate clearly the importance of ensuring that correlations between costs and effects are adequately captured in whatever method is being used to represent uncertainty.

11.3.3 Parametric confidence interval estimation: Fieller's theorem

The ellipse approach has clear advantages over the confidence box method, and can be a useful way of graphically displaying the distribution of cost/effect differences, but it still only gives an approximate measure of uncertainty. Publications describing the ellipse approach revived interest in Fieller's theorem, a well-established exact parametric method for confidence interval estimation around ratios (Chaudhary and

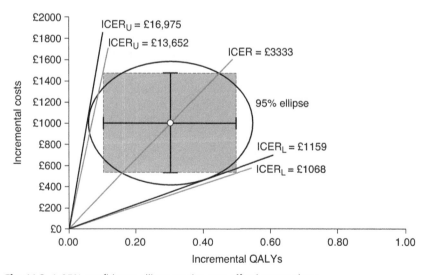

Fig. 11.3 A 95% confidence ellipse on the cost-effectiveness plane.

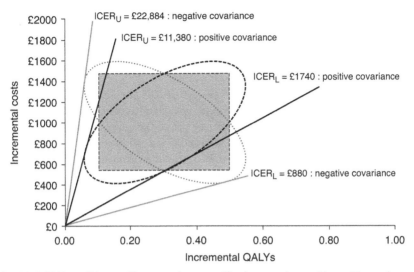

Fig. 11.4 95% confidence ellipses on the cost-effectiveness plane with positive and negative covariance between cost and effect differences.

Stearns 1996; Willan and O'Brien 1996). Fieller's theorem is based on the idea that while ratio statistics themselves do not necessarily follow a well-behaved distribution, it is often reasonable to assume that the numerator and denominator of the ratio follow a joint normal distribution.

The algebra of Fieller's theorem is reproduced in the Technical Appendix. Although the equation itself is quite complex, its component parts are easily estimated from sample information in the two groups of interest, and it is straightforward to calculate in a software package such as Microsoft Excel. As long as the assumption of joint normality holds, and the cost and effect differences are located in the north-east quadrant, Fieller's theorem will provide a precise confidence interval (Polsky *et al.* 1997a).

Using the dataset summarized in Table 11.2, Fieller's theorem gives confidence intervals of £1486 and £9813 around the ICER. A worked example showing how these are derived is given in the Technical Appendix.

11.3.4 **Bootstrapping**

Although Fieller's theorem has the attractions of being quick to use and giving precise estimates, it depends on the assumption of joint normality, and as we have already seen, particularly with reference to costs, this may not be the case. An initial response to this was to suggest the use of the non-parametric approach of bootstrapping. Typically, we draw one sample from a real-world population, calculate the statistic of interest (usually the mean) from that sample, and then infer how the value of that statistic might vary if the sampling procedure were to be repeated. In the bootstrap world, we treat the observed sample as a proxy for the population of interest and resample from it to estimate empirically the distribution around the statistic of interest.

The use of the bootstrap in relation to the analysis of costs has already been examined in Chapter 7. Although the bootstrap has been proposed as an alternative to standard parametric methods when the assumption of normality does not hold, or at least as a check on the robustness of standard parametric methods in the presence of skewness (Barber and Thompson 2000; Thompson and Barber 2000), it is not clear that bootstrap results in the presence of severe skewness are likely to be any more or less valid than parametric results. As O'Hagan and Stevens (2003) argued, when the variable of interest is skewed and sample size is relatively small, the sample mean is not an ideal estimator of the population mean; bootstrap and parametric methods both rely on sufficient sample sizes and are likely to be valid or invalid in similar circumstances.

Instead, interest in the bootstrap has increasingly focused on its usefulness in dealing simultaneously with issues such as censoring, missing data, multiple statistics of interest such as costs and effects, and non-normality. Use of the bootstrapping procedure with cost-effectiveness data has been well documented (Efron and Tibshirani 1993; Chaudhary and Stearns 1996; Willan and O'Brien 1996; Briggs *et al.* 1997, 1999; Obenchain *et al.* 1997; Polsky *et al.* 1997b; Severens *et al.* 1999) and involves the following steps, which follow the original sampling process:

1 A bootstrap resample of the control group is created by re-sampling with replacement cost–effect pairs from the original control group data (equivalent to selecting 'patients'). By sampling pairs of costs and effects for the same patient, we retain the covariance between cost and effect within the control group. The mean costs and effects for the control group resample are then calculated.

2 In an identical fashion, a bootstrap resample of the treatment group is created by re-sampling cost–effect pairs from the original treatment group data. The mean costs and effects for the treatment group resample are then calculated.

3 The bootstrap estimate of the difference in costs, difference in effects, and ICER are calculated based on the bootstrapped means of the costs and effects in each group.

4 The whole process is repeated until a large number of bootstrap ICERs have been recorded, thus building up an accurate estimate of the ICER sampling distribution. Note that increasing the number of bootstrap replications only improves the estimate of the sampling distribution and does not make the point estimate itself more precise.

Once a sufficient number of bootstrap ICERs (e.g. 1000) have been recorded, each cost and effect difference can be plotted on the cost-effectiveness plane to give a non-parametric estimate of the joint density of cost and effect differences. Moreover, if we rank-order the full set of ICER values we can then identify the 2.5% of ICERs at each end of the distribution to obtain an estimate of the confidence limits for the ICER, with 95% of the estimated joint density falling within these confidence limits.

Figure 11.5 shows the sample dataset again, now with 1000 cost–effect pairs plotted, each based on a bootstrap sample of 150 patients in each of the control and treatment groups. Note that the bootstrap confidence limits for this dataset (£1383 and £9878) are inside the intervals approximated by the box or the ellipse methods, but are very close to those reported above using Fieller's theorem (95% CI: £1,486, £9,813).

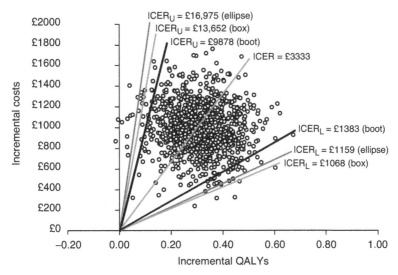

Fig. 11.5 Bootstrap replications on the cost-effectiveness plane with percentile confidence limits.

Another point of interest in Figure 11.5 is that several cost–effect pairs are very close to the vertical and so have very high cost-effectiveness ratios (in fact two points are to the left of the vertical in the north-west quadrant of the cost-effectiveness plane). These phenomena illustrate some other problems with the cost-effectiveness ratio: even when staying within the north-east quadrant, as the numerator (cost difference) becomes very small the ratio becomes very large, and as the denominator of the ratio (effect difference) tends towards zero the ICER tends to infinity. This raises a basic problem: the formula for the variance of a ratio statistic is intractable whenever there is a chance that the denominator of the ratio (i.e. the incremental effects) may equal zero To address these problems, we now need to relax the assumption made up until now, and move beyond the north-east quadrant.

11.4 **Moving out of the north-east quadrant**

So far we have assumed that treatment has significantly higher costs and significantly higher effects than its comparator, but this is just one of nine possible combinations of significant or non-significant cost and effect differences. These nine combinations are illustrated on the cost-effectiveness plane in Figure 11.6. For simplicity, boxes are used to indicate the area bounded by individual confidence limits on cost and effect; statistically significant differences in cost (or effects) occur where the box does not cross the x (or y) axis.

Situations 1 and 2 represent positions of dominance as discussed in Chapter 2: one intervention is significantly more effective and significantly cheaper than the other, and therefore is clearly the treatment of choice. Situations 7 and 8 are positions of clear trade-off, when one treatment is significantly more costly, but also significantly

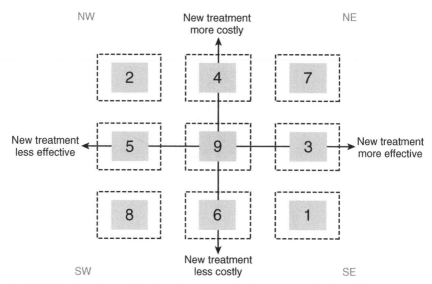

Fig. 11.6 Combinations of significant and non-significant cost and effect differences on the cost-effectiveness plane. Reproduced from Briggs and O'Brien (2001) with permission.

more effective, than the alternative. In these situations it will clearly be appropriate to estimate an ICER, as seen in section 11.2 above.

Where either the cost difference (situations 3 and 5) or the effect difference (situations 4 and 6) is not statistically significant, a number of problems arise. It is tempting in these circumstances to focus only on the dimension where a difference has been shown: for example, to report a cost-minimization analysis where there is no significant difference in effects but a significant cost difference exists. However, as discussed in Chapter 2, this is inappropriate; it is based on simple sequential tests of hypotheses concerning costs and effects separately when in fact we are interested in their joint distribution (Briggs and O'Brien 2001). This apparent non-difference may result in falsely interpreting absence of evidence of a difference as evidence of absence of a difference in circumstances where in fact there is insufficient power to be able to establish the existence of equivalence.

Finally in situation 9, no statistically significant difference is observed either in costs or effects.

In fact it is not difficult to devise situations (particularly when the point estimate of incremental cost and effect is in the dominant or south-east quadrant) in which the individual cost and effect differences are non-significant, but more than 97.5% of the cost–effect joint density is located on the cost-effective side of the ceiling ratio line. This reinforces a recurring theme: we are interested in the **joint** distribution of costs and effects and must be very careful about dismissing results on the basis of individual tests of significance. The primary objective of economic evaluation should not be hypothesis testing, but rather the estimation of the central parameter of interest—the incremental cost-effectiveness ratio—along with appropriate representation of the uncertainty surrounding that estimate.

However, while confidence intervals for cost-effectiveness ratios are a valid approach to addressing uncertainty in cost-effectiveness analysis in some of the situations set out in Figure 11.6 (e.g. boxes 7 and 8), problems will arise when the uncertainty is such that the ICER could be negative. For example, cost–effect pairs in the south-east quadrant will have negative ICERs because they are more effective and less costly than the alternative. However, cost–effect pairs in the north-west quadrant will also have negative ICERs for precisely the opposite reason—they are more costly and less effective than the alternative. Clearly, these are radically different situations, but could have identical ICERs.

The interpretation of the ICER also differs between the south-west and north-east quadrants. In the north-east quadrant, the ICER indicates the additional amount that we must pay to gain one unit of health gain, and treatments with ICERs *below* the ceiling ratio are considered cost-effective. By contrast, in the south-west quadrant, the ICER indicates the savings that we can gain for a one-unit loss of health; subsequently, treatments with high ICERs are preferable to those with lower ICERs (as we will save more money for the same loss of health) and only those treatments with ICERs *above* the ceiling ratio should be adopted. Subsequently, a treatment with an ICER of £5000/QALY may be considered cost-effective if it lay within the north-east quadrant, but not if it lay in the south-west quadrant.

Fortunately, these problems can be overcome either by adapting the way we interpret the ICER or by using the net-benefit framework, which does not suffer from the problems associated with the ICER in situations where negative ratios arise (Stinnett and Mullahy 1998). Before discussing these in detail, let us return to our example in Table 11.2, but make things more difficult for our analysis by assuming that treatment remains more expensive and more effective than the control, but not significantly so. Table 11.3 summarizes the new situation.

Figure 11.7 illustrates this new situation, showing clearly that we are now in the situation described by box 9 in Figure 11.6, with no significant differences in costs or effects and a chance that the true difference in costs and effects could lie in any of the four quadrants.

In this situation it is no longer possible to define confidence intervals based on either the confidence box or the ellipse. The origin of the figure lies within the box and

Table 11.3 Summary statistics for example dataset

	Control group (C) (n = 150)		Treatment group (T) (n = 150)		Difference (T – C)	
	Cost (£s)	Effect (QALYs)	Cost (£s)	Effect (QALYs)	Cost (£s)	Effect (QALYs)
Mean	4000	7.50	4250	7.65	250	0.15
Standard deviation	1763	0.78	1918	0.88	–	–
Standard error	144	0.06	157	0.07	213	0.10
Correlation	0		0		0	

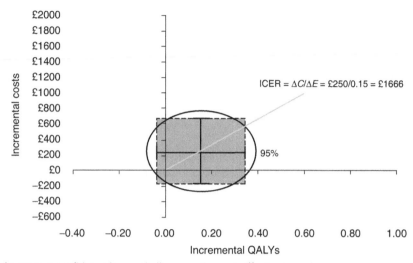

Fig. 11.7 A confidence box and ellipse on the cost-effectiveness plane.

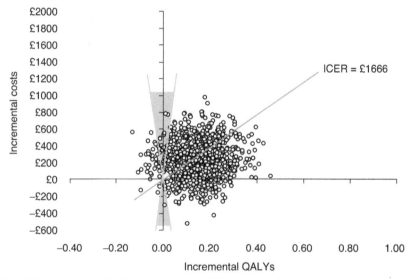

Fig. 11.8 Bootstrap replications on the cost-effectiveness plane with percentile confidence limits and with no significant differences in costs or effects.

ellipse and there can be no upper or lower lines of tangency. A possible alternative would be to use the bootstrap approach, adopting the percentile method to define the confidence intervals. Figure 11.8 shows the result. The confidence intervals have been defined by rank-ordering the 1000 bootstrapped ICERs as before, and then identifying the smallest 2.5% and the largest 2.5% of values, which fall in the 'bow-tie' or shaded triangles between the intervals.

However, this approach treats negative ratios in same way whether they are arising because costs are greater and effects are less (north-west quadrant) or because costs are less and effects are greater (south-east quadrant), despite the fact that these represent radically different situations from any decision-making perspective. Similarly, low positive cost-effectiveness ratios in the north-east quadrant are favourable to the new treatment, indicating that it gives large amounts of health gain for small added costs, but in the south-west quadrant the lower the positive cost-effectiveness ratio the less favourable it is to the new treatment, indicating that the denominator is becoming larger (the new treatment becoming less and less effective) and/or the numerator is becoming smaller (the new treatment is saving less and less) compared with the existing treatment. Therefore the ICERs are not helpful in differentiating between desirable and undesirable outcomes, and consequently the confidence intervals for the ICERs are not informative.

11.5 **The cost-effectiveness acceptability curve**

To find a solution to this problem, consider the line running through the origin in Figure 11.8 that identifies the point estimate of the cost and effect difference: the intervention costs £250 more, for an additional 0.15 QALYs, giving an ICER of £1666. Assuming a joint normal distribution, this line divides the bootstrap replicates into two equal halves: the 50% of bootstrap replications above the line are all less cost-effective than the point estimate, and the 50% below the line are all more cost-effective. In other words the bootstrap procedure has given us a reasonable approximation of the cost–effect joint density: we can simply count how many bootstrap replications fall on the cost-effective side of the line and divide by the total number of replications to obtain an estimate of the proportion of the joint density falling in the cost-effective half of the plane.

Pursuing this, if a decision-maker looking at these data had a maximum willingness to pay of £1666 per QALY gained, there would be a 50–50 chance that this new treatment was cost-effective (i.e. it was below this ceiling ratio). However, if the decision-maker was prepared to pay more than £1666 per QALY gained (let us say £10,000 per QALY gained), we could simply rotate the line through the origin that represents this ceiling ratio until it had a slope equivalent to £10,000 per QALY gained, and then recalculate how many of the bootstrap replicates are below this line and how many are above. The proportion of replicates lying below the line equals the probability that the intervention will be cost-effective, i.e. below the decision-maker's ceiling ratio.

At this point the reader may recall the discussion in Chapter 2, where we acknowledged that we do not always know the decision-maker's maximum willingness to pay for health gain. However, we know that it must lie somewhere between zero and positive infinity. If it was zero, the line representing the ceiling ratio would be horizontal and lie on the x-axis. At that point, as the decision-maker is not prepared to pay anything for health gains, the new treatment would be cost-effective only if it was less costly than its comparator, measured by the proportion of bootstrap replicates falling below the x-axis. However, if the decision-maker was prepared to pay positive infinity for health gains, the line representing the ceiling ratio would lie vertically along the y-axis. Now costs have become of no concern, and the probability of treatment being 'cost-effective' will be determined entirely by the probability that the new treatment is more effective than the existing treatment, i.e. the proportion of bootstrap replicates falling to the right of the y-axis. Figure 11.9 shows the result of exactly this procedure for the bootstrap data we have been considering.

The ceiling ratio R_c is set at zero on the x-axis and at infinity on the y-axis. When R_c is zero, 123 of the 1000 replications on the figure lie below the line, i.e. they are cost-saving. In other words there is a 12.3% probability that the new treatment will be cost-effective if the decision-maker's willingness to pay for health gain is zero. At the other extreme, when R_c is infinity and therefore lies along the x-axis, only 57 of the replications are to the left of the line and 943 are to the right, i.e. they are more effective. This indicates that there is a 94% probability that the new treatment is cost-effective when the decision-maker has an infinite willingness to pay for health gain.

From the information in Figure 11.9, it is a small additional step to plot a curve that traces the probability that this intervention is cost-effective as the ceiling ratio is rotated all the way round from $R_c = 0$ to $R_c = \infty$. Figure 11.10 shows this way of presenting information, first set out by van Hout *et al.* (1994) and described as a cost-effectiveness acceptability curve (CEAC). The CEAC shows the likelihood that the intervention will be acceptable to a decision-maker, whatever value is placed on the ceiling ratio. (Note that the figure shows two curves: the dashed line is based on the bootstrapping replications, and the smoothed line (which is virtually identical) is based on a parametric approach, which will be discussed in section 11.6.)

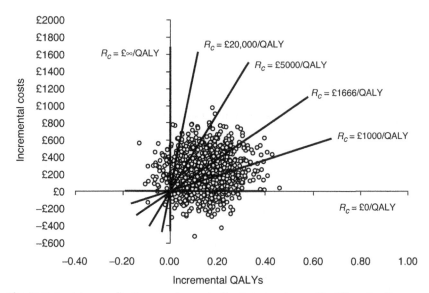

Fig. 11.9 Bootstrap replications on the cost-effectiveness plane with different ceiling ratios.

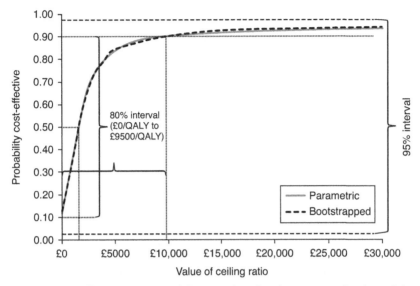

Fig. 11.10 Cost-effectiveness acceptability curve based on bootstrap replications of data in Table 11.3, and a parametric estimate of the same curve.

The x-axis gives the value of the ceiling ratio, and the y-axis gives the proportion of the estimated joint density which falls in the cost-effective half of the plane, i.e. the probability that the intervention is cost-effective. If we read across from the 50% point on the y-axis until we reach the curve and then trace down to the x-axis, we reach the point estimate of £1666 per QALY gained (as the incremental costs and effects are normally distributed in this example), exactly in line with Figures 11.8 and 11.9.

There are some other notable features of the acceptability curve. First, it cuts the y-axis at the one-sided P-value for the cost difference ($P = 0.12$) and asymptotes to 1 minus the one-sided P-value on the effect difference, in this case $P = 0.06$ or $P = 0.94$ on the y-axis. The figure also shows, as dotted horizontal lines, the 0.025 and 0.975 points on the vertical axis indicating the 95% confidence limits. If we trace these across the figure we find that they do not cut the curve at any point, indicating that in this particular instance the 95% confidence limits on the cost-effectiveness do not exist. However, it is possible to define an 80% interval on cost-effectiveness by tracing from the 0.1 and 0.9 points on the vertical axis across to the curve and down to the horizontal axis; in this instance, the curve is entirely above the 0.1 point, and at 0.9 cuts the curve at £9500, giving an 80% interval of approximately £0/QALY to £9500/QALY.

In summary, displaying uncertainty in cost-effectiveness by means of a cost-effectiveness acceptability curve provides several pieces of useful information. The curve can be used to find the point estimate of cost-effectiveness, the significance of the cost difference, the significance of the effect difference, or any level of confidence interval that we choose, without encountering any of the problems of negative ratios identified above. Finally, and perhaps most importantly, a decision-maker who knows their maximum willingness to pay for health gain can use the curve to find the strength of evidence in support of the intervention's being cost-effective.

11.6 **The net-benefit framework**

The cost-effectiveness acceptability curve offers one way of resolving many of the problems associated with the incremental cost-effectiveness ratio, particularly in representing uncertainty. Another approach, originally set out by Claxton and Posnett (1996) and subsequently developed by others (Stinnett and Mullahy 1998; Zethraeus *et al.* 2003), offers the advantages of the acceptability curve approach but can also facilitate statistical and economic analysis of patient-level data: the **net-benefit framework**.

The net-benefit framework is based on a simple but powerful insight into the fundamental cost-effectiveness decision rule: a decision-maker will consider an intervention worthwhile if its cost-effectiveness ratio is less than their maximum willingness to pay, represented here as λ: $\Delta C/\Delta E < \lambda$. The insight behind the net benefit approach is that by placing a value on λ it is straightforward to rearrange this into a linear expression:

$$\text{net monetary benefit (NMB)} = \Delta E \, \lambda - \Delta C.$$

For example, if ΔC was £8000, ΔE was 0.5 QALYs, and λ was £20,000, we could multiply the gain in health (0.5) by the maximum willingness to pay (£20,000) and subtract the incremental cost (£8000) to obtain the NMB. As long as the result was greater than zero, we could say that treatment was cost-effective. In this example, $0.5 \times 20,000 - 8000 = +2000$, indicating that there is indeed a positive NMB. However, if NMB is negative, it will not be cost- effective (i.e. the benefits of the intervention are outweighed by its costs).

Alternatively we could undertake a similar rearrangement, but in terms of the net health benefit (NHB):

$$\text{NHB} = \Delta E - \Delta C/\lambda.$$

Using the same simple example as above, we could take the gain in health (0.5) and then subtract from it the incremental cost (£8000) divided by the maximum willingness to pay (£20,000). Now, as long as the result was greater than zero, we could say that treatment was cost-effective and that there is a positive NHB. In this example, $0.5 - 8000/20,000 = 0.5 - 0.4 = 0.1$, indicating that there is indeed a positive NHB. Therefore, in general we can say that if NHB is positive it will be cost-effective, but if it is negative it will not be cost-effective.

There are a number of advantages to using the NMB or NHB. First, we do not need to worry about ambiguous interpretations of positive or negative ICERs: larger NHBs or NMBs are unambiguously better and smaller are unambiguously worse.

Secondly, by turning the decision rule into a linear expression, the sampling distribution of the net benefits will be much closer to a normal distribution than is the case for incremental cost-effectiveness ratios, which tend towards infinity when ΔE is very small. Therefore it becomes straightforward to calculate the variance for the NMB or NHB, which will be the sum of the variances of incremental costs and effects minus twice their covariance:

$$\text{var(NMB)} = \lambda^2 \, \text{var}(\Delta E) + \text{var}(\Delta C) - 2\lambda \, \text{cov}(\Delta E, \Delta C)$$

$$\text{var(NHB)} = \text{var}(\Delta E) + \text{var}(\Delta C)/\lambda^2 - 2/\lambda \, \text{cov}(\Delta E, \Delta C)$$

From here, it becomes straightforward to calculate a confidence interval for net benefits using standard methods and assuming a normal distribution.

Of course, the net monetary benefit or net health benefit statistic both rely on placing a value on the ceiling ratio λ when in practice this may be unknown or uncertain. However, this can be resolved in the same way as with acceptability curves, by plotting the net benefit as a function of different values of λ. Figure 11.11 shows such a graph obtained using the data from Table 11.3, but rearranged in terms of net monetary benefits. The solid line shows the central estimate of net monetary benefit on the y-axis as the decision-maker's willingness to pay (λ or R_c) varies along the x-axis from zero up to £30,000. The dashed lines in the figure show the upper and lower 80% confidence intervals around the central estimate.

As with the acceptability curve, there are a number of interesting and useful things to note in Figure 11.11. First, the net benefit curve crosses the x-axis at the point estimate of the cost-effectiveness of the intervention, in this case £1666 per QALY gained. The intuition behind this is that at the point where the decision-maker is prepared to spend £1666 for each QALY gained, the net monetary benefit of the intervention will be zero because £1666 is precisely how much each QALY costs with this intervention. When the value of λ is less than £1666, the net monetary benefit will be negative, as the amount that the decision-maker is willing to pay for each QALY is less than the cost of obtaining it. At a willingness to pay of zero, the net monetary benefit will be –£250, which is simply the difference in cost between the treatment and the intervention; the treatment costs £250 more and the decision-maker is placing no value on the health benefits, so this is a straightforward loss. Notice that the 80% confidence limits cut the

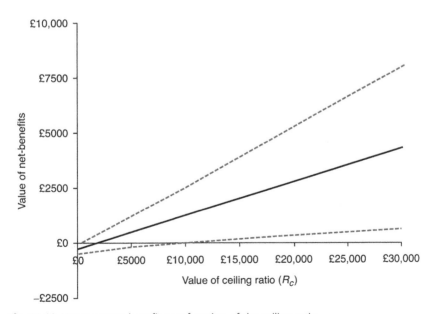

Fig. 11.11 Net monetary benefit as a function of the ceiling ratio.

x-axis at approximately the same points as those calculated using bootstrapping in the previous section: £0 to £9500/QALY.

We can also use the net benefit approach to calculate an acceptability curve. Using only summary information from Table 11.3 on mean difference in effect and cost, variance and covariance, the probability that the intervention is cost-effective can be calculated parametrically for each value of λ and then plotted. The resulting acceptability curve is shown by the solid line in Figure 11.10, and it is clear that the result is almost identical to the curve derived from the bootstrap replications. It would be worrying if this was not the case, as we are deploying the same decision rule in both approaches and our data are normally distributed. The net benefit approach also simplifies estimation of the CEAC from bootstrapping in situations where some bootstrap replicates lie in different quadrants from the point estimate. Rather than having to consider the interpretation of the CEAC in each quadrant, we can simply calculate the net benefit for each bootstrap replicate and calculate the proportion of replicates with positive net benefits.

The net benefit approach also has advantages when dealing with patient-level data. With cost-effectiveness ratios, we must always be careful to observe that the average of two ratios is not the same as the ratio of two averages: the average of the ratios £4000/2QALYs and £6000/1QALY is

$$(2000 + 6000)/2 = £4000$$

but the ratio of the averages is

$$(4000 + 6000)/(2 + 1) = 10,000/3 = £3333.$$

ICERs must always be based on the ratio of mean incremental costs over mean incremental effects, and never the average of ICERs across bootstrap replicates or probabilistic simulations (Stinnett and Mullahy 1998). However, this difficulty disappears with the net benefit approach; the difference between two average net benefits is equal to the incremental net benefit. This makes it easier to find the most cost-effective option when there are multiple treatment comparisons, as we only need to calculate the average net benefit for each option and choose the one with the greatest average net benefit. It also avoids the issues of extended dominance discussed in Chapter 2. Again, it is simply a case of identifying the option with the greatest average net benefits, which will automatically correspond to the treatment that lies on the frontier which generates the most health and can be afforded within the health-care budget.

11.7 **Heterogeneity**

The statistically well-behaved properties of the net benefit statistic also make it tempting to employ it directly in patient-level analyses, such as multiple regression, and to use it to deal with other stochastic issues, for example heterogeneity in the population of interest. Cost-effectiveness could be analysed within a regression framework by formulating a net-benefit value for each patient from the observed effects and costs for each patient, and then constructing a regression model with a treatment variable and covariates such as age, sex, and disease severity. The magnitude and significance of the coefficients on the interaction between the covariates and the treatment variable might then provide an estimate of cost-effectiveness by subgroup. The net-benefit framework also permits the use of standard methods for model selection and diagnostic statistics.

However, despite these potential advantages, a number of limitations and problems should be noted. First, covariates could impact costs and effects differently, and such a differential impact could not easily be dealt with in a net-benefit regression framework; in fact combining cost and effect data into a single statistic could reduce explanatory power in these circumstances. Secondly, and related to the previous point, the regression model cannot necessarily be assumed to be the same across different values of willingness to pay. As willingness to pay falls towards zero, so cost differences and hence variables which are related to these differences become more important. Conversely, as willingness to pay increases, effect differences and the variables that affect these become more important (for a discussion of this see Hoch *et al.* 2002). Thirdly, dealing with subgroups by means of indicator variables or covariates does not resolve the inherent limitations of subgroup analysis (Hoch *et al.* 2002).

Therefore other methods may be required to deal with patient heterogeneity. One example, based on analysis of patient-level data in a within-trial analysis of the Heart Protection Study, started by establishing that the relative effect of treatment (40 mg simvastatin daily for 5 years compared with placebo) on the risk of major vascular events was similar in every subcategory of participant studied (Mihaylova *et al.* 2005). This permitted a precise estimate of the relative treatment effect to be made, drawing on the statistical power of all trial participants. As the trial participants were heterogeneous with respect to their absolute risk of major vascular events at entry to the study, it was possible to apply the overall relative treatment effect to different groups stratified by risk to derive estimates of absolute effect. Likewise, a similar proportional reduction in hospitalization costs for vascular events across the entire study resulted in different absolute reductions in vascular event costs per person allocated to 40 mg simvastatin daily. As a result, the study was able to demonstrate that cost-effectiveness varied substantially between different groups of patients, while avoiding the danger of spurious differences in treatment effects in subgroups due to the play of chance. Table 11.4 shows some results from this analysis.

The 5-year risk of a major vascular event is seen to vary from 12% in the lowest risk group quintile to 42% in the highest risk group quintile. This results in a strong gradient across risk groups in the absolute number of major vascular events and vascular deaths avoided, and similarly large differences in the absolute cost of these events. In consequence, the overall trial estimate of cost per vascular death avoided of £66,000 is not particularly informative, as this ranged from £21,400 in the highest risk group to £296,300 in the lowest risk group. An advantage of the analytical method adopted—applying overall trial estimates of relative effect to the absolute risk in each subgroup—is that the confidence intervals around the reported cost-effectiveness ratios (which were derived from bootstrapping) are substantially narrower than if estimates had been derived from results only within each subgroup. For example, the discounted cost per major vascular event avoided for the lowest risk quintile was estimated from the overall results to be £31,100 with a 95% CI of £22,900–42,500, whereas an estimate

Table 11.4 Discounted incremental costs, effects, and cost-effectiveness during a 5-year mean follow-up of Heart Protection Study patients by risk group and overall

Risk group (5-year MVE risk)	Incremental cost (SE) (£)*	MVE avoided per 1000 persons (SE)	Cost per MVE avoided (95% CI) (£)	Vascular deaths avoided per 1000 persons (SE)	Cost per vascular death avoided (95% CI) (£)
1 (12%)	1164 (45)	37 (5)	31,100 (22,900–42,500)	4 (1)	296,300 (178,000–612,000)
2 (18%)	1062 (61)	58 (7)	18,300 (13,500–25,800)	7 (2)	147,800 (92,000–292,200)
3 (22%)	987 (71)	80 (9)	12,300 (8900–17,600)	13 (3)	78,900 (48,800–157,400)
4 (28%)	893 (83)	93 (11)	9600 (6700–13,900)	18 (5)	49,600 (30,800–100,700)
5 (42%)	630 (126)	141 (16)	4500 (2300–7400)	29 (7)	21,400 (10,700–46,100)
Overall	947 (72)	82 (9)	11,600 (8500–16,300)	14 (4)	66,600 (42,600–135,800)

*Discounted at 3·5% per annum; MVE=major vascular event

Reproduced from Mihaylova *et al.* (2005) with permission from Elsevier.

derived from the results within that subgroup only had a 95% CI of £10,700–44,600. As a consequence, clear trends are apparent in the cost-effectiveness estimates across different underlying levels of vascular risk, which would not have been apparent if subgroups had been analysed independently.

11.8 **Methodological uncertainty**

Finally, let us briefly consider uncertainty that is unrelated to sampling variation, in particular methodological uncertainty.

Standard sensitivity analysis still has a role to play when addressing the possible impact on results of different methodological approaches, such as the range of costs being included, discount rates for costs and/or effects, or assumptions about likely patterns of care, drug prices, or future technological innovations. However, it is worth noting that we would still be interested in capturing and presenting uncertainty under the different scenarios being considered in a sensitivity analysis by plotting CEACs for each scenario, as well as reporting changes in the point estimate of the ICER.

An example of this is shown in Figure 11.12, which is derived from an early empirical application of the cost-effectiveness acceptability curve approach to data from the UK Prospective Diabetes Study (UKPDS Group 1998). In this instance, the objective was to estimate the cost-effectiveness of tighter blood pressure control for people with type 2 diabetes compared with less tight control. In addition to presenting the main results, it was considered important to give some sense of the impact of different discount rates, as effects were being extrapolated over a lifetime horizon in some analyses.

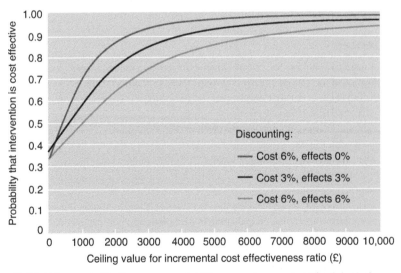

Fig. 11.12 Using cost-effectiveness acceptability curves to report methodological uncertainty. The effect of different discount rates on the probability that tight blood pressure control for patients with type 2 diabetes is cost-effective. Reproduced from UKPDS Group (1998) with permission from the BMJ Publishing Group Ltd.

Rather than simply reporting the point estimate of the ICER under different discount rate assumptions, the analysts presented acceptability curves for each scenario.

With this method of presentation, it is possible not only to look at the effect of different discount rates on the results, but also to consider the effect of these on the probability that the intervention is cost-effective, thus presenting the uncertainty due to sampling variation alongside that due to methodological uncertainty.

11.9 **Summary**

This chapter and Chapter 10 both began from the position that it is not acceptable simply to present point estimates of cost-effectiveness. Informed decision-making requires full knowledge of the degree of uncertainty surrounding the results of an analysis, whether it is model-based (Chapter 10) or based on patient-level data (this chapter).

Although the incremental cost-effectiveness ratio is the primary focus of cost-effectiveness analysis, we have seen that this ratio is subject to a number of limitations which restrict statistical analysis and hinder interpretation, even when interpreting the point estimate, but especially when considering uncertainty. Cost-effectiveness acceptability curves can be used to summarize uncertainty on the cost-effectiveness plane. They also have the advantage of directly addressing the study question: Is a particular intervention cost-effective at a given willingness to pay for health gain? The net-benefit framework also offers the advantages of acceptability curves, with the additional merit of facilitating other forms of patient-level analysis such as regression methods.

Finally, while non-sampling variation such as methodological uncertainty should be handled using sensitivity analysis, this should still be combined with sampling variation, for example through the use of acceptability curves.

References

Barber, J.A. and Thompson, S.G. (2000). Analysis of cost data in randomized trials: an application of the non-parametric bootstrap. *Statistics in Medicine*, **19**, 3219–36.

Briggs, A. and Fenn, P. (1998). Confidence intervals or surfaces? Uncertainty on the cost-effectiveness plane. *Health Economics*, **7**, 723–40.

Briggs, A.H. and O'Brien, B.J. (2001). The death of cost-minimisation analysis? *Health Economics*, **10**, 179–84.

Briggs, A.H., Wonderling, D.E., and Mooney, C.Z. (1997). Pulling cost-effectiveness analysis up by its bootstraps: a non-parametric approach to confidence interval estimation. *Health Economics*, **6**, 327–40.

Briggs, A.H., Mooney, C.Z., and Wonderling, D.E. (1999). Constructing confidence intervals for cost-effectiveness ratios: an evaluation of parametric and non-parametric techniques using Monte Carlo simulation. *Statistics in Medicine*, **18**, 3245–62.

Chaudhary, M.A. and Stearns, S.C. (1996). Estimating confidence intervals for cost-effectiveness ratios: an example from a randomized trial. *Statistics in Medicine*, **15**, 1447–58.

Claxton, K. and Posnett, J. (1996). An economic approach to clinical trial design and research priority-setting. *Health Economics*, **5**, 513–24.

Efron, B. and Tibshirani, R. (1993). *An Introduction to the Bootstrap*. Chapman & Hall, New York.

Gold, M.R., Siegel, J.E., Russell, L.B., and Weinstein, M.C. (1996). *Cost-effectiveness in Health and Medicine*. Oxford University Press, New York.

Hoch, J.S., Briggs, A.H., and Willan, A.R. (2002). Something old, something new, something borrowed, something blue: a framework for the marriage of health econometrics and cost-effectiveness analysis. *Health Economics*, 11, 415–30.

Mihaylova, B., Briggs, A., Armitage, J., Parish, S., Gray, A., and Collins, R. (2005). Cost-effectiveness of simvastatin in people at different levels of vascular disease risk: economic analysis of a randomised trial in 20,536 individuals. *Lancet*, 365, 1779–85.

NICE (2008). *Guide to the Methods of Technology Appraisal*. National Institute for Health and Clinical Excellence, London.

Obenchain, R.L., Melfi, C.A., Croghan, T.W., and Buesching, D.P. (1997). Bootstrap analyses of cost effectiveness in antidepressant pharmacotherapy. *Pharmacoeconomics*, 11, 464–72.

O'Brien, B.J., Drummond, M.F., Labelle, R.J., and Willan, A. (1994). In search of power and significance: issues in the design and analysis of stochastic cost-effectiveness studies in health care. *Medical Care*, 32, 150–63.

O'Hagan, A. and Stevens, J.W. (2003). Assessing and comparing costs: how robust are the bootstrap and methods based on asymptotic normality? *Health Economics*, 12, 33–49.

Polsky, D., Glick, H.A., Willke, R., and Schulman, K. (1997a). Confidence intervals for cost-effectiveness ratios: a comparison of four methods. *Health Economics*, 6, 243–52.

Polsky, D., Glick, H.A., Willke, R., and Schulman, K. (1997b). Confidence intervals for cost-effectiveness ratios: a comparison of four methods. *Health Economics*, 6, 243–52.

Severens, J.L., De Boo, T.M., and Konst, E.M. (1999). Uncertainty of incremental cost-effectiveness ratios: a comparison of Fieller and bootstrap confidence intervals. *International Journal of Technology Assessment in Health Care*, 15, 608–14.

Stinnett, A.A. and Mullahy, J. (1998). Net health benefits: a new framework for the analysis of uncertainty in cost-effectiveness analysis. *Medical Decision Making*, 18, S68–80

Thompson, S.G. and Barber, J.A. (2000). How should cost data in pragmatic randomised trials be analysed? *British Medical Journal*, 320, 1197–1200.

UKPDS Group (1998). Cost effectiveness analysis of improved blood pressure control in hypertensive patients with type 2 diabetes: UKPDS 40. UK Prospective Diabetes Study Group [see comments]. *British Medical Journal*, 317, 720–6.

van Hout, B., Al, M.J., Gordon, G.S., and Rutten, F.F. (1994). Costs, effects and C/E-ratios alongside a clinical trial. *Health Economics*, 3, 309–19.

Willan, A.R. and O'Brien, B.J. (1996). Confidence intervals for cost-effectiveness ratios: an application of Fieller's theorem. *Health Economics*, 5, 297–305.

Zethraeus, N., Johannesson, M., Jonsson, B., Lothgren, M., and Tambour, M. (2003). Advantages of using the net-benefit approach for analysing uncertainty in economic evaluation studies. *Pharmacoeconomics*, 21, 39–48.

Presenting cost-effectiveness results

Overview

Note that in this exercise we will be working with costs and outcomes for each patient that have not been adjusted for censoring. The main reason for this is that the methods used in previous exercises to adjust for censoring give results for the group rather than for individual patients, but here we want to begin with patient-level data and demonstrate the importance of distinguishing between individual patients and group means. Parametric and non-parametric methods do exist for dealing with combined group-level cost and effect data that are censor-adjusted, but these are quite complex to deal with in a spreadsheet-based exercise.

If you go to the website www.herc.ox.ac.uk/books/applied you will find an Excel file ***Present Results Exercise2.xlsm***. On loading this file you will find a dataset of observations recorded for two groups of patients: a Control Group and a Treatment Group. These are the patient datasets you have already worked with in the Cost and Outcomes exercises.

The spreadsheet includes a macro that will generate 1000 bootstrap replications of the cost and effect differences from this dataset. The aim of this exercise is for you to analyse the data from the study and present the results. The following list aims to guide you through the stages you should cover, but the overall aim of the exercise is for you to become comfortable with analysing and presenting cost-effectiveness information. To aid you, all cells that you have to complete are coloured yellow. A detailed step-by-step guide to the exercise follows this summary.

- Start by testing whether the individual cost and effect differences are significant.
- Go on to estimate the bootstrap confidence intervals for the ICER. What method did you use? Are any adjustments to this interval required?
- Employ the bootstrap replications to produce a cost-effectiveness acceptability curve.
- Choose a possible value of the ceiling ratio and use this value to estimate the net-benefit statistic from the data. Estimate the confidence interval for this statistic.
- Using the same bootstrap information on cost and effect differences, calculate replicates of the net-benefit statistic.
- Calculate the bootstrap estimate of variance of the net-benefit statistic and compare this with the parametric variance.
- Plot the distribution of net-benefits. Does it look normal?

- Estimate the cost-effectiveness acceptability curve parametrically from the net-benefit statistic.

Step-by-step guide

If you go to the website www.herc.ox.ac.uk/books/applied you will find the file *Present Results Exercise2.xlsm*. This workbook provides the raw data for the exercise and will give labels and headings for the summary information that you will be asked to complete as part of the exercise. All cells which require you to complete information are coloured yellow. Each stage of the exercise is given by the steps below.

Step 1. Getting to know the data

Spreadsheet commands required: AVERAGE, STDEV, SQRT, NORMINV

On the **Raw data** sheet of the exercise workbook you will find data from a hypothetical clinical trial which compared a Treatment Group with a Control Group. The trial recruited 100 patients in each arm and the cost–effect pairs for each of the patients in each of the arms is listed.

(a) On the sheet marked 'Summary statistics' use the appropriate spreadsheet commands to estimate the mean and standard deviation for the cost and effect data in the treatment and control groups from the **Raw data** worksheet.

(b) Go on to calculate the standard error for these data (recall that the standard error is equal to the standard deviation divided by the square root of the sample size).

(c) Now calculate the differences in mean cost and mean effect between the treatment and control arms of the trial.

(d) Calculate the standard error of these differences (recall that the variance of a sum or difference is equal to the sum of the variances).

(e) Calculate the 95% confidence intervals for these differences.

(f) Finally, calculate the incremental cost-effectiveness ratio (ICER). (Ignore the correlation statistics for now.)

Although we are clearly interested in the point estimate of the ICER statistic for the drug intervention over placebo, we are also interested in a confidence interval estimate. Unfortunately, confidence intervals for ratio statistics pose particular problems for parametric techniques (notice that we cannot estimate the variance of a ratio directly). Hence this exercise shows how we can use the non-parametric bootstrapping technique to estimate the confidence interval for this ICER.

Step 2. Running the bootstrap simulation

Spreadsheet commands employed: VLOOKUP

Now turn to the **Bootstrapping** worksheet. To save you time, the bootstrap process has been written for you and is instigated by pressing the 'Run bootstrap macro' button at the top of the **Bootstrapping** worksheet. However, before running the macro, make sure that you understand the structure of the spreadsheet given on this worksheet.

On the left of the worksheet a bootstrap resample of the treatment and control groups is generated using a random number generator and the VLOOKUP command (refer to the exercise in Chapter 7 for more detail on this command). The random numbers are generated in columns A and E, referring to the Control Group and the Treatment Group, respectively. These random numbers are generated to take an integer value between 1 and 100 for the Control Group and between 101 and 200 for the Treatment Group, and they refer to the patient number on the **Raw data** sheet. The VLOOKUP command then 'looks up' the cost and effect pairs corresponding to this patient number from the **Raw data** sheet. Try selecting one of the cells in this range to see what is happening.

At the bottom of 100 of these resamples (corresponding to the number of patients in each group in the original sample), the average cost and effect of the resamples are calculated. This is the bootstrap replication of the original data. The macro simply takes these average values and pastes them into the bootstrap resample part of the worksheet on the right. The macro repeats this 1000 times (i.e. for 1000 different bootstrap resamples).

(a) When you are happy with this process, press the 'Run bootstrap macro' button. The macro will take a few minutes to complete the 1000 resamples. When it is finished, you should be left with 1000 replications of the mean costs and effects from the bootstrap resamples corresponding to each arm of the trial.

(b) Use these bootstrap data to calculate the cost and effect differences in each of the 1000 replications.

(c) Now use these differences to estimate the vector of 1000 bootstrapped ICERs.

Step 3. Plotting the data

Plotting the cost and effect data on the cost-effectiveness plane is a good way of 'eye-balling' the bootstrap estimate of the dispersion of the cost and effect differences.

(a) Select the **CE plane** worksheet. This worksheet is blank. However, it contains the formatting of the appropriate $(x$–$y)$ chart. Users of MS Excel 97–2003 click the right-hand mouse button and choose 'Source data' from the pop-up menu. Users of MS Excel 2007 click the right-hand mouse button and choose 'Select data' from the pop-up menu.

(b) The 'Source data' dialogue should now pop up and the cursor should be in the 'Data range' part of the 'Data range' tab. Press the button with the red arrow, then select the effect and cost vectors of bootstrapped differences (columns R and S) from the **Bootstrap results** worksheet that you calculated in step 2(b) above. Press 'Enter' to return to the dialogue box; then press OK and the chart should appear.

NB. For users of MS Excel 2007: a bug in the programme means that Excel joins up the dots on the cost-effectiveness plane. To correct for this and remove these lines we need to change the chart type. To do this, right click on the plane, and then select 'Change series chart type'. In the window that opens, select the *x–y* scatter chart that plots only the data points (this is the first of the five chart types shown under XY (scatter)).

What is the relationship between each of the cost and effect pairs and the ICERs that you calculated in terms of the cost-effectiveness plane?

Step 4. Plotting the ICER sampling distribution

Spreadsheet commands required: MEDIAN, MIN, MAX, PERCENTILE

We can use the vector of bootstrapped ICERs to estimate summary information concerning the ICER statistic and, most importantly, to estimate confidence intervals. First, calculate the summary statistics indicated in column W for the ICER. Use the histogram wizard to plot the bootstrap estimate of the sampling distribution of the ICER. The vector of 1000 bootstrap estimates of the ICER that you calculated above is the bootstrap estimate of the sampling distribution of the ICER statistic, and the shape of this distribution is clearly shown by the histogram. Turn back to the **Bootstrapping** worksheet.

(a) In column X of the worksheet, calculate the mean, median, standard deviation, and minimum and maximum values of the bootstrap vector. Use the PERCENTILE command to calculate the 2.5th and 97.5th percentile values of the bootstrap vector. These are the bootstrap estimates of the confidence interval.

(b) To generate frequency data for a histogram of the bootstrap ICERs, use the histogram wizard. (In MS Excel 97–2003, the wizard is found through Tools, Data Analysis, Histogram. In MS Excel 2007, it can be found through Data, Analysis, Data Analysis, Histogram). In the histogram dialogue box, you are required to enter three items of information.

(i) The 'Input range'—this is the vector of bootstrapped ICERs. Select the button with the red arrow. Now highlight the ICER vector and press 'Enter' to return to the dialogue box.

(ii) The 'Bin range'—this is the values at which Excel will evaluate the frequency of the data. Press the red arrow adjacent to 'Bin range' and select the values from –20,000 to 60,000 in column W (note that the full range of values is too wide for us to plot, so we will concentrate on the centre of the distribution).

(iii) The final information required is the output range. Press the button next to output range. Then press the red arrow and select the single cell X17 and press 'Enter' to return to the dialogue box. Now press OK to start the histogram calculation. In a few seconds, Excel will generate a frequency table.

(c) To plot the histogram of frequencies, first select the **ICER histogram** worksheet. Again, the formatting of the histogram has been done for you. MS Excel 97–2003 users click the right-hand mouse button and choose the 'Source data' option from the pop-up menu. MS Excel 2007 users click the right-hand mouse button and choose 'Select Data'.

(i) Press the red arrow next to 'Data range' and select the frequency data that you have just calculated for the ICER (column Y).

(ii) Press 'Enter' to return to the dialogue box.

(iii) We now need to set appropriate labels for the x-axis of the histogram.

- ◆ To do this in MS Excel 97–2003 select the 'Series' tab in the dialogue box and press the red arrow next to the 'Category (X) axis labels'. Now select the values adjacent to the frequency data labelled 'Bin' (column X) and press 'Enter' to return to the dialogue box.

- ◆ To do this in MS Excel 2007, click on the 'Edit' button in the box labelled 'Horizontal (Category) Axis Labels'. In the dialogue box that opens, press the red arrow next to 'Axis label range'. Now select the values adjacent to the frequency data labelled 'Bin' (column X) and press Enter' to return to the dialogue box.

(iv) Finally, press 'OK' to enter the information and generate the chart.

What do you notice about the bootstrap estimate of the ICER sampling distribution? Although the summary information you calculated for the bootstrapped ICERs is useful for descriptive purposes, the mean of the bootstrap replications will not equal the ICER calculated from the original data. It is the original ICER, not the mean of the bootstrapped ICERs, which is the best estimate.

Similarly, care should be taken when interpreting the standard deviation of the bootstrap replications. In particular, this standard deviation should not be used to calculate confidence intervals. (Why?) How useful are the estimated confidence intervals for the ICER in this case?

Step 5. Generating a cost-effectiveness acceptability curve

Spreadsheet commands required: IF

As was argued in this chapter, confidence limits on ICERs do not give the information required when there is a non-negligible probability that the ratio could take a negative value. Instead, cost-effectiveness acceptability curves show the proportion of the joint density of costs and effects falling in the 'cost-effective' portion of the plane, conditional on a particular value for the ceiling ratio.

Use a nested 'IF' statement to determine, for each bootstrapped cost–effect pair, whether that point on the cost-effectiveness plane represents a cost-effective point ($1 =$ yes, $0 =$ no) using the value of R_C given in cell AA2. Then work out the proportion of cost-effective bootstrap replications and enter in the cell AA3. Change the value of R_C and see the proportion change.

The 'Run CEA curve macro' button can be used to produce results for the proportion of bootstrap replicates that are cost-effective for different values of R_C. Once the macro has finished running, plot the results on the **CE curve** worksheet.

Turn back to the **Bootstrapping** worksheet.

(a) The cells to be completed in column AA should indicate whether the bootstrap cost–effect pair in that row represents a cost-effective point on the plane ($1 =$ yes, $0 =$ no) in relation to the given value of the ceiling ratio (R_C) in cell AA2. Cell AA2 has been named R_C so you can refer to it quickly. To get the correct answer you must use three 'IF' statements in combination to sort out the issue of negative ratios. We cannot use a simple statement like 'IF(AA10<AA2,1,0)' because negative ratios in the north-west quadrant of the plane will satisfy such a statement but are clearly not cost-effective. The key is first to establish whether the difference in effects is less than zero . If it is, a point will be cost-effective if costs are also <K0 and the ICER is *above* the ceiling ratio. If the effect difference is greater than zero, a point will be cost-effective if the ICER is *below* the ceiling ratio.

(b) Once you have successfully generated the indicator in column AA, calculate the proportion of replicates that are cost-effective and enter this result in cell AA3.

(c) A macro is provided that takes the value of R_C from column AC, puts the value it cell AA2, and records the result in column AD. Run this macro in order to generate the data for the acceptability curve.

(d) Now plot the acceptability curve. Select the **CEA curve** worksheet and use the right mouse button to get 'Source data' ('Select Data' for MS Excel 2007 users). Choose the data in columns AC and AD for the 'Data range' field to plot the CEA curve.

Step 6. Non-parametric net-benefit estimation

We can use the bootstrap replicates of cost and effect differences to calculate the net-benefit statistic instead of the ICER. For each of the 1000 bootstrap replications, calculate the net-benefit statistic using a decision rule $R_C = £10,000$. Now complete the summary statistics for net benefits and, using the values given, plot a histogram on the **Net ben histogram** worksheet showing the distribution of net benefits.

Compare this distribution with that for the ICER based on the same bootstrap replications. Is the net-benefit statistic roughly normally distributed?

Calculate the proportion of replicates for which the intervention is cost-effective based on the bootstrap net benefits. How easy is this compared with the same approach based on the cost-effective plane?

(a) The net-benefit replicates are obtained by multiplying the bootstrap estimate of the effect difference by the decision rule ($R_C = £10,000$) and subtracting the bootstrap estimate of the cost difference. Make sure you change cell AA2 to £10,000.

(b) Complete the summary statistics for net benefits. Note how much better behaved the statistic is. Is the bootstrap estimate of the standard error close to what you would expect using the parametric formula?

(c) Using the histogram wizard, produce a frequency table for the net-benefit statistic using the 'Bin range' provided. Plot this histogram on the *<Net Ben Histogram>* worksheet.

(d) Complete the CE? column by noting that the replication is cost-effective if the net benefit is positive. Hence you can use a simple IF statement without any nesting, which will be much simpler than the previous approach based on ICERs and the cost-effective plane. The replication will be cost-effective if the net monetary benefit is greater than zero.

Step 7. Parametric net benefits and acceptability curves

Spreadsheet commands required: *NORMDIST*

Having demonstrated that the net-benefit statistic follows a roughly normal distribution, we can now be more confident in employing the parametric assumptions in order to generate cost-effectiveness acceptability curves.

Switch to the **Parametric** worksheet.

$$\text{var}(NB) = R_c^2 \, \text{var}(\Delta E) + (\Delta C) - 2R_c \, \text{cov}(\Delta E, \Delta C)$$

Using the formulae for net-benefit and the standard error of net-benefit given in Chapter 11, complete columns B and C of the worksheet, using the values of R_C given between zero and £50,000 (for simplicity assume that the correlation between cost and effect differences is zero). Standardize the net-benefit statistic in column D, and using this value and the NORMDIST function calculate the probability that the intervention is cost-effective in column E.

Finally, plot these data on the CEA curve chart to give the parametric estimate of the acceptability curve. How do the parametric and non-parametric curves compare?

(a) Calculate the net-benefit statistic for the values of R_C given between zero and £50,000 using the cost and effect differences from the **Summary Statistics** worksheet.

(b) Also calculate the corresponding standard error of net-benefits, employing the simplifying assumption that the correlation between costs and effects is zero (which is almost correct for this dataset).

(c) Reminder: In column D, calculate the standardized value of net-benefit by dividing the statistic through by its standard error. Note that this effectively gives the test-statistic for testing net-benefits as significantly different from zero.

(d) We now use the test-statistic from the previous step as an input to the NORMDIST function in order to estimate the probability that net-benefits is positive (i.e. that the intervention is cost-effective) . The NORMDIST function has four arguments. Use the test statistic from the previous step as the first, set the mean and the standard deviation to 0 and 1, respectively, and choose the cumulative distribution by entering the logical value 1.

(e) Finally, add the data that you have just calculated to the CEA curve figure and compare the parametric and non-parametric estimated curves.

Step 8. Including correlation between costs and effects

Spreadsheet commands required: CORREL

In Step 7, we used a simplifying assumption that costs and effects were not correlated. However, in general we do need to allow for potential covariation between costs and effects in the parametric method (see the formula in Chapter 11 and the Technical Appendix).

(a) From Chapter 11 and the Technical Appendix, calculate the correlation between costs and effects in the raw data, and add this to the **Summary statistics** worksheet.

(b) Now calculate the correlation between the cost and effect differences and again add to the **Summary statistics** worksheet.

(c) Finally, recalculate the standard error of the net-benefit statistic in column C of the **Parametric** worksheet including a covariance term.

A completed version of this exercise is available from the website www.herc.ox.ac. uk/books/applied in the Excel file *Outcomes2 solutions.xlsx*

Technical appendix

The first section of this appendix gives a brief summary of how Fieller's theorem is derived, and the second provides a worked example of how it is used to calculate confidence intervals.

Theoretical basis behind Fieller's Theorem confidence intervals

In Fieller's approach, it is assumed that the cost and effect differences (represented by ΔC and ΔE, respectively) follow a joint normal distribution. The standard cost-effectiveness ratio calculation of $R = \Delta C/\Delta E$ can be expressed as $R\Delta E - \Delta C = 0$ with known variance $R^2 \operatorname{var}(\Delta E) + \operatorname{var}(\Delta C) - 2R \operatorname{cov}(\Delta E, \Delta C)$. Therefore we can generate a standard normally distributed variable by dividing the reformulated expression through by its standard error:

$$\frac{R\Delta E - \Delta C}{\sqrt{R^2 \operatorname{var}(\Delta E) + \operatorname{var}(\Delta C) - 2R \operatorname{cov}(\Delta E, \Delta C)}} \sim N(0,1)$$

Setting this expression equal to the critical point from the standard normal distribution, $z_{\alpha/2}$ for a $(1-\alpha)100\%$ confidence interval, yields the following quadratic equation in R:

$$R^2 \left[\Delta E^2 - z^2_{\alpha/2} \operatorname{var}(\Delta E) \right] - 2R \left[\Delta E \cdot \Delta C - z^2_{\alpha/2} \operatorname{cov}(\Delta E, \Delta C) \right] + \left[\Delta C^2 - z^2_{\alpha/2} \operatorname{var}(\Delta C) \right] = 0$$

The roots of this equation give the Fieller confidence limits R for the ICER. This equation is solved using the standard quadratic formula

$$\frac{-b \pm \sqrt{b^2 - 4ac}}{2a}$$

where

$$a = \Delta E^2 - z^2_{\alpha/2} \operatorname{var}(\Delta E)$$
$$b = -2 \left[\Delta E . \Delta C - z^2_{\alpha/2} \operatorname{cov}(\Delta E, \Delta C) \right]$$
$$c = \Delta C^2 - z^2_{\alpha/2} \operatorname{var}(\Delta C).$$

Substituting these values into the expression above simplifies only slightly with the 2's cancelling to give

$$\frac{\left[\Delta E . \Delta C - z_{\alpha/2}^2 \operatorname{cov}(\Delta E, \Delta C)\right]}{\Delta E^2 - z_{\alpha/2}^2 \operatorname{var}(\Delta E)}$$

$$\pm \frac{\sqrt{\left[\Delta E . \Delta C - z_{\alpha/2}^2 \operatorname{cov}(\Delta E, \Delta C)\right]^2 - \left[\Delta E^2 - z_{\alpha/2}^2 \operatorname{var}(\Delta E)\right] . \left[\Delta C^2 - z_{\alpha/2}^2 \operatorname{var}(\Delta C)\right]}}{\Delta E^2 - z_{\alpha/2}^2 \operatorname{var}(\Delta E)}$$

Worked example of Fieller's theorem

The five pieces of information required to calculate the Fieller's theorem confidence intervals are (1) the estimated effect difference, (2) the estimated cost difference, (3, 4) their respective variances, and (5) the covariance between them. $z_{\alpha/2}$ is the critical value from the normal distribution at the significance level of interest. At the conventional significance level of $\alpha = 0.05$, $z_{\alpha/2} \approx 1.96$. With control and treatment interventions indicated by subscripts C and T, respectively, we have

1. $\Delta E = \bar{E}_T - \bar{E}_C = \dfrac{1}{n_T}\sum_{i=1}^{n_T} E_{Ti} - \dfrac{1}{n_C}\sum_{j=1}^{n_C} E_{Cj}$

2. $\Delta C = \bar{C}_T - \bar{C}_C = \dfrac{1}{n_T}\sum_{i=1}^{n_T} C_{Ti} - \dfrac{1}{n_C}\sum_{j=1}^{n_C} E_{Cj}$

3. $\operatorname{var}(\Delta E) = \operatorname{var}(\bar{E}_T) + \operatorname{var}(\bar{E}_C) = \dfrac{1}{n_T(n_T-1)}\sum_{i=1}^{n_T}(\bar{E}_T - E_{Ti})^2 - \dfrac{1}{n_c(n_c-1)}\sum_{j=1}^{n_c}(\bar{E}_C - E_{Cj})^2$

4. $\operatorname{var}(\Delta C) = \operatorname{var}(\bar{C}_T) + \operatorname{var}(\bar{C}_C) = \dfrac{1}{n_T(n_T-1)}\sum_{i=1}^{n_T}(\bar{C}_T - C_{Ti})^2 - \dfrac{1}{n_c(n_c-1)}\sum_{j=1}^{n_c}(\bar{C}_C - C_{Cj})^2$

5. $\operatorname{cov}(\Delta E, \Delta C) = \operatorname{cov}(\bar{E}_T, \bar{C}_T) + \operatorname{cov}(\bar{E}_c, \bar{C}_c) = \rho_T\sqrt{\operatorname{var}(\bar{E}_T)\operatorname{var}(\bar{C}_T)} + \rho_C\sqrt{\operatorname{var}(\bar{E}_C)\operatorname{var}(\bar{C}_C)}$

where E and C represent effect and cost, respectively, and ρ is the correlation coefficient between costs and effects in each group.

Note that the correlation ρ_Δ between the incremental costs and effects is given by

$$\rho_\Delta = \frac{\operatorname{cov}(\Delta E, \Delta C)}{\sqrt{\operatorname{var}(\Delta E)\operatorname{var}(\Delta C)}}$$

and that (by rearrangement)

$$\operatorname{cov}(\Delta E, \Delta C) = \rho_\Delta \sqrt{\operatorname{var}(\Delta E)\operatorname{var}(\Delta C)}.$$

In the example shown in Table 11.2, these five pieces of information take the following values:

$$\Delta C = £1000 \quad \text{var}(\Delta C) = se_{\Delta C}^2 = 239.2^2 = 57{,}218$$

$$\Delta E = 0.3023 \quad \text{var}(\Delta E) = se_{\Delta E}^2 = 0.0993^2 = 0.00986$$

$$\text{cov}(\Delta E, \Delta C) = \rho_\Delta \sqrt{\text{var}(\Delta E)\text{var}(\Delta C)} = 0.\sqrt{57218 * 0.00986} = 0$$

Using the derivation above, Fieller's theorem confidence intervals around the ICER can be calculated using the formula:

$$\frac{\left[\Delta E.\Delta C - z_{\alpha/2}^2 \text{cov}(\Delta E, \Delta C)\right]}{\Delta E^2 - z_{\alpha/2}^2 \text{var}(\Delta E)}$$

$$\pm \frac{\sqrt{\left[\Delta E.\Delta C - z_{\alpha/2}^2 \text{cov}(\Delta E \cdot \Delta C)\right]^2 - \left[\Delta E^2 - z_{\alpha/2}^2 \text{var}(\Delta E)\right].\left[\Delta C^2 - z_{\alpha/2}^2 \text{var}(\Delta C)\right]}}{\Delta E^2 - z_{\alpha/2}^2 \text{var}(\Delta E)}$$

Substituting the values for this example into this formula, Fieller's theorem confidence limits for this example are

$$\frac{\left[0.3023 \cdot 1000 - 1.96^2 \cdot 0\right]}{0.3023^2 - 1.96^2 \cdot 0.00986}$$

$$\pm \frac{\sqrt{\left[0.3023 \cdot 1000 - 1.96^2 \cdot 0\right]^2 - \left[0.3023^2 - 1.96^2 \cdot 0.00986\right].\left[1000^2 - 1.96^2 \cdot 57{,}218\right]}}{0.3023^2 - 1.96^2 \cdot 0.00986}$$

Lower 95% limit = 5650 − 4324 = £1486

Upper 95% limit = 5650 + 4324 = £9813.

Chapter 12

Summing up and future directions

In this book we set out to provide the reader with a reasonably detailed and practical description of the methods and steps required to perform a cost-effectiveness analysis of a health intervention. We began in Chapter 2 by describing the different types of economic evaluation, the use of presentation devices such as the cost-effectiveness plane, and ways of trying to quantify willingness to pay for health gains. Chapters 3 and 4 focused on methods of quantifying and extrapolating changes in life expectancy and quality-adjusted life expectancy, and Chapter 5 considered how quality adjustment can be undertaken. Chapters 6 and 7 set out methods for defining, measuring, valuing, and analysing costs. Chapters 8, 9, and 10 considered the rationale for modelling, the construction and analysis of decision tree and Markov models, and methods to take account of uncertainty in cost-effectiveness models. Chapter 11 then brought together the cost, outcome, and modelling chapters and demonstrated appropriate ways of presenting cost-effectiveness results.

We did not intend to give a fully comprehensive treatment of the methodological principles of economic evaluation in health care. This can be obtained elsewhere in general textbooks (e.g. (Gold *et al.* 1996; Drummond *et al.* 2005) or in texts dealing with specific aspects of the subject such as measurement and valuation of health benefits (e.g. Brazier *et al.* 2007). Rather, our intention was to produce a more practical handbook, in line with other volumes in the *Handbooks in Health Economic Evaluation* series of which this is a part (Briggs *et al.* 2006; Glick *et al.* 2007; McIntosh *et al.* 2010) and also reflecting the philosophy underlying the 'Advanced Methods of Cost-Effectiveness Analysis' short course which forms the foundation of this book.

In Chapter 2 we considered at some length the different ways of trying to ascertain the maximum value that decision-makers might place on their willingness to pay for health gain. In recent years, these debates have largely taken place in the relatively benign climate of steadily expanding real health expenditure during the first decade of the 21st century in which reimbursement agencies such as NICE operated. If this climate becomes more inclement, as seems likely, debates on willingness to pay may become much more pointed. In particular, quite apart from the different techniques being used, it is evident that some such studies are mainly trying to estimate the opportunity cost of adopting new technologies, for example by looking at cost-effectiveness at the margin of existing levels of care, while others are focusing primarily on the social value placed on a life, a life-year, or a quality-adjusted life-year. Clearly, problems could arise if these conceptually separate questions become confused, for example if social valuations of willingness to pay for health gain are used to estimate the opportunity cost of introducing new technologies to the existing health-care budget. In an era of tightly constrained public spending, the opportunity cost of adopting new technologies, and of retaining existing interventions that have weak evidence of cost-effectiveness, will become ever more pressing considerations.

One theme running through the book has been the advantages of having access to individual patient data. This has come up in many contexts, such as survival analysis techniques, model construction and validation, event-based costing and quality-of-life analysis, and addressing heterogeneity. Our emphasis on individual patient data reflects in part the research orientation of the Health Economics Research Centre at the University of Oxford, where we have developed close collaborations with a number of leading clinical trial groups. We are of course well aware of the limitations of trial-based economic evaluations, which have been clearly outlined (Sculpher *et al.* 2006): truncated time horizons, limited comparators, lack of relevance to the decision context in a specific country, etc. We are also fully aware that trial-based and model-based approaches are often complements rather than alternatives (Buxton *et al.* 1997). That said, we remain convinced that there are a number of advantages to trial-based studies. In part these pertain to the ability of randomized studies to produce unbiased estimates of effect, the correspondingly higher value that clinicians tend to place on their results, and the fact that they have often been commissioned precisely because of an absence of reliable evidence. A strong move in recent years towards the use of randomized studies in other areas such as development economics is worth noting (Duflo and Kremer 2004), although here, as in health economics, it is clear that it is not appropriate in all circumstances and needs to be seen alongside other econometric and statistical methods (Deaton 2009; Imbens 2009).

However, trials also make available to researchers a wealth of data on individual participants: their characteristics and history at entry; their risk factors at entry and often over time; the frequency, timing, and sequence of endpoints; the reliable clinical ascertainment of these endpoints; patient treatments, co-medications, and adherence; their resource use; and their quality of life. Because these are available for the same individuals over time, the full structure of covariance can be estimated.

Throughout the book we have used many examples based on these types of data which would have been hard to obtain in any other way. In Chapter 4 we referred to the UK Prospective Diabetes Study Outcomes Model, a probabilistic discrete-time simulation model based on an integrated system of parametric proportional hazards risk equations estimated from patient-level data and including time-varying risk factors (Clarke *et al.* 2004). While not a specific focus of the book, we have aimed to show the link between such simulation models and parametric survival analysis methods. The complex interactions between risk factors, individual characteristics, and disease history would be extremely hard to capture reliably without access to patient-level data, suggesting that this approach, in which key aspects of diseases are modelled using systems of equations estimated using individual patient data, will or at least should become more common in health economic models in coming years.

Data from the same study permitted estimation of the quality of life and cost impact of a set of diabetes-related complications at the time and subsequently, again controlling for other characteristics (Clarke *et al.* 2002, 2003). Participant data from the Heart Protection Study (HPS) (Mihaylova *et al.* 2005), referred to in Chapters 10 and 11, allowed a full exploration of heterogeneity and the adoption of robust methods to deal with it. The extrapolation model constructed as part of the HPS analysis to assess cardiovascular events over a lifetime also demonstrated the advantages of individual patient data in modelling: for example, internal validation of the model on the overall population and subgroups, the ability to observe the emergence of the treatment effect over time, and the ability to address uncertainty without having to assume distributions around parameter values (Mihaylova *et al.* 2006).

In short, to view the value of conducting economic evaluations alongside clinical trials purely in terms of the generation of a single-trial-based estimate of cost-effectiveness is to take too narrow a view of their potential research outputs and benefits. Moreover, access to patient-level data permits use of a much wider range of statistical and econometric techniques.

Preparation of a handbook such as this, with the required searches for good examples and relevant citations, makes authors very aware of the distribution of the existing literature. Some areas, such as handling uncertainty or valuation of health-related quality of life, have attracted an extensive literature in recent years. However, it is apparent that other areas have been relatively neglected. For example, an important focus of this book has been measuring outcomes using both life-table methods and survival analysis. This is the quantity dimension of quality-adjusted life expectancy and therefore must be a crucial component of outcome measurement, but health economists appear to have neglected this area of research and instead have relied heavily on other disciplines such as demography, biostatistics, and actuarial science for the methods and empirical estimates of outcomes such as life expectancy. However, as we have shown, the issues raised when modelling outcomes for cost-effectiveness analysis throw up unique challenges which increasingly mean that tools such as life-tables need to be understood, used, and adapted by health economists.

For example, a key difference between economic and clinical outcome assessment is that the latter is generally confined to focusing on how an intervention impacts on the relative risk of a predefined outcome observed within a follow-up period. Economists, on the other hand, need measures such as life expectancy and QALYs which generally need to be measured over a patient's life time. This almost inevitably means that economists must focus on both absolute and relative risk and tackle issues surrounding the extrapolation of outcomes. Similarly, clinicians are often mainly interested in the time to a first event, whereas economists have to be interested in multiple events and their timing and sequence. Therefore life-table methods (Chapter 3) and parametric survival analysis (Chapter 4) can provide a useful toolbox, but must be used with caution and always checked against external sources. As we showed in Chapter 4, use of some parametric forms in survival analysis predict a sizable proportion of people living well beyond 100 years, which (at least currently) seems highly implausible.

Another area that has attracted surprisingly little attention concerns methods of collecting data, particularly in the context of prospective economic evaluations alongside clinical trials. As noted in Chapter 6, although there are a small number of studies on, for example, optimal recall period, empirical or theoretical research into data collection issues such as frequency, recall period, the detail requested, and the cost of different collection strategies is seriously lacking with respect to both resource use and quality of life. Research into data collection methods in multi-centre studies is especially lacking.

The chapters on modelling (Chapters 8–10) were able to draw on a substantial body of recently published work for at least some of the topics covered there, including the handling of uncertainty. Again, preparation of this book helped to identify lacunae in the literature. For example, although many models are expressly designed to extrapolate from the end of a clinical trial over a longer analytical horizon, and therefore the analysis will involve combining within-trial results with modelled results, there is a relatively sparse literature on how within-trial observed data and lifetime predicted data should be appropriately and robustly combined. The modelling chapters also identified that, while model uncertainty is likely to be substantial, there are very few practical examples of how it might be addressed. One possible way forward, mentioned in Chapter 8, is the example of the Mount Hood Challenge, where an international gathering of different diabetes modelling groups tried systematically to compare model predictions on the basis of specified risk factor changes, and agreed in advance to publish the results (Mount Hood 2007). This approach to assessing both predictive validity and cross-model agreement has been used in other subject areas, including environmental science, but is uncommon in health economics despite the extensive use of model-based evaluation. One possible extension of this is to incorporate an agreed model in the reference case for particular disease areas, so that the cost-effectiveness of interventions can be assessed while holding analytical methods and disease progression assumptions constant.

Cost-effectiveness analysis is increasingly required by trial funders and for reimbursement. Despite the many methodological developments identified in this handbook, there is still lack of agreement on many design issues, such as methods of efficient data collection, reliable measurement of patient outcomes, methods of extrapolation, handling uncertainty and analysing multi-centre and multi-country studies. We need more methodological work on these topics, but these are not problems which will be solved only by theorists working in isolation from the data. Continued advance requires more empirical research, continued close involvement with trialists, clinicians, and decision-makers, and, not least, more evidence.

The short course on which this book was initially based has evolved considerably since it was first designed, and it seems certain that the methodological foundations, the evidence base, and the policy context will continue to develop in ways that are impossible to anticipate. Therefore we cannot prevent this handbook from becoming out of date in certain respects, but rather than apologizing in advance we should perhaps celebrate this as a tribute to the continued vigour of health economics.

References

Brazier, J., Ratcliffe, J., Tsuchiya, A., and Salomon, J. (2007). *Measuring and Valuing Health Benefits for Economic Evaluation*. Oxford University Press, New York.

Briggs, A.H., Claxton, K., and Sculpher, M.J. (2006). *Decision Modelling for Health Economic Evaluation*. Oxford University Press.

Buxton, M.J., Drummond, M.F., Van, H.B., *et al.* (1997). Modelling in economic evaluation: an unavoidable fact of life [editorial]. *Health Economics*, **6**, 217–27.

Clarke, P., Gray, A., and Holman, R. (2002) Estimating utility values for health states of type 2 diabetic patients using the EQ-5D (UKPDS 62). *Medical Decision Making*, **22**, 340–9.

Clarke, P., Gray, A., Legood, R., Briggs, A., and Holman, R. (2003). The impact of diabetes-related complications on healthcare costs: results from the United Kingdom Prospective Diabetes Study (UKPDS Study No. 65). *Diabetic Medicine*, **20**, 442–50.

Clarke, P., Gray, A., Briggs, A., *et al.* (2004). A model to estimate the lifetime health outcomes of patients with type 2 diabetes: the United Kingdom Prospective Diabetes Study (UKPDS) Outcomes Model (UKPDS 68). *Diabetologia*, **47**, 1747–59.

Deaton, A. (2009). *Instruments of Development: Randomization in the Tropics, and the Search for the Elusive Keys to Economic Development*. NBER Working Paper No. 14690, National Bureau of Economic Research, Cambridge, MA.

Drummond, M.F., Sculpher, M.J., Torrance, G.W., O'Brien, B.J., and Stoddart, G.L. (2005). *Methods for the Economic Evaluation of Health Care Programmes* (3rd edn). Oxford University Press.

Duflo, E. and Kremer, M. (2004). Use of randomization in the evaluation of development effectiveness. In: Feinstein, O., Ingram, G.K., and Pitman, G.K. (eds), *Evaluating Development Effectiveness*, pp. 205–32. Transaction Publishers, Piscataway, NJ.

Glick, H., Doshi, J.A., Sonnad, S.S., and Polsky, D. (2007). *Economic Evaluation in Clinical Trials*. Oxford University Press.

Gold, M.R., Siegel, J.E., Russell, L.B., and Weinstein, M.C. (1996). *Cost-Effectiveness in Health and Medicine*. Oxford University Press, New York.

Imbens, G.W. (2009). *Better LATE Than Nothing: Some Comments on Deaton (2009) and Heckman and Urzua (2009)*. NBER Working Paper No.14896, National Bureau of Economic Research, Cambridge, MA.

McIntosh, E., Louviere, J.J., Frew, E., and Clarke, P.M. (2010). *Applied Methods of Cost–Benefit Analysis in Health Care*. Oxford University Press.

Mihaylova, B., Briggs, A., Armitage, J., Parish, S., Gray, A., and Collins, R. (2005). Cost-effectiveness of simvastatin in people at different levels of vascular disease risk: economic analysis of a randomised trial in 20,536 individuals. *Lancet*, **365**, 1779–85.

Mihaylova, B., Briggs, A., Armitage, J., Parish, S., Gray, A., and Collins, R. (2006). Lifetime cost effectiveness of simvastatin in a range of risk groups and age groups derived from a randomised trial of 20,536 people. *British Medical Journal*, **333**, 1145.

Mount Hood (2007). Computer modeling of diabetes and its complications: a report on the Fourth Mount Hood Challenge Meeting. *Diabetes Care*, **30**, 1638–46.

Sculpher, M.J., Claxton, K., Drummond, M., and McCabe, C. (2006). Whither trial-based economic evaluation for health care decision making? *Health Economics*, **15**, 677–87.

Index

Printed and bound by CPI Group (UK) Ltd, Croydon, CR0 4YY